Nursing-Sensitive Outcomes:
State of the Science

Jones and Bartlett Nursing Research Titles

Nursing-Sensitive Outcomes: State of the Science

Editor

Diane Doran, RN, PhD
Faculty of Nursing
University of Toronto

Authors

Joan Almost, RN, MScN
Faculty of Health Sciences
University of Western Ontario

Diane Doran, RN, PhD
Faculty of Nursing
University of Toronto

Linda McGillis Hall, RN, PhD
Faculty of Nursing
University of Toronto

Heather Laschinger, RN, PhD
Faculty of Health Sciences
University of Western Ontario

Claire Mallette, RN, PhD (c)
Faculty of Nursing
University of Toronto

Dorothy Pringle, RN, PhD
Faculty of Nursing
University of Toronto

Souraya Sidani, RN, PhD
Faculty of Nursing
University of Toronto

Judy Watt-Watson, RN, PhD
Faculty of Nursing
University of Toronto

Peggy White, RN, MN
Ministry of Health & Long-Term Care
Province of Ontario

JONES AND BARTLETT PUBLISHERS
Sudbury, Massachusetts
BOSTON   TORONTO   LONDON   SINGAPORE

World Headquarters
Jones and Bartlett Publishers
40 Tall Pine Drive
Sudbury, MA 01776
978-443-5000
info@jbpub.com
www.jbpub.com

Jones and Bartlett Publishers Canada
2406 Nikanna Road
Mississauga, ON L5C 2W6
CANADA

Jones and Bartlett Publishers International
Barb House, Barb Mews
London W6 7PA
UK

Library of Congress Cataloging-in-Publication Data not available at time of printing.

ISBN: 0-7637-2287-1

Acquisitions Editor: Penny M. Glynn
Production Manager: Amy Rose
Associate Production Editor: Karen C. Ferreira
Associate Editor: Karen Zuck
Production Assistant: Jenny McIsaac
Senior Marketing Manager: Alisha Weisman
Associate Marketing Manager: Joy Stark-Vancs
Manufacturing Buyer: Amy Bacus
Cover Design: Philip Regan
Interior Design: Chiron, Inc.
Composition: Chiron, Inc.
Printing and Binding: Courier Stoughton
Cover Printing: Courier Stoughton

Printed in the United States of America
07 06 05   10 9 8 7 6 5 4 3 2

Contents

Preface

With the increasing demand for professional and financial accountability, nurses are challenged to identify and delineate their contributions within the healthcare system by demonstrating that the care they provide is of high quality. Such high-quality care refers to the delivery of services that are appropriate, efficient, and effective, resulting in the best health outcomes for patients (Donabedian, 1982).

The types of nurse quality indicators discussed in the literature are outcome, process of care, and structure of care indicators (American Nurses' Association, 1995). In this book we will concentrate on the outcome indicators. "Outcome indicators focus on how patients, and their conditions, are affected by their interaction with nursing staff" (ANA, p. viii). The challenge of demonstrating nurses' contributions has led many scholars to identify nursing-sensitive outcomes. These refer to outcomes for which individual nurses are held accountable. Outcomes that are identified as sensitive to nursing are those that are relevant, based on nurses' scope and domain of practice, and for which there is empirical evidence linking nursing inputs and interventions to the outcome. They represent the consequences or effects of interventions delivered by nurses and are manifested by changes in the patient's health-related state, behavior, or perception, and/or by the resolution of the presenting problem for which the nursing intervention is given (Hegyvary, 1993; Johnson & Maas, 1998; Martin & Scheet, 1992).

The outcomes that have been consistently considered as sensitive to nursing care provided across the continuum of healthcare settings (that is, acute, community or home, and long-term care settings) can be classified as follows: (a) clinical, which include symptom control or symptom management; (b) functional, which include physical and psychosocial functioning and self-care abilities; (c) safety, which include adverse incidents and complications, such as decubitus ulcers; and (d) perceptual, which include satisfaction with nursing care and with the results of care (American Nurses' Association, 1995; Brooten & Naylor, 1995; Doran, Sidani, Keatings, & Doidge, 2002; Gillette & Jenko, 1991; Hegyvary, 1993; Johnson & Maas, 1997; Lang & Marek, 1990).

In order to demonstrate their contributions towards achieving these outcomes, nurses working in acute, community, complex continuing, and long-term care settings need to build clinical databases documenting the care they provide, as well as the outcomes achieved as a result of that care. The development of a database for recording and monitoring nursing outcomes requires a clear definition of the outcome concepts and use of standardized instruments to measure and quantify the outcomes achieved by patients.

The literature on nursing-sensitive outcomes is expanding. Several articles and books propose frameworks or models for identifying and evaluating nursing-sensitive outcomes or classifications of these outcomes (e.g., Johnson & Maas, 1997; Martin & Scheet, 1992). Others present conceptual definitions of outcome concepts. Various instruments are used to measure the outcomes in research or program evaluation studies. An increasing number of studies are evaluating the impact of different nursing care delivery models or of specific nursing interventions on clinical, functional, safety, and perceptual outcomes (e.g., Brooten & Naylor, 1995; Heater, Becker, & Olson, 1988; Kovner & Gergen, 1998; Marek, 1989; Needleman, Buerhaus, Mattke, Stewart, & Zelevinsky, 2002; Smith, Holcombe, & Stullenbarger, 1994).

The authors of this book offer a synthesis of the state of the science on nursing-sensitive outcomes. Specifically, the book provides a critical review and analysis of the literature on outcomes considered to be indicators of nursing care effectiveness. The authors of the first chapter discuss the importance of building knowledge about nursing-sensitive outcomes for policy, practice, and research. The chapter concludes with a discussion of the specific objectives and methodology for the critical review. In the next six chapters, the quality of the evidence linking functional status, self-care, symptom control, pain control, patient safety, and patient satisfaction is critically examined. A separate chapter is dedicated to a review of the evidence for pain as an outcome of nursing care because of the centrality of pain management to processes of nursing care. Chapter Nine provides a review of the minimum data sets for acute care, long-term care, and home care, with a particular focus on their use for nursing resource planning and outcomes assessment. Because of the growing recognition that nurse quality indicators are integrally linked to the quality of nurses' work life and the work environment, we have included, as Chapter Eight, a critical review of the literature on the relationship between nurses' job satisfaction and patient outcomes, and approaches to the measurement of nurses' job satisfaction.

The primary goal of this book is to present a comprehensive and critical analysis of the evidence concerning nursing-sensitive outcomes by reviewing the conceptual and empirical literature. Each chapter includes a concept analysis of the outcome concept; then defining characteristics are identified and a conceptual definition is proposed. Factors that influence the outcome concept are discussed, as well as the consequences for clients' health and well-being. The strength of the evidence is reviewed concerning the sensitivity of the outcome concept to nursing structure variables and nursing process/interventions. A secondary goal of this book is to review the different methods and tools used to measure the outcome concepts, and to review critically the evidence of their reliability, validity, and sensitivity to nursing structure and process variables.

This book will interest graduate and undergraduate students who are concerned with the state of the science for nursing-sensitive outcomes and their measurement. In particular, this book will provide a valuable resource to master's and doctoral students who are developing the methodology for their graduate research. Researchers will also value the book because it offers a comprehensive synthesis of the literature, critically reviews the quality of the evidence, and provides direction for the selection of outcome variables and approaches to measurement. The book will be valuable to policy-makers and decision-makers who are building clinical databases for quality monitoring and quality improvement.

Diane Doran, RN, PhD
Editor

References

American Nurses Association. (1995). *Nursing report card for acute care.* Washington, DC: American Nurses Publishing.

Brooten, D., & Naylor, M. D. (1995). Nurses' effect on changing patient outcomes. *Image: The Journal of Nursing Scholarship, 27,* 95–99.

Donabedian, A. (1982). Quality, cost and health: An integrative model. *Medical Care, 20,* 975–992.

Doran, D. M., Sidani, S., Keatings, M., & Doidge, D. (2002). An empirical test of the Nursing Role Effectiveness Model. *Journal of Advanced Nursing, 38,* 29–39.

Gillette, B., & Jenko, M. (1991). Major clinical functions: A unifying framework for measuring outcomes. *Journal of Nursing Care Quality, 6,* 20–24.

Heater, B. S., Becker, A. M., & Olson, R. K. (1988). Nursing interventions and patient outcomes: A meta-analysis of studies. *Nursing Research, 37,* 303–307.

Hegyvary, S. T. (1993). Patient care outcome related to management of symptoms. *Annual Review of Nursing Research, 11,* 145–168.

Johnson, M., & Maas, M. (Eds.). (1997). *Nursing outcome classification (NOC).* St. Louis, MO: Mosby.

Johnson M., & Maas, M. (1998). The nursing outcome classification. *Journal of Nursing Care Quality, 12*(5), 9–20.

Kovner, C., & Gergen, P. (1998). Nurse staffing levels and adverse events following surgery in U.S. hospitals. *Image: The Journal of Nursing Scholarship, 30*(4), 315–321.

Lang, N. M., & Marek, K. D. (1990). The classification of patient outcomes. *Journal of Professional Nursing, 6,* 153–163.

Marek, K. (1989). Outcome measures in nursing. *Journal of Nursing Quality Assurance, 4*(1), 1–9.

Martin, K. S., & Scheet, N. J. (1992). *The Omaha system: Applications for community health nursing.* Philadelphia: W. B. Saunders.

Needleman, J., Buerhaus, P., Mattke, S., Stewart, M., & Zelevinsky, K. (2002). Nurse-staffing levels and the quality of care in hospitals. *New England Journal of Medicine, 346,* 1715–1722.

Smith, M. C., Holcombe, J. K., & Stullenbarger, E. (1994). A meta-analysis of intervention effectiveness for symptom management in oncology nursing research. *Oncology Nursing Forum, 21,* 1201–1209.

Acknowledgements

This book is based on work funded by the Ministry of Health and Long-Term Care, Ontario, Canada, in response to a request for a critical analysis of the literature on nursing-sensitive outcomes and approaches to their measurement. The request arose from the Expert Panel on Nursing and Health Outcomes, chaired by Dr. Dorothy Pringle, and the research was undertaken by Dr. Doran (principal investigator), Dr. Sidani, Dr. McGillis Hall, Dr. Laschinger, Dr. Watt-Watson, and Ms. Mallette (co-investigators). The opinions, results, and conclusions are those of the authors; no endorsement by the Ministry of Health and Long-Term Care is intended or should be inferred.

The authors would like to thank Barbara Bauer for her role in directing the initial copyediting. We would like to acknowledge the contribution of Barbara Bauer and Jean Bacon to the preliminary copyediting. We would like to thank Kristin Vanderstelt for her role in formatting the text.

The authors would like to acknowledge the contributions of the following members of the Expert Panel on Nursing and Health Outcomes for their vision in commissioning the original literature synthesis and for their review of the final report on which this book is based: Dorothy Pringle, Duncan Hunter, Heather Laschinger, John McIntosh, Linda O'Brien Pallas, Peggy White, Christine Fitzgerald, Diane Doran, Lynn Nagle, George Pink, Ann-Marie Strapp, Anton Basinski, Jacqueline Gerlach, Margaret Harrison, and Frank Markel.

List of Tables

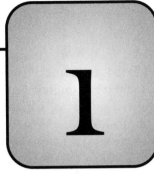

Patient Outcomes as an Accountability

Dorothy Pringle, RN, PhD

Diane M. Doran, RN, PhD

1.1 Introduction

Outcomes have been of interest to health science researchers for decades. The earliest work concentrated on the outcomes of medical and nursing practice. Nurse researchers were interested in the effects of specific nursing interventions on such things as patient symptoms (with pain being of particular interest), patient sense of well-being, and rapidity of recovery. Physicians examined the effects on patients of new surgical techniques in contrast to existing ones, and drug companies invested billions of dollars in testing whether new drugs improve patient symptoms when compared to either no treatment or currently available ones. The increasing prominence of the randomized controlled trial as the research design of choice for testing many new interventions has accelerated the identification of outcomes. This research, accumulated over 40 or 50 years, has produced a rich legacy of information on a wide range of patient outcomes, including their definitions and measurement.

Donabedian's now classic framework of structure, process, and outcomes, proposed in 1966, introduced outcomes to the lexicon of health service researchers (Donabedian, 1966). His interest was in identifying factors in health care organizations that affected quality of patient care. Hospital structures and processes were the focus of most of the early research based on this framework, but more recent work has moved to a focus on outcomes (Mitchell, Ferketich, & Jennings, 1998; Scherb, 2002). The outcomes that dominate the research emanating from this framework are cost, length of stay, patient mortality, and patient satisfaction. When nursing has been the focus of studies, outcomes have included nurses' job satisfaction and retention rates (Aiken, Sochalski, & Lake, 1997).

Aiken and her colleagues (Aiken et al., 1997) noted that up until the mid-1990s little attention had been paid to the relationship between organizational attributes and patient outcomes. This picture is rapidly changing, and one of the driving forces behind the change is the work done by the American Academy of Nursing Expert Panel on Quality Health Care. When preparing in 1994 for a planned conference on the relevance of outcomes to nursing, this group developed a conceptual model that linked patient outcomes to organizational structures and patient attributes, as well as to health care interventions (Mitchell et al., 1998). The group entertained a revolutionary idea. Perhaps interventions did not directly affect outcomes but rather worked through one of the systems in which the individual is embedded: the physiologic system of the individual, organizational systems, or groups (Mitchell, 2001). The resultant Quality Health Outcomes Model integrated functional, social, psychological, and physical/physiologic factors along with patients' experiences, in contrast to the exclusively physiological outcomes that were the usual indicators of care. Five outcomes were proposed: achievement of appropriate self-care, demonstration of health-promoting behaviors, health-related quality of life, patient perception of being well cared for, and symptom management to criteria (Mitchell et al., 1998).

A conference on outcome measures and care delivery systems, to which health services researchers, insurance company representatives, and nurse researchers were invited, was held in 1996 in Washington, D.C., under the sponsorship of the American Academy of Nursing and the Agency for Health Care Policy and Research. The proceedings from this conference were reported in *Medical Care Supplement, 35* (11). Participants heard and debated papers that summarized the state of knowledge on each of the outcomes of interest. They also explored theoretical and methodological issues involved in linking organizations and outcomes. This conference and the planning that preceded it have had a profound influence on nursing's approach to the study of nursing-sensitive patient outcomes. No longer were mortality and length of stay the only considerations when examining how patients fared in an encounter with the health care system.

The Quality Health Outcomes Model deliberately provides a multidisciplinary view of the relationship between patient outcomes and the health care system (Mitchell, 2001). Irvine, Sidani and McGillis Hall (1998) developed an equally deliberate but nurse-specific model that was subsequently tested (Doran et al., 2002). In this model the nurses' independent, dependent, and interdependent roles are treated as the processes linking the nurse, organizational and patient structures, and patient outcomes and team functioning. The patient outcomes of interest are symptom control, freedom from complications, functional status/self-care, knowledge of disease and treatment, and satisfaction with care and costs.

Aiken et al. (1997) developed a theoretical framework based on the premise that organizational models that provide nurses with substantial autonomy and more control of resources at the unit level, and encourage better relations between nurses and physicians, will result in better patient outcomes, including higher satisfaction and reduced complications and mortality. This team is particularly interested in understanding the relationship between nurses and patient mortality. A number of studies have shown correlations between better nursing staffing ratios and lower patient mortality (Aiken, Smith, & Lake, 1994; Al-Hader & Wan, 1991; Hartz et al., 1989; Van Servellen & Schultz, 1999; Shortell & Hughes, 1988) but why this occurs is poorly understood (Aiken et al., 1997). The concept of "failure to rescue" that Silber and his colleagues at the University of Pennsylvania (Silber et al., 1992) originally proposed to explain medical effectiveness has been co-opted by Aiken and her team as a potential explanatory factor in nursing. Failure to rescue means that patients die subsequent to complications from their condition, but from which they have a chance to recover if the complication is detected and treated in time (Silber et al., 1992). In nursing, this situation may result when there are insufficient registered nurses available to monitor patients and intervene when something goes wrong (Aiken et al., 1997) These three models/frameworks, among others, provide a strong basis for testing relationships between a variety of organizational structures; nursing interventions and processes; and patient, nurse, and organizational outcomes.

1.1.1 Categorizing Patient Outcomes

Many nursing-sensitive patient outcomes have been examined over the last 15 years of research on the topic, and a number of typologies exist to categorize them. Lohr (1985) proposed a list of six categories based on the continuum of care: mortality, adverse events and complications during hospitalization, inadequate recovery, prolongation of the medical problem, decline in health status, and decline in quality of life. Clearly, they are all negative in orientation and do not provide for the possibility that patients might benefit from their health care episode. Using a different approach, Hegyvary (1991) suggested four categories of outcome assessment from the patients', providers', and purchasers' perspectives: (a) clinical (patients' responses to interventions), (b) functional (improvement or decline in physical functioning), (c) financial (cost and length of stay), and (d) perceptual (patient satisfaction with care received and persons providing the care).

Jennings, Staggers, and Brosch (1999) reviewed the nursing, medical, and health services research literature from 1974 forward to locate all indicators of outcomes. These were classified as patient-focused, provider-focused, or organization-focused. The patient-focused category was further subdivided into diagnosis-focused and holistically focused outcomes. Examples of the diagnosis-specific outcomes are laboratory values, Apgar scores, and vital signs. The holistically oriented outcomes include health status, health-related quality of life, patient satisfaction ratings, assessments of patient knowledge, and symptom management. Care provider-focused outcomes include complication rates, appropriate use of medications, provider profiling, and, when a family caregiver is involved, a measure of caregiver burden. Adverse events such as falls, deaths, and unplanned readmission are categorized as organization-focused outcomes. Jennings et al. recommended that a battery of outcomes include both diagnostic and holistic outcomes, using rationale supplied by Guyatt, Feeny, & Patrick (1993).

Although derived and categorized very differently, there is considerable overlap in the actual outcomes recommended by Hegyvary(1991) and Jennings et al. (1999). When the various classification systems and the outcomes included in them are integrated, it is possible to propose a simple three-class system: adverse events, patient well-being, and patient satisfaction. The adverse events include nosocomial infections such as those occurring in the blood stream or urinary tract, pneumonia, falls, medical complications such as gastro-intestinal (GI) bleeding, deep vein thrombosis (DVT) and shock, skin breakdown, and unanticipated death. Outcomes that can be classified as patient well-being include functional status, ability to perform self-care, control of symptoms, performance of health-promoting activities, and health-related quality of life. Patient satisfaction is a subjective rating of nursing care received and can include assessments of the nurses providing the care, the way symptoms were managed, and any education received.

Although not a patient outcome, nursing job satisfaction is of interest when patient satisfaction is an outcome. In a number of studies, increased patient satisfaction with nursing care has been associated with higher levels of nurses' job satisfaction (Atkins, Marshall, & Javagli, 1996; Kaldenberg, 1999; Weisman & Nathanson, 1985).

1.1.2 Major Nursing Research Efforts on Outcomes

It is possible to identify five major research initiatives developed in the 1990s that examined the linkages between selected nursing components of organizations and a variety of patient outcomes. These are the American Nurses Association (ANA) Patient Safety and Nursing Quality Initiative, the Harvard School of Public Health Study, the Kaiser Permanente Medical Care Program Northern California Region (KPNCR) Project, the Nursing Staff Mix Outcomes Study in Ontario, and an international study under the overall leadership of Aiken that explored the failure to rescue phenomenon (Aiken et al., 2001).

The ANA study is an excellent example of the use of adverse events as outcomes. A central database was constructed using information supplied by 200 acute care hospitals participating in the studies; at the same time, nine individual state nursing organizations focused on outcomes of specific interest to them. Patient diagnostic-related groups (DRGs) that were conceptually related to nursing were included, and the New York State Nursing Intensity Weights was used to adjust for complexity across patients. The five outcomes included were urinary tract infections (UTIs), postoperative infections, pneumonias, pressure ulcers, and length of stay. The analyses showed a significant statistical relationship between all five outcomes and nursing staffing, that is, overall increased number of nurses and/or increased numbers of registered nurses as part of the nursing staff (ANA, 2000; Lichtig, Knauf & Milholland, 1999; Rowell, 2001).

Another study that focused on complications as outcomes was conducted by the Harvard School of Public Health (Needleman et al., 2002). Using administrative data from 799 hospitals in 11 American states, they measured 12 adverse outcomes and length of stay: UTIs, pressure ulcers, hospital-acquired pneumonias, shock or cardiac arrest, upper-GI bleeding, hospital-acquired sepsis, DVT, central nervous system complications, in-hospital death, wound infection, pulmonary failure, and metabolic derangment. When death resulted from pneumonia, shock, upper-GI bleeding, sepsis, or DVT, it was treated as failure to rescue. Significant statistical relationships were found between a higher proportion of hours of care by RNs and a larger number of hours of care by RNs and some of the adverse outcomes, among them lower rates of UTIs, pneumonia, and failure to rescue (Needleman et al.)

Aiken and a large team of associates (Aiken et al., 2001) from five countries (United States, Canada, Germany, England, and Scotland) examined the effects nurse staffing, other organizational features in hospitals, and nurses' job satisfaction had on patient outcomes of mortality and failure to rescue. Patient discharge data from 713 hospitals were included; 45,300 nurses completed surveys on their perceptions of their workloads, their satisfaction with their jobs, their intention to remain in their positions, relationships between nurses and management, and their views of the adequacy of the care provided on their units. Hospitals that rated highly in the level of staffing as reported by the nurse survey had lower mortality rates and lower rates of failure to rescue (Jackson et al., 2002).

Lush (2001) and her colleagues at the Kaiser Permanente Medical Care Program Northern California Region undertook a project that contrasted in several ways with the three projects just described. Rather than adverse events, the patient outcomes that they focused on included functional status, health care engagement (both knowledge and involvement in care), and mental and social well-being. Included in the latter were fear, anxiety, individual coping, altered role performance, family/caregiver role strain, and family coping. After some experience with this set of outcomes, the group decided to collect additional information about skin breakdown, symptom distress, nosocomial infections, and UTIs (Lush, 2001). Another difference resulted from the fact that Kaiser Permanente is a health system, and patients receiving home care and ambulatory care as well acute hospital care were included. Finally, this project was not being conducted as a research study. Rather, a database was being established that will allow Kaiser Permanente to benchmark best practices, that is, the practice patterns associated with better patient outcomes, shortest length of stay, and lowest costs (Crawford et al., 1996; Lush & Jones, 1995). Using this database, the organization was able to identify differing patterns of care across various elements of its service delivery system and to match these against readmissions, number of provider visits after hospital discharges, and the number of visits to the ER (Lush, 2001).

The fifth project was conducted in all 17 teaching hospitals in Ontario, Canada. A total of 2,046 patients admitted to hospitals with a select number of diagnoses and 1,116 nurses who cared for them participated in this Nursing Staff Mix Outcomes Study (NSMOS), which developed in response to the major restructuring efforts taking place across the province. The mix of skills in nursing staff was being changed, and nonprofessional workers were introduced to the hospital environment for the first time (McGillis Hall et al., 2001). Consequently, there was an interest in knowing what the impact of these changes were on the nurses, the system, and the patients. The patient outcomes selected were a combination of patient well-being, patient satisfaction, and adverse events. Included among the first two outcomes were functional status and pain control, and among the latter, falls, medication errors, wound infections, and UTIs. This group also investigated the social costs to patients of their hospital episode: the number of days of lost income, the number of days post-discharge required to return to gainful employment, whether they were able to return to their previous position of work or to a modified one, and caregiver burden. Nurses in the study reported their levels of job stress, role tension, and job satisfaction. Higher proportions of regulated workers, that is, RNs and registered practical nurses (RPNs), in the staff mix were associated with better patient outcomes at discharge, but not at the six-week follow-up (McGillis Hall et al., 2001).

The latter two projects come reasonably close to operationalizing the Quality Health Outcomes Model (Mitchell et al., 1998) in their inclusion of at least most of the five recommended types of outcomes. The one exception is a direct measure of patient quality of life. Neither project team incorporated this into their range of patient outcomes, perhaps because of the conceptual and measurement difficulties inherent in doing so (Anderson & Burckhardt, 1999; Harrison, Juniper, & Mitchell-DiCenso, 1996).

Kaiser Permanente Medical Care is the only example to date of an organization actively building a database to reflect nursing's input and selecting outcomes that specifically reflect this. These data are not collected on a one-time-only basis, but reflect an ongoing assessment and inputting of information about each patient admitted to their health system. This practice permits year-to-year analysis of how well patients are being cared for from the perspective of the patients and the nursing staff, as well as an examination of the factors that are influencing those perspectives. It represents an important future direction for outcomes research, but one that is dependent on the emergence of relevant variables that have demonstrated relationships with nursing inputs and processes and that are measured with reliable and valid instruments.

1.1.3 Issues in Outcomes Research

Among the many issues confronting the rapidly developing field of patient outcomes research are what outcomes to include, how to measure them, where and when to measure them, how nursing-centric to be, and how to move to database construction. Establishing databases that house information about nursing's contribution to patient care and patient outcomes that are known to be reflective of that contribution is critical if we are to further our understanding of how to use nursing resources to their best effect. It is simply too expensive and not sufficiently comprehensive to rely on individual research studies involving the primary collection of data to answer all of nursing's and the health care system's questions about what nursing-related factors lead to better patient outcomes. Among these factors are skill mix and configuration of nursing personnel; staffing levels; assignment patterns (primary, functional, or team); shift patterns; levels of nursing education, experience, and expertise; ratios of full and part-time nurses; level and type of nursing leadership available centrally and on the units; cohesion and communication among the nursing staff and between nurses and physicians; the implementation of clinical care maps for all patients with selected diagnoses; and the interrelationships of these factors.

Databases that capture the care of all patients in a given hospital, region, or system provide a huge resource both in terms of the number of patients and the amount of information about those patients. The sheer size of this resource cannot be duplicated in primary research efforts. This is important because huge numbers of patients may be needed to examine relationships between nursing factors and subgroups of patients who share certain characteristics. For example, in some research that has already been undertaken, different relationships have been found for medical patients versus surgical patients, and for patients sharing similar diagnoses (Diagnostic Related Groups [DRGs] in the United States and Case Mix Groups [CMGs] in Canada) when compared to other groups (Lichtig, Knauf, & Milholland, 1999; McGillis Hall et al., 2001; Needleman et al., 2002). However, database establishment is complex (Hegyvary, 1991; Jones, 1993) and "getting it wrong" in terms of what variables are included and what is omitted can be very expensive in terms of cost of nurses' time for assessments and recording information, abstracting the information from the patients' charts, and entering it into the database. If information that is not related to outcomes is collected, it becomes an expensive irrelevancy. Alternatively, if something that is highly relevant is omitted from the model that guides the data collection, it is expensive in terms of what questions cannot be asked and answered. In order for databases that house information relevant to nursing to be established for a region or a health care system, there must be consensus among nurses as to (a) what inputs, processes, and outcomes to include; (b) how to define and measure them; and (c) agreement on the timing of their measurement, recording, and abstraction. As important as these dimensions of database establishment are, they are matched by the technical dimensions of the availability of electronic systems, the location of and access to the databases for research, and the security systems that must be in place to ensure patient privacy is protected.

Despite the complexity of database establishment, it is a crucial next step in order for nursing to develop an understanding of how to use its resources to best meet patients' needs. The Ministry of Health and Long-Term Care in Ontario is committed to establishing databases that will house nursing-relevant information for the acute care, home care, complex continuing care, and long-term care sections of the provincial health care system. The appraisal of potential outcomes and their measurement that are the subject of this book were commissioned as part of the development of these databases.

The issue of what to include as an outcome is dependent on the strength of primary research that examines relationships between the myriad of possible effects of nursing care on patients. There are at least four factors that influence this research: (a) the availability of theoretical explanations to link various nursing inputs and processes to outcomes, (b) the need for access to large samples to detect relationships that may be subtle or exist only between subgroups of patients and nursing factors, (c) the ease of accessing these large samples, and (d) appropriate measures that are congruent with the theory supporting the research and that have demonstrated reliability and validity. These are difficult criteria to achieve. There is still little theory linking patient outcomes and antecedent nursing factors. Most of the patient outcomes included in models are empirically rather than theoretically derived and then tested (Mitchell & Shortell, 1997). Failure to rescue (Aiken et al., 1997; Silber et al., 1992) is an exception because it is a theory that links nursing and adverse patient outcomes, specifically mortality. As such, it is of particular interest. However, it is still in the early days of its theoretical life. Some small-scale research studies that demonstrate a statistically significant relationship between a variety of hospital-acquired infections and these adverse outcomes have been replicated in several large-scale studies using clinical databases as the sources of data (Jackson et al., 2002). However, in the failure to rescue research to date, the researchers have taken quite different approaches in how they have tested for the phenomenon. Aiken and her team followed Silber et al.s' (1992) approach and defined failure to rescue as the percentage of patients who died relative to the number who either had a complication and died or died without complication. They also used length of stay greater than expected for a given CMG/DRG as an alternative way of examining rates of failure to rescue (Personal communication, C.A. Estabrooks, August 7, 2002). Needleman et al. (2002) defined failure to rescue as in-hospital death from six specific complications. Significant statistical relationships were found between some of these complications and nursing factors that suggest that the theory may have explanatory potential and should be further tested. It will be interesting to see how the definition of failure to rescue evolves with further testing.

A concern with adverse outcomes has dominated outcomes research, as exemplified by three of the five projects described in this chapter. One reason for this is their accessibility. Patient complications are recorded on their charts and abstracted into clinical databases. This process allows the researchers to include thousands of patients without the expense and complexity of contacting all of the patients and eliciting information from them directly. Similarly, records are kept of adverse events such as patient falls, medication errors, and skin breakdown which, as such, are reasonably easy to retrieve. However, these types of events are plagued by definitional problems; for example, in some institutions a fall is not recorded unless the patient sustains an injury, whereas in others a fall is any situation that results in a patient unintentionally arriving on the floor. Mark and Burleson (1995) examined the availability and consistency with which five adverse events were measured across 16 hospitals from 10 states. Information was available on medication errors and patient falls, but not on nosocomial infections, decubitus ulcers, and unplanned readmissions. However, the descriptions of what constituted a fall and a medication error differed from one hospital to another, and the location of the data varied (for example, on patients' charts, in incident reports, and in quality assurance reports) across even these two outcomes. When more than one institution is involved and hospital discharge records or administrative databases are the sources of data, it is imperative that common definitions across the institutions are assured.

When measuring an outcome of interest requires a scale, as with all research, issues of validity and reliability are highly relevant. A good example of this is found in the work of the Kaiser Permanente group, who elected to construct their own 14-item instrument, the Health Status Outcomes Dimensions, to measure all the outcomes of interest. They refined it until they were satisfied with its reliability and validity before using it as the basis for assessment and subsequent database development (Lush et al., 1997; Lush & Jones, 1995). In the NSMOS study, the investigator group chose to use established instruments to measure all the outcomes of interest. These included the Functional Independence Measure (FIM) and the Medical Outcome Study SF-36 to measure functional status in medical surgical patients, and the Inventory of Functional Status after Childbirth (IFSAC) to measure the same outcome in obstetrical patients. To assess the effect of illness on role performance across all patient groups, they used the Functional Status II (R). The Brief Pain Inventory- Short Form (BPI-SF) was used to measure the severity of pain and how it affects patients' functioning, and the Caregiver Load Scale was used to assess caregiver burden (McGillis Hall et al., 2001).

There is merit to using established scales if they exist and are valid for assessing the outcomes of interest. This practice is recommended for all research, but it may be a particularly important principle when databases to house outcomes are being created. When established scales are used, results from analyzing the databases can be compared with benchmarks where they exist. Many more explanations may be generated and questions raised when the outcomes of the population represented in the database can be compared with similar and different populations represented in other studies.

Another issue in outcomes research is timing: When should measurements be taken and with what frequency (Hegyvary, 1991; Jones, 1993)? These questions cannot be answered in a vacuum, but are dependent on the nature of the outcome of interest. Furthermore, if the outcomes are to be housed in databases, then the number of times an outcome will be abstracted over a specific time period must be established. For example, if the outcome of interest is falls, then a summary score of all falls experienced during an episode of care may be sufficient. If functional status is the outcome, assessments on admission and discharge from hospital and/or home care may provide sufficient information for comparisons. However, if the outcome of interest is pain control, a number of assessments of pain at predetermined intervals may have to be established and a decision made as to how many of these will be abstracted for the purposes of research of database housing. When database development is the objective, it is important that the measurement be useful to staff nurses in their ongoing assessment and delivery of care to patients, as well as to the capture of the outcome for the database.

Should nursing develop nursing-specific models and select outcomes whenever possible that are unique to nursing? It is hard to find support for a nursing-centric approach to the study of outcomes; rather, the importance of acknowledging the multidisciplinary nature of health care is emphasized, as is the need to select outcomes that reflect the contributions of the team of providers as opposed to a discipline within the team (Crawford et al., 1996; Jennings et al., 1999; Jones, 1993; Mitchell et al., 1998). Frankly, it is difficult to identify any outcome that nursing can claim as uniquely reflective of its contribution alone. Selecting outcomes to which many providers can claim partial contribution is more efficient and realistic than seeking nursing-specific variables. Although the Nursing Role Effectiveness Model (Irvine et al., 1998) seeks to represent nursing's unique contribution to patient outcomes, the outcomes themselves are not unique to nursing. They include symptom control, functional status, and self-care knowledge; although evidence links all of them to nursing inputs and processes (Irvine et al.), other disciplines also make contributions to their achievement. Also, there is likely to be more trust across disciplines if established instruments that are recognized by a number of disciplines are used to measure outcomes.

1.1.4 Why Study Outcomes?

Mitchell (2001) searched Medline from 1978–1989 using outcomes as a key word; no references were elicited. But when the same exercise was undertaken for the years 1997–2000, over 700 citations were listed. Why have outcomes generated so much interest in the nursing and health services research communities over the last decade? The explanation seems to be accountability. Outcomes are "in" because accountability has become an important expectation of the health care system and they provide evidence for accountability exercises. All components of the health care system are now asked to demonstrate their value, whereas their value was taken for granted in the decades preceding the 1990s. Nursing has had little to offer in terms of "hard" evidence when asked to demonstrate that nurses make a difference to patient care. Consequently, over the last decade there has been increasing activity to fill this gap by identifying outcomes that demonstrate that nurses do make a difference to patients and their experience of illness. The next major breakthrough will be establishing databases that will house these outcomes collected from all patients in a system who receive the services of nursing personnel. These databases can then serve as the source of data for research studies with policy and practice implications. For example, if the research shows that patients achieve better outcomes when specific proportions of registered nurses are present to care for them or when specific organizational structures are in place, the foundations for policy recommendations are laid (Sovie & Jawad, 2001). If other research demonstrates that patients are leaving hospitals or home care programs with insufficient understanding of their health condition to care for themselves safely, the practice implications are obvious.

There is no guarantee that having evidence demonstrating nursing's direct effect on how well patients achieve outcomes that are important to their recovery from illness and to the financial well-being of the health care system will influence how nursing is valued, respected, and heard in political and administrative circles. However, we have years of experience indicating that not having this evidence is seriously damaging nursing as a profession and eroding the quality of care available to society.

1.1.5 Purpose of this Review of the State of Science on Nursing-Sensitive Outcomes

In order to establish the databases that will house outcomes from all patients who receive the services of nursing personnel, we need an evidenced-based understanding of which outcomes have demonstrated sensitivity to nursing care.

In addition, we need evidence upon which to make decisions about how to measure these outcomes in a valid and reliable manner. This book seeks to address this need by critically reviewing the state of the evidence on nursing-sensitive outcomes and approaches to their measurement. The outcomes included in this review were selected based on the theoretical/conceptual work undertaken to categorize nursing-sensitive patient outcomes and on the recommendations of members of the Nursing and Health Outcomes Task Force, Ministry of Health and Long-Term Care, Ontario. The outcomes included in this review are *functional status, self-care, symptom management, patient safety,* and *patient satisfaction.* A review of the literature on minimum data sets for nursing and health care services is included in the book because these data sets have been developed as a way to standardize the assessment and recording of health outcomes data across settings and countries. A critical review and analysis of the literature on nurse job satisfaction measures was conducted because of the growing recognition that patient outcomes are related to quality work environments. The goal of the analysis is to provide sound information for building a clinical database to document the quality and effectiveness of nursing care in acute, community or home, and long-term care settings.

The specific objectives of this literature analysis are:

- To identify the essential characteristics or attributes defining each outcome concept. This objective was critical for developing a clear conceptual definition of the concepts.

- To determine the extent to which each outcome has demonstrated sensitivity to nursing care. This was accomplished by examining structure and process variables that influence or contribute to the achievement of the functional, symptom, safety, and perceptual outcomes within acute, community, and long-term care settings.

- To identify the instruments that have been used to measure each outcome concept in acute, community, and long-term care settings.

- To review the content of the instruments and assess their congruence/consistency with the essential attributes of each outcome concept (i.e., to determine the content validity of the instruments).

- To critically review the instruments for reliability, validity, responsiveness to change, and sensitivity to nursing care.

1.2 Framework

The literature review on nursing-sensitive outcomes was guided by two frameworks: (a) the Nursing Role Effectiveness Model (Irvine, Sidani, & McGillis Hall, 1998), which was used as a guide to identify the structure, process, and outcome variables to be included in the review; and (b) a measurement framework (Sidani & Irvine, 1998), which informed and structured the review of the psychometric properties and clinical utility of the instruments measuring the outcomes of interest. An overview of the frameworks is presented in this section.

1.2.1 The Nursing Role Effectiveness Model

The Nursing Role Effectiveness Model was developed by Irvine et al. (1998) to identify the contribution of nurses' roles to outcome achievement. The model is based on the structure-process-outcome model of quality care (Donabedian, 1980). It has been reformulated for the purposes of this book, based on empirical testing (Doran et al., 2002) (see Figure 1.1).

The structure component consists of nurses, patients, and organizational variables that influence the processes and outcomes of care. Nurse variables entail professional characteristics such as experience, knowledge, and skill levels, which can influence the quality of nursing care. Patient variables include personal and health- or illness-related characteristics, such as age, type and severity of illness, and co-morbidities, that affect either the delivery of care or the achievement of

Figure 1.1. The Nursing Role Effectiveness Model

Structure	Process	Outcomes
Patient Age, gender, education, type and severity of illness, co-morbidities	**Independent role** Nursing interventions	**Nursing-sensitive patient outcomes** Functional status, self-care, symptom control, safety/adverse occurrences, patient satisfaction
Nurse Education, experience	**Medical care-related role** Medically directed care, expanded scope of nursing practice	
Organizational Staffing, staff mix, workload, work environment	**Interdependent role** Team communication, coordination of care, case management	

Note: Based on the original Nursing Role Effectiveness model (Irvine, Sidani, & McGillis Hall, 1998). From "Linking Outcomes to Nurses' Role in Health Care," by D. Irvine, S. Sidani, & L. M. McGillis Hall, 1998, *Nursing Economic$, 16*(2), 58–64, 87. Copyright 1998 by Nursing Economic$. Reprinted with permission of the publisher.

outcomes. Organizational variables focus on staffing and nursing assignment patterns, which directly affect the delivery of nursing care.

The process component consists of the nurses' independent, medical care-related, and interdependent roles. The independent role concerns functions and activities initiated by professional nurses. They refer to autonomous actions initiated by the nurse in response to the patients' problems; they do not require a physician's order. The medical care-related role concerns functions and activities initiated by nurses in response to a medical order. They include the nurse's clinical judgment, implementation of medically directed care, and evaluation of the patient's response to the care. The interdependent role concerns functions and activities in which nurses engage that are shared by other members of the health care team. They include activities such as interdisciplinary team communication, care coordination, and health system maintenance and improvement.

The outcome component consists of nursing-sensitive patient outcomes. These are classified into six categories: (a) prevention of complications like injury or nosocomial infections; (b) clinical outcomes such as symptom control; (c) knowledge of the disease, its treatment, and management of side effects; (d) functional health outcomes such as physical, social, cognitive, mental functioning, and self-care abilities; (e) satisfaction with care; and (f) cost.

Irvine et al. (1998) proposed that the structure variables influence the process and outcome variables, and that the process affects the outcome variables. They supported the propositions with empirical evidence synthesized from the literature (Irvine et al.) and with an empirical validation of the proposed relationships in an acute-care setting (Doran et al., 2002).

This model guided the selection of variables to be included in the review of the state of the science on nursing-sensitive outcomes. The following structure and process variables that influence the functional, self-care, symptom, safety, and perceptual outcomes of interest were examined:

Structure variables:

- Nurse variables: Education and position, which are often reported in published articles, were used as "proxy" indicators of nurses' knowledge and skill levels.

- Patient variables: Age, gender, and type of illness are frequently reported in published articles. Accumulating evidence is showing that these characteristics influence the patients' responses to some nursing interventions, particularly psychoeducational interventions (Brown, 1992; Hentinen, 1986; Sidani, 1994; Sidani & Braden, 1998).

- Organizational variables: Staffing and staff mix is a variable that has been extensively investigated recently, and was found to affect the quality of communication with patients (Doran et al., 2001), adverse occurrences in the hospital (Needleman et al., 2002), and patient satisfaction with care (Lengacher et al., 1996). Evidence is growing that the environment in which nurses work influences the quality of their practice and patient outcome achievement (Aiken, Smith, & Lake, 1994; McGillis Hall et al., 2002).

Process variables:

- Nursing independent role functions: Patient education is, by far, the independent nursing activity that has been most commonly investigated in acute, community, and long-term care settings, as evidenced by the number of published meta-analytic studies conducted to synthesize the literature and/or to estimate its effects on various outcomes (e.g., Brown, 1992; Devine & Cook, 1986; Hathaway, 1986). Patient education is usually focused on self-care and symptom management strategies.

- Nursing medical care-related role functions: Nurses are assuming direct medical care-related activities with the development of advanced practice roles, such as nurse practitioners (Aiken et al., 1993; Garrard et al., 1990). Furthermore, some practice settings are experimenting with nurse-led inpatient units as a way to provide cost-effective care for less resource-intensive patient populations (Griffiths et al., 2001).

- Nursing interdependent role functions: Coordination of discharge planning and nurse-led case management are two examples of the interdependent functions assumed by nurses in acute, community, and long-term care settings. Their impact on clinical and functional patient outcomes (e.g., Braden et al., 1989, Piette et al., 2000) has been less frequently investigated than their impact on perceptual outcomes (e.g., Moher et al., 1992; Naylor et al., 1999).

Outcome variables:

- Clinical outcomes: Symptom control has been extensively investigated in post-surgical patients with a particular focus on pain control (Tuman et al., 1991) and in oncology in- and outpatient settings (Smith et al., 1994).

- Functional outcomes: Physical and psychosocial functioning and self-care abilities were outcomes of concern for patients with chronic and acute illness (Gillette & Jenko, 1991; Doran et al., 2002).

- Patient safety outcomes: These have been the foci of nursing report cards (American Nurses Association, 1995, 1996, 1997, 2000; Pierce, 1997) and studies involving secondary databases (Needleman et al., 2002).

- Perceptual outcomes: Satisfaction with nursing care has been examined in a multitude of studies investigating nursing care delivery models (ANA, 1997; Gillette & Jenko, 1991; Lang & Marek, 1990).

1.2.2 Measurement Framework

This literature review and analysis is aimed at providing information that will guide the development of a database for monitoring outcomes of nursing care. Building this database rests on the availability of standardized measures of the outcomes that have the ability to collect accurate data with minimal error. Instruments that have been used to measure the outcomes of interest were identified, and their ability to obtain valid data was critically analyzed. The following framework guided the critical review of the outcome measures. The framework was based on the premise that for an instrument to be useful in accurately measuring or monitoring outcomes, it should demonstrate acceptable reliability, validity, responsiveness, and clinical utility.

Reliability
Reliability refers to the dependability of measurement. It concerns the extent to which measurements are consistent and reproducible across items, individuals, or occasions, that is, it introduces minimal error. Three types of reliability can be assessed:

- Internal consistency: refers to the degree to which the items comprising the instrument are interrelated and able to measure a single concept or domain/dimension of a concept with minimal error. Internal consistency is most commonly assessed with the Cronbach's alpha coefficient (Streiner & Norman, 1995). It is based on the average correlations among the items. An alpha coefficient value of .70 is considered the minimal acceptable level of internal consistency for newly developed instruments, and .80 is the minimum for established instruments (Nunnally, 1978).

- Stability or test-retest: refers to the degree to which the instrument reproduces similar scores for the same individuals when measured at different occasions. Stability is frequently evaluated with a correlation coefficient. A coefficient ≥ 0 indicates an acceptable level of stability (Streiner & Norman, 1995).

- Equivalence or inter-rater: refers to the degree of agreement between raters/observers. It is examined using any of the following statistical tests: percent of agreement among the raters, Cohen's Kappa coefficient, Pearson's correlation coefficient, or intra-class correlation coefficient. A coefficient value $\geq .80$ indicates acceptable inter-rater reliability.

Validity

Validity is concerned with whether an instrument measures what it is supposed to measure, that is, it should accurately reflect all the domains and dimensions of the concept. Different types of validity can be assessed:

- Content validity: refers to the degree to which the content of the items comprising the instrument covers all the domains of the concept it is supposed to measure. It is evaluated by having experts or judges rate the extent to which the items capture all the domains and the relevance of the items' content to their corresponding domain. A content validity index $\geq .80$ represents an acceptable level of agreement among the experts, which supports content validity (Lynn, 1986).

- Criterion or concurrent validity: refers to the correspondence between a measure and a criterion (i.e., another instrument measuring the same concept) administered at the same or different points in time. This type of validity is assessed by computing a correlation coefficient or by conducting sensitivity and specificity analyses. A correlation coefficient $\geq .50$ and sensitivity and specificity values $\geq 90\%$ provide empirical support for an instrument's criterion or concurrent validity (Beutler, Wakefield, & Williams, 1994).

- Construct validity: assesses whether a measure is related to other variables in a way that is consistent with theoretically derived predictions. It is evaluated one of two ways: first, by examining the difference in the mean score on the measure between two groups of individuals known to differ on the concept of interest, using a *t-test* or *F-ratio*. A statistically significant difference supports the construct validity of the measure. The second way to evaluate construct validity is by examining the correlation coefficients between the measure of the concept of interest and the measures of related concepts. Statistically significant correlations between the measures of the hypothesized direction and magnitude provide evidence of construct validity (Waltz et al., 1991).

Responsiveness

Responsiveness refers to the instrument's sensitivity to changes in the level of the concept being measured. Evidence for responsiveness includes significant differences in the mean scores obtained at different points in time, such as before and after treatment. The evidence for responsiveness is strengthened when changes in the scores are correlated with other indicators of change, such as clinically assessed changes. No specific criteria indicating responsiveness are well established (Guyatt et al., 1989).

Clinical Utility

Instruments to be used by clinicians in their everyday practice must be useful. To be clinically useful, an instrument needs to be simple, that is, it does not take much time to complete, it is easy to use or does not require a special technique to administer, it is easy to score, and the scores are easy to interpret (Corcoran & Fischer, 1987; Sidani & Irvine, 1998). Although there are no well-defined criteria for evaluating clinical utility, the following information was reported for the instruments: number of items comprising it, amount of time to complete it, and availability of cut-off scores or normative values that could be used as a reference for interpreting the obtained scores (i.e., determining clinically meaningful categories for classifying patients).

1.3 Methodology for Conducting the Literature Review

The literature review was conducted through a series of consecutive steps. Two general categories of references were included: theoretical (or conceptual) and empirical, in order to address all the objectives set for the review. Theoretical/conceptual references discussed a perspective of how the clinical, functional, safety, or perceptual outcomes are viewed. That is, they presented theoretical and/or operational definitions of the outcomes. The definitions identify the essential characteristics of the outcome concept and point to its domains and indicators. Empirical articles reported the results of descriptive-correlation or experimental studies that examined the relationships among structure, process, and outcome variables; assessed the psychometric properties of outcome measures; or evaluated the effectiveness of nursing interventions in achieving the desired outcomes.

1.3.1 Step 1: Literature Search

The first step of the literature review consisted of identifying conceptual and empirical references that discussed or investigated the clinical, functional, and perceptual outcomes of interest in acute, community, and long-term care settings. The literature search involved four strategies:

- A comprehensive list was generated of relevant articles, book chapters, books, or other documents that the research team members have accumulated through their involvement in previous work on any of the structure, process, or outcome variables of interest to this review.

- A computerized literature search was conducted to update and obtain a comprehensive list of references on the variables of interest in the acute, community, and long-term care patient populations. The following computerized literature databases were used in this step: CINHAL, HEALTH PLANNING, MEDLINE, CANCERLIT, SOCIOFILE, and PSYCHLIT. The Virginia Henderson library was also checked for additional references. The Virginia Henderson Library is an electronic database that holds reports of completed and in-progress research studies, dissertations, and conference presentations. It is maintained by Sigma Theta Tau International-Honor Society of Nursing (www.stti.iupui.edu/library).

- The literature search strategy entailed using specific key words relevant to the outcomes under review. Examples include functional status, nausea, fatigue, pain, and self-care. These specific key words were paired with common key words that were used for each search. The following common key words were used: nursing-sensitive patient outcomes, nursing interventions, nursing care, quality of nursing care, nursing outcomes, patient, and quality of care. A separate key word search was conducted to identify articles to include in the chapters on nursing job satisfaction and minimum data sets. With regard to nursing job satisfaction, the focus of the search was to identify studies that investigated the relationship between nursing job satisfaction and a patient outcome.

- The references reported within the articles, in particular those reporting the results of meta-analytic studies or integrative literature reviews/syntheses (e.g., Heater et al., 1986; Smith et al., 1994) were traced to identify additional references.

1.3.2   Step 2: Literature Selection

The references identified were included in the literature review if they met the following criteria:

For theoretical/conceptual references:

- They discussed the definition and the domains/dimensions of the functional, self-care, symptom, safety, patient, and nurse job satisfaction outcome concepts of interest.

- They presented the findings of a concept analysis or literature review performed to identify the essential characteristics, domains, and dimensions, as well as the empirical indicators or manifestations, of the outcome concepts of interest.

- They reported the results of a qualitative study conducted to explore the understanding or perception of the functional, self-care, symptom, safety, or satisfaction outcomes in acute, community, or long-term care settings.

For empirical references:

- They described the development of an instrument used to measure the outcomes of interest in patients and nurses in acute, community, or long-term care settings.

- They reported the results of testing the psychometric properties of the instrument in the patient and nurse populations of interest.

- They described the instrument in detail and discussed its clinical utility and its applicability or use in practice settings.

- They reported the results of studies that examined the relationships among the structure, process, and outcome variables selected for this review (as identified in the framework section).

- They reported the results of studies that examined the effects of interdependent, independent, or medical care-related nursing functions/interventions (as delineated in the framework section) on the functional, self-care, symptom, safety, and satisfaction outcomes in acute, community, or long-term care settings.

Studies with experimental or quasi-experimental designs were included. Including quasi-experimental studies was important for two reasons: (a) it increased the number of references for the comprehensive literature review, particularly studies that were conducted in the context of actual/everyday practice where randomization may not have been feasible or possible; and (b) it provided evidence for determining the extent to which the outcomes are responsive to change. Differences in research designs were accounted for when synthesizing the findings across studies to address the objectives set for this literature review.

1.3.3 *Step 3: Literature Compilation*

A list of references was generated for each of the functional, self-care, symptom, safety, patient satisfaction, and nursing job satisfaction outcomes of interest. Each author assumed primary responsibility for reviewing the literature pertinent to an outcome. With the exception of the nursing minimum data set chapter, a standardized framework and tables for extracting the relevant data were used in order to promote a consistent approach to the review among all authors. As the editor of the book, Dr. Doran oversaw and coordinated the activities of all members of the team. The results of the critical analysis of the literature are presented in the chapters that follow.

Each chapter provides a discussion of how the particular outcome concept has been conceptualized in the nursing literature. A conceptual definition is proposed based on this evidence. The empirical evidence linking patient outcome to nursing inputs or processes is critically examined. The approaches to measurement are reviewed with regard to the reliability, validity, and sensitivity of the outcome instrument to nursing variables. Recommendations are proposed related to the strength of the evidence concerning the relationship between nursing practice and patient outcomes. Then recommendations are also made about approaches to the measurement of the outcome concept. The chapters conclude with directions for further research.

References

Aiken, L. H., Clarke, S. P., Sloane, D. M., Sochalski, J. A., Busse, R., Clarke, H., et al. (2001). Nurses' reports on hospital care in five countries. *Health Affairs, May–June,* 43–53.

Aiken, L. H., Lake, E. T., Semaan, S., Lehman, H. P., O'Hare, P. A., Cole, C. S., et al. (1993). Nurse practitioner managed care for persons with HIV infection. *Image, Journal of Nursing Scholarship, 25,* 172–177.

Aiken, L. H., Smith, H. L., & Lake, E. T. (1994). Lower medical mortality among a set of hospitals known for good nursing care. *Medical Care, 32,* 171–187.

Aiken, L. H., Sochalski, J., & Lake, E. T. (1997). Studying outcomes of organizational change in health services. *Medical Care, 35*(Suppl.), NS6-NS18.

Al-Hader, A. S., & Wan, T. T. (1991). Modeling organizational determinants of hospital mortality. *Health Services Research, 26,* 303–323.

American Nurses Association. (1995). *Nursing report card for acute care.* Washington, DC: American Nurses Publishing.

American Nurses Association. (1996). *Nursing quality indicators.* Washington, DC: American Nurses Publishing.

American Nurses Association. (1997). *Implementing nursing's report card.* Washington, DC: American Nurses Publishing.

American Nurses Association. (2000). *Nurse staffing and patient outcomes in the inpatient hospital setting.* Washington, DC: American Nurses Publishing.

Anderson, K. L., & Burckhardt, C. S. (1999). Conceptualization and measurement of quality of life as an outcome variable for health care intervention and research. *Journal of Advanced Nursing, 29,* 298–306.

Atkins, P. M., Marshall, B. S., & Javagli, R. G. (1996). Happy employees lead to loyal patients. *Journal of Health Care Marketing, 16*(4), 15–23.

Beutler, L. E., Wakefield, P., & Williams, R. E. (1994). Use of psychological tests/instruments for treatment planning. In M. E. Maruish (Ed.), *The use of psychological testing for treatment planning and outcome assessment* (pp. 55–74). Hillsdale, NJ: Lawrence Erlbaum.

Braden, C. J., Mishel, M. H., Longman, A., & Burns, L. R. (1989). *Nurse interventions promoting self-help response to breast cancer.* Washington, DC: National Cancer Institute.

Brown, S. A. (1992). Meta-analysis of diabetes patient education research: Variations in intervention effects across studies. *Research in Nursing & Health, 15,* 409–419.

Corcoran, K., & Fischer, J. (1987). *Measures for clinical practice: A sourcebook.* New York: The Free Press.

Crawford, B. L., Taylor, L. S., Seipert, B. S., & Lush, M. (1996). The imperatives of outcomes analysis: An integration of traditional and nontraditional outcomes measures. *Journal of Nursing Care Quality, 10*(2), 33–40.

Devine, E. C., & Cook, T. D. (1986). Clinical and cost-saving effects of psychoeducational interventions with surgical patients: A meta-analysis. *Research in Nursing and Health, 9,* 89–105.

Donabedian, A. (1966). Evaluating the quality of medical care. *Milbank Quarterly, 44* (Suppl.), 166–206.

Donabedian, A. (1980). *Exploration in quality assessment and monitoring: The definition of quality and approaches to its assessment.* Ann Arbor, MI: Health Administration Press.

Doran, D. M., McGillis Hall, L., Sidani, S., O'Brien-Pallas, L., Donner, G., Baker, G. R., et al. (2002). Nursing staff mix and patient outcome achievement: The mediating role of nurse communication. *The Journal of International Nursing Perspectives, 1,* 74–83.

Doran, D. I., Sidani, S., Keatings, M., & Doidge, D. (2002). An empirical test of the Nursing Role Effectiveness Model. *Journal of Advanced Nursing, 38,* 29–39.

Garrard, J., Kane, R. L., Radosevich, D. M., Skay, C. L., Arnold, S., Kepferle, L., et al. (1990). Impact of geriatric nurse practitioners on nursing-home residents' functional status, satisfaction, and discharge outcomes. *Medical Care, 28,* 271–283.

Gillette, B., & Jenko, M. (1991). Major clinical functions: A unifying framework for measuring outcomes. *Journal of Nursing Care Quality, 6,* 20–24.

Griffiths, P., Harris, R., Richardson, G., Hallett, N., Heard, S., & Wilson-Barnett, J. (2001). Substitution of a nursing-led inpatient unit for acute services: Randomized control trial of outcomes and cost of nursing-led intermediate care. *Age and Aging, 30,* 483–488.

Guyatt, G. H., Deyo, R. A., Charlson, M., Levine, M. N., & Mitchell, A. (1989). Responsiveness and validity in health status measurement: A clarification. *Journal of Clinical Epidemiology, 42,* 403–408.

Guyatt, G. H., Feeny, D. H., & Patrick, D. L. (1993). Measuring health-related quality of life. *Annals of Internal Medicine, 118,* 622–629.

Harrison, M. B., Juniper, E. F., & Mitchell-DiCenso, A. (1996). Quality of life as an outcome measure in nursing research. *Canadian Journal of Nursing Research, 28*(3), 49–68.

Hartz, A. J., Krakauer, H., Kuhn, E. M., Young, M., Jacobsen, S. J., Gay, G., et al. (1989). Hospital characteristics and mortality rates. *New England Journal of Medicine, 321,* 1720–1725.

Hathaway, D. (1986). Effect of preoperative instruction on postoperative outcomes: A meta-analysis. *Nursing Research, 35,* 269–275.

Heater, B.S., Becker, A. K., & Olson, R. K. (1988). Nursing interventions and patient outcomes: A meta-analysis of studies. *Nursing Research, 37,* 303–307.

Hegyvary, S. T. (1991). Issues in outcomes research. *Journal of Nursing Quality Assurance, 5* (2), 1–6.

Hentinen, M. (1986). Teaching and adaptation of patients with myocardial infarction. *International Journal of Nursing Studies, 23*(2), 125–138.

Irvine, D., Sidani, S., & McGillis Hall, L. (1998). Linking outcomes to nurses' roles in health care. *Nursing Economic$, 16*(2), 58–64, 87.

Jackson, M., Chiarello, L. A., Gaynes, R. P., & Gerberding, J. L. (2002). Nurse staffing and healthcare-associated infections. *Journal of Nursing Administration, 32,* 314–322.

Jennings, B. M., Staggers, N., & Brosch, L. R. (1999). A classification scheme for outcome indicators. *Image: Journal of Nursing Scholarship, 31,* 381–88.

Jones, K. (1993). Outcomes analysis: Methods and issues. *Nursing Economic$, 11,* 145–52.

Kaldenberg, D. (1999). Patient satisfaction and the role of choice. *Marketing Health Services, 19* (3), 39–42.

Lang, N. M., & Marek, K. D. (1990). The classification of patient outcomes. *Journal of Professional Nursing, 6,* 153–163.

Lengacher, C. A., Mabe, P. R., Heinenmann, D., VanCott, M. L., Swymer, S., & Kent, K. (1996). Effects of the PIPC model on outcome measures of productivity and costs. *Nursing Economics, 14,* 205–212.

Lichtig, L. K., Knauf, R. A., & Milholland, D. K. (1999). Some impacts of nursing on acute hospital outcomes. *Journal of Nursing Administration, 29*(2), 25–33.

Lohr, K. N. (1985). *Impact of Medicare prospective payment on the quality of medical care: A research agenda.* Santa Monica, CA: The Rand Corporation.

Lush, M. (2001). Continuity across sectors. In *Invitational Symposium, Nursing and Health Outcomes Project, March 15 and 16, 2001, Toronto, Ontario, Canada.* Retrieved from http://www.gov.on.ca/health/nursing.

Lush, M. T., Henry, S. B., Foote, K., & Jones, D. L. (1997). Developing a generic health status measure for use in a computer-based outcomes infrastructure. In U. Gerdin, M. Tallberg, & P. Wainwright (Eds.), *Nursing informatics* (pp. 229–234). Amsterdam: IOS Press.

Lush, M. T., & Jones, D. L. (1995). Developing an outcomes infrastructure for nursing. *Journal of the American Medical Informatics Association Symposium Supplement, SCAMC Proceedings.* Philadelphia: Hanley & Belfus.

Lynn, M. R. (1986). Determination and quantification of content validity. *Nursing Research, 35,* 382–385.

Mark, B. A., and Burleson, D. L. (1995). Measurement of patient outcomes. *Journal of Nursing Administration, 25*(4), 52–59.

McGillis Hall, L., Doran, D. I., Baker, G. R., Pink, G. H., Sidani, S., O'Brien-Pallas, L., et al. (2001). *The impact of nursing staff mix models and organizational change strategies on patient, system and nursing outcomes.* Toronto, Ontario, Canada: University of Toronto, Faculty of Nursing.

Mitchell, P. (2001). The evolving world of outcomes. In *Invitational Symposium, Nursing and Health Outcomes Project, March 15 and 16, 2001, Toronto, Ontario, Canada.* Retrieved from http://www.gov.on.ca/health/nursing.

Mitchell, P. H., Ferketich, S., & Jennings, B. M. (1998). Quality health outcomes model. *Image: Journal of Nursing Scholarship, 30,* 43–46.

Mitchell, P. H. & Shortell, S. M. (1997). Adverse outcomes and variations in organization of care delivery. *Medical Care, 35*(Suppl.), NS19-32.

Moher, D., Weinberg, A., Hanlon, R., & Runnalls, K. (1992). Effects of a medical team coordinator on length of hospital stay. *Canadian Medical Association Journal, 146,* 511–515.

Naylor, M. D., Brooten, D., Campbell, R., Jacobson, B. S., Mezey, M. D., Pauly, M. V., et al. (1999). Discharge planning and home follow up by advanced practice nurses reduced hospital readmissions of elderly patients. *Journal of the American Medical Association, 281,* 613–620.

Needleman, J., Buerhaus, P., Mattke, S., Stewart, M., & Zelevinsky, K. (2002). Nursing-staffing levels and the quality of care in hospitals. *New England Journal of Medicine, 346,* 1715–1722.

Nunnally, J. C. (1978). *Introduction to psychological measurement.* New York: McGraw-Hill.

Pierce, S. F. (1997). Nurse-sensitive health care outcomes in acute care settings: An integrative analysis of the literature. *Journal of Nursing Quality, 11*(4), 60–72.

Piette, J. D., Weinberger, M., & McPhee, S. J. (2000). The effect of automated calls with telephone nurse follow-up on patient-centered outcomes of diabetes care. A randomized, controlled trial. *Medical Care, 38,* 218–230.

Rowell, P. A. (2001). ANA study on nursing-sensitive outcomes. In *Invitational Symposium, Nursing and health Outcomes Project, March 15 and 16, 2001, Toronto, Ontario, Canada.* Retrieved from http://www.gov.on.ca/health/nursing.

Scherb, C. A. (2002). Outcomes research: Making a difference in practice. *Outcomes Management, 6,* 22–26.

Shortell, S., & Hughes, E. (1988). The effects of regulation, competition, and ownership on hospital rates among hospital inpatients. *New England Journal of Medicine, 318,* 1100–1107.

Sidani, S. (1994). Empirical testing of a conceptual model to evaluate psychoeducational interventions. Unpublished Doctoral Dissertation, University of Arizona, Tucson.

Sidani, S., & Braden, C. J. (1998). *Evaluating nursing interventions. A theory-driven approach.* Thousand Oaks, CA: Sage.

Sidani, S., & Irvine, D. (1998). *Defining and operationalizing clinical utility of instruments.* Paper presented at the Nursing Research Conference, Edmonton, June 14–15.

Silber, J. H., Williams, S. V., Krakauer, H., & Schwartz, J. S. (1992). Hospital and patient characteristics associated with death after surgery: A study of adverse occurrence and failure to rescue. *Medical Care, 30,* 615–629.

Smith, M. C., Holcombe, J. K., & Stullenbarger, E. (1994). A meta-analysis of intervention effectiveness for symptom management in oncology nursing research. *Oncology Nursing Forum, 21,* 1201–1210.

Sovie, M. D., & Jawad, A. (2001). Hospital restructuring and its impact on outcomes: Nursing staff regulations are premature. *Journal of Nursing Administration, 31,* 588–600.

Streiner, D. L., & Norman, G. R. (1995). *Health measurement scales. A practical guide to their development and use* (2nd ed.). Oxford, England: Oxford University Press.

Tuman, K., McCarthy, R., March, R., Delaria, G., Patel, R., & Ivankovich, A. (1991). Effects of epidural anesthesia and analgesia on coagulation and outcome after vascular surgery. *Anesthesia Analgesia, 73,* 696–704.

Van Servellen, G., & Schultz, M. A. (1999). Demystifying the influence of hospital characteristics on inpatient mortality rates. *Journal of Nursing Administration, 29*(4), 39–47.

Waltz, C. F., Strickland, O. L., & Lenz, E. R. (1991). *Measurement in nursing research* (2nd ed.). Philadelphia: F. A. Davis.

Weisman, C. S., & Nathanson, C. A. (1985). Professional satisfaction and client outcomes: A comparative organizational analysis. *Medical Care, 23,* 1179–1192.

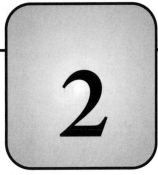

Functional Status

Diane M. Doran, RN, PhD

2.1 Introduction

"Functional health status has emerged as an important patient outcome because (a) it captures patients' perceptions of their day-to-day functioning, and (b) it adds another perspective to more traditional outcomes such as adverse occurrences and physiological clinical data" (Ramler et al., 1996). Maintaining and enhancing the individual's ability to achieve functional independence in personal care, mobility, and social activities has been identified as a goal of nursing in many of the nursing theoretical frameworks (e.g., Orem, 1980; Olson, 2001; Roy & Roberts, 1981). Furthermore, it has been included as a concept in most of the outcome classifications for nursing (Gillette & Jenko, 1991; Johnson & Maas, 1997) and has been suggested as a relevant outcome of care for staff nurses (Brown & Grimes, 1995; Kline Leidy, 1994) and advanced practice nurses (Mill Barrell, Irving Merwin, & Poster, 1997). Several empirical studies have demonstrated that nursing interventions can have an effect on functional status outcomes (Brown & Grimes, 1995; McCorkle et al., 1989). In a meta-analysis examining the effect of nursing interventions on patient outcomes, Heater, Becker, & Olson (1988) reported a mean effect size of 0.63 for behavioral outcomes and 0.54 for psychosocial outcomes. Both types of outcomes reflect aspects of human functioning.

In this chapter, the way in which functional status has been conceptualized as an outcome of nursing care is examined, and then a conceptual definition of functional status is proposed based on this evidence. The empirical evidence linking patients' functional status outcomes to nursing inputs or processes is critically examined. The approaches to measurement are reviewed with regard to the reliability, validity, and sensitivity of the functional status instrument to nursing variables. Recommendations are proposed, related to the strength of the evidence concerning the relationship between nursing practice and functional health outcomes and approaches to the measurement of functional status. The chapter concludes with directions for further research.

The methodology used to identify the relevant literature, as well as the criteria for the literature selection and systematic review, were discussed in Chapter 1. A systematic search of the nursing and health databases yielded a total of 237 sources that were either empirical or conceptual papers addressing the concept of functional status. Ninety-six of these met the inclusion criteria and are reviewed in this chapter.

2.2 Theoretical Background: Definition of the Concept

Knight (2000) published a paper on two concepts—cognitive ability and functional status—that offered a very nice overview of the development of functional status as a concept. She noted that in the early literature, discussion of functional status focused on an individual's ability to engage in activities of daily living (ADL) such as bathing, dressing, feeding, and motor performance (Knight, 2000). In the middle to late 1980s, as providers became more focused on shorter hospital stays and outcomes that reflected an individual's ability to live at home, measures began to emerge that addressed common daily activities other than activities of daily living (Knight, 2000). Functional status became a descriptor for instrumental activities of daily living (IADL) such as shopping, cooking, and cleaning. In addition, functional status was used to describe broad functioning in major aspects of living, such as the social, occupational, and psychological aspects (Knight, 2000). According to Knight (2002), Moinpour, McCorkle, and Saunders (1988) proposed one the earliest comprehensive definitions of functional status in nursing. They defined functional status measurement as "any systematic attempt to measure the level at which a person is functioning in a variety of areas, such as physical health, quality of self-maintenance, quality of role activities, intellectual status, social activity, attitude toward the world and toward self, and emotional status."

In her conceptual analysis, Knight (2000) noted that the conceptualization of functional status must include cognitive, behavioral, and psychological dimensions. The behavioral dimension typically has been operationally defined as performance of activities of daily living and instrumental activities of daily living. Knight suggested that the psychological dimension might include components such as mood, affect, and motivation. The cognitive dimension might include components such as attention, concentration, memory, and problem solving. Fawcett, Tulman, and Samarel (1995) identified a psychological dimension and a social dimension to functional status. The psychological element of function included mental, cognitive, emotional, and spiritual activities. The social element included activities associated with roles taken on at various stages of development, as well as activities associated with interpersonal relationships (Fawcett et al., 1995).

Cooley (1998) defined functional status as the individual's actual performance of normal day-to-day role activities. These included performance of (a) basic activities of daily living, such as bathing, dressing, eating, and walking; and (b) carrying out role responsibilities both in and out of the house, such as cleaning, cooking, shopping, and working. Richmond, McCorkle, Tulman, and Fawcett (1997) defined the term "function" as how people perform activities that are relevant to them.

Many terms have been used interchangeably in the literature to refer to functional status. Among them are function, functioning, functional ability, functional capacity, functional status, functional performance, physical function, impairment, handicap, functional assessment, activities of daily living, health status, and quality of life (Fawcett et al., 1995; Richmond et al., 1997). Ouellet and Rush (1996), for example, conducted a qualitative study of nurses' perceptions of client mobility that yielded results very similar to those of studies in which functional status had been conceptualized. Nurses in their study described mobility as having three dimensions: physical, cognitive, and social. The physical dimension was expressed as movement of the body, performance of activities of daily living, and performance of instrumental activities of daily living. Nurses defined mobility as "the ability ... to move ... either by walking or by moving a joint.... Ability to move through space from point A to point B." Under categories related to activities of daily living or self-care, nurses included references to instrumental activities such as, "Can they use the phone, do they do their own affairs, do they do their banking ... can they make out their grocery list, can they phone the grocery store, can they order...." The social dimension was described by the nurses as movement of an affiliative nature that enabled one to initiate and maintain contact with others through social events and activities. The cognitive dimension was defined as movement of the mind that seeks to keep it active. Cognitive mobility was reflected in such references as keeping "up with what's going on like at the movie theatre or even if it's bingo ...," stimulating the mind, and having an active mind. Critical qualities of mobility emerged from the qualitative data. These included ease of movement, independence, and safety. In a more recent study, Bourret, Bernick, Cott, and Kontos (2002) investigated the meaning of mobility for residents and staff in long-term care facilities. The qualitative results indicated that "the dimensions of mobility for residents included not only the independent performance of physical tasks and activities of daily living, but also the ability to get out of bed and get around the institution on one's own." Independence was an important defining characteristic of mobility.

The way in which functional status has been operationally defined within the nursing literature reflects its multidimensional nature. Within the empirical literature, functional status outcomes have been operationally defined as physical and social functioning (Lang & Clinton, 1984), role functioning (Naylor et al., 1991), cognitive and mental functioning (Aydelotte, 1962; Naylor et al., 1991; Waltz & Strickland, 1988), continence and mobility (McCormich, 1991; Johnson & Maas, 1997), self-care (Gillette & Jenko, 1991; Hover & Zimmer, as cited in Johnson & Maas, 1997; Johnson & Maas, 1997), and home functioning (Lang & Marek, 1990).

Several theorists have drawn a distinction between functional status and functional ability (Knight, 2000; Richmond et al., 1997). For them, functional ability refers to the actual or potential capacity to perform biological, psychological, and social activities normally expected of an individual at a particular age and developmental stage (Knight, 2000; Nagi, 1991; Richmond et al., 1997). Functional status refers to individuals' actual performance of activities and tasks associated with their current life roles. These include basic, instrumental, and advanced activities of daily living (e.g., working, traveling, engaging in hobbies, and participating in social and religious groups) (Richmond et al., 1997).

Kline Leidy (1994) offers an analytic framework for understanding the concept of functional status. She defines it as "a multidimensional concept characterizing one's ability to provide for the necessities of life; that is, those activities people do in the normal course of their lives to meet basic needs, fulfill usual roles, and maintain their health and well-being.... Necessities include, but are not limited to, physical, psychological, social, and spiritual needs that are socially influenced and individually determined."

Furthermore, Kline Leidy (1994) suggested that functional status had four dimensions: capacity, performance, reserve, and capacity utilization. Functional capacity referred to "one's maximum potential to perform those activities people do in the normal course of their lives to meet basic needs, fulfill usual roles, and maintain their health and well-being." She defined *Functional performance* as "the physical, psychological, social, occupational, and spiritual activities that people actually do in the normal course of their lives to meet basic needs, fulfill usual roles, and maintain their health and well-being." These activities are the outcome of individual choice, subject to the limits imposed by capacity. The physical component of functional performance consists of activities motivated by personal bodily needs, that is, activities of daily living (ADL), such as dressing, eating, and bathing, and intermediate activities (IADL) that enable meeting those needs (Kline Leidy, 1994). Kline Leidy suggested that the psychological component consists of activities involving mental health and personal growth, including hobbies or favorite pastimes, such as music, reading, or gardening; and sharing personal concerns with another. The social component includes activities involving interaction with the community and family, such as attending parties or organizational meetings, visiting friends, or phoning relatives. Work activities are included in occupational task performance. The spiritual component encompasses those activities involved in developing spiritual perspective, including devotional activities, meditation, attendance at religious ceremonies or worship services, and volunteer work (Kline Leidy, 1994).

According to Kline Leidy (1994), *functional reserve* is defined as "the difference between capacity and performance, one's functional latency or dormant abilities that can be called upon in time of perceived need." *Functional capacity utilization* refers to "the extent to which functional potential is called upon in the selected level of performance."

In summary, the early definitions of functional status were narrower in their defining characteristics than what is reflected in the recent literature. Theorists in the literature reviewed in this chapter recognized that functional status includes the basic and instrumental activities of daily living, as well as social, work-related, and spiritual dimensions. Moreover, they considered it important to differentiate the term "functional ability," which encompasses the capacity to perform, from that of "functional status," which refers to the actual performance of an activity or behavior. The latter is more often the focus of interest when functional status is investigated as an outcome of nursing care.

2.3 Conceptual Definition

Based on the theoretical review, functional status is viewed as a multidimensional construct that consists of, at least, behavioral (e.g., performance of activities of daily living), psychological (e.g., mood), cognitive (e.g., attention, concentration), and social (e.g., activities associated with roles at various stages of development) components. A distinction is made between functional status (the actual performance of an activity) and functional ability (the capacity to perform a given function or activity) (Knight, 2000).

2.4 Factors that Influence Functional Status

Individuals' performance of activities of daily living, work, social, and family role activities is influenced by internal, external, and cultural factors (Fawcett et al., 1995). The individual's health status, attitude, and demographic characteristics are some of the internal influences on functional status (Bourret et al., 2002; Fawcett et al., 1995; Tulman & Fawcett, 1990). For example, functioning is influenced by a positive attitude (Bourret et al., 2002), physical energy, (Tulman

& Fawcett, 1990), and the existence of "acute illness (e.g., pneumonia) and chronic illnesses (e.g., diabetes, cancer, and bipolar disease)" (Fawcett et al., 1995). The normative beliefs and values that govern role expectations and behaviors are examples of the cultural determinants of functional status (Fawcett et al., 1995). The physical characteristics of the environment and access to mobility aids such as canes and wheelchairs are examples of external factors that influence functional status (Bourret et al., 2002). Other external influences include social supports individuals have in their environment and financial resources (Fawcett et al., 1995; Zemore & Shepel, 1989). These internal, external, and cultural factors need to be taken into consideration when assessing functional status. Furthermore, when planning and evaluating a nursing intervention, it is important to consider the role of these factors in affecting outcome achievement.

2.5 Issues in Assessing Functional Status

Several important issues concerning the assessment of functional status emerged from the review of the literature. These included (a) who should assess functional status; (b) what constitutes good outcomes with regard to functional status; (c) how one controls for the impact of aids, adaptations, and helpers (Kaufert, 1983); (d) how one controls for situational variation and motivation factors (Kaufert, 1983); (e) whether one should control for the patient's role expectation in the performance of certain functions (Kaufert, 1983); (f) the advantages and disadvantages of ADL versus IADL scales to measure functional status (Rubenstein et al., 1984); and (g) whether one can use secondary sources to assess functional status.

2.5.1 *Whose Perspective Should Be Considered When Functional Status Is Assessed?*

Clinicians and patients often have differing perspectives of the patients' functional ability, with the latter being more optimistic in their view than the clinicians. Reiley et al. (1996) found that nurses' predictions about patients' functional status two months after discharge were significantly more pessimistic than warranted. The nurses often overestimated the functional disability of their patients. Rubenstein et al. (1984) found that patients rated themselves higher on ADL and IADL items than nurses who, in turn, rated patients higher than a community proxy, such as a spouse or child. The items most likely to show incongruence between the patient and the nurse were those of ambulation, dressing, bathing, and grooming.

2.5.2 What Constitutes a Good Outcome with Regard to Functional Status?

Although improvements in functional status constitute a good outcome for many patient populations, this is not the case for all of them. Hirdes and Carpenter (1997) noted that for the frail elderly, if restoration of complete independence is not possible, preventing decline and maintaining a stable level of function could be indicative of a successful intervention. In the case of inevitable decline, it may be reasonable to focus on slowing its rate. Moreover, it may not be possible to affect all aspects of functioning, but optimizing specific areas (e.g., cognition) and avoiding pain may have a profound effect on well-being (Hirdes & Carpenter, 1997).

2.5.3 How Does One Control for the Impact of Aids, Adaptations, and Helpers?

Kaufert (1983) observed that not all approaches to the assessment of functional status account for the fact that some individuals may successfully use an assistive device or helper, without which they could not attain the same level of function. One approach to control for variation in the effect of the use of aids and helpers is to develop more complex systems for summarizing functional status, which also control for the level of difficulty encountered and for consistency of performance (Kaufert, 1983).

2.5.4 How Does One Control for Situational Variation and Motivation Factors?

Situational factors may influence functional performance and thus be a source of variation in performance ratings. Kaufert (1983) also noted that "subjects being assessed by clinicians who are directly involved in their treatment, for example, may attempt to maximize secondary gains by over- or under-representing their level of disability. Additionally, validity comparisons must distinguish between a subject's potential physical ability to perform a function and his actual performance." To minimize the impact of volitional factors, many indices ask, "Do you perform a function?" instead of "Are you able to perform the function?" Kaufert suggests "to minimize situational variation, alternate measurement should be made in similar situations."

2.5.5 *Should One Control for the Patient's Role Expectation in the Performance of Certain Functions?*

Cultural expectations about the roles of men and women are important to consider when assessing functional status outcomes (Kaufert, 1983). Furthermore, it is important to establish whether the individual activities being assessed are relevant to the independent functioning of the population being studied or treated (Kaufert, 1983).

2.5.6 *The Advantages and Disadvantages of ADL versus IADL Measures*

The behavioral component of functional status has been measured with ADL and IADL scales. Rubenstein et al. (1984) argued that IADL scales possess several limitations not shared by ADL scales. These include a lack of Guttman scalability, a greater sensitivity of score to variations in mood and emotional health, a greater difficulty in measuring IADLs in institutional settings, and an overemphasis on traditional women's tasks (such as cooking, cleaning, and laundering) (Rubenstein et al., 1984). Confirming the lack of sensitivity of IADL items in institutional settings, Meissner, Andolsek, Mears, and Fletcher (1989) found significant improvements on Katz's ADL items between admission and discharge for patients admitted to a dedicated geriatric unit with specialized nursing, but no significant change over time in the instrumental activities of daily living items.

2.5.7 *Assessing Functional Status Based on Secondary Sources*

One approach to assessing outcomes, including functional status outcomes, is through using data from secondary sources, such as the patient record. This method is economical and unobtrusive because it capitalizes on data that have already been collected for another purpose and does not burden the patient with additional data collection. Burns et al. (1992) evaluated the congruence between self-report and a medical record-derived measure of functional status. Data were collected on 2,504 patients over 65 years of age who were discharged from the hospital alive. A personal interview conducted two days before hospital discharge recorded the patient's self-reported ability to perform activities of daily living. Medical record abstraction was used to determine the patient's ability to perform the same activities of daily living. The amount of missing medical record functional status data varied by function, from 20% for bathing to 50% for dressing. Within each function, the amount of missing information was least for patients with a hip fracture and most for patients with chronic obstructive lung disease (COPD) and congestive heart failure (CHF). Overall, the medical record tended to document less dependence than patients reported. On dressing, for example, the medical record contained documentation that 40% of the total population was dependent, but 73% of the population reported themselves as dependent (Burns et al., 1992). Sensitivity of the medical record ranged from 48% for dressing to 68% for transferring. Specificity ranged from 64% for bathing to 83% for feeding. Patients consistently reported more dependencies than were documented in the medical record (Burns et al., 1992)

In summary, there are a number of issues that need to be considered when assessing functional status. The research evidence suggests that patients have a different view of their functional ability than clinicians do. Therefore, it is important to clarify whose perspective is the focus of assessment. Second, maintaining functional performance or slowing the rate of decline may be a good outcome for some populations, such as older persons. Third, instruments used to assess functional status should account for the level of difficulty encountered in the activity and the ability to perform with physical aids. Furthermore, instruments assessing functional status need to be sensitive to cultural norms and role expectations for different patient populations. ADL measures are probably more sensitive to functional status change in the institutional setting than IADL measures. To date, there is not good evidence that functional status can be reliably and validly assessed from secondary sources.

2.6 Evidence Concerning the Relationship between Nursing and Patients' Functional Status Outcomes

Thirty-four empirical studies were identified and are reviewed in Table 2.1. Twenty-two of these studies evaluated a nursing intervention in which functional status was an outcome measure. The other 12 studies described the development and/or testing of a functional status instrument that was used within a nursing context. Nineteen of the studies were conducted in an acute-care hospital setting, 12 in a community setting, 2 in a long-term care setting, and one in a rehabilitation setting. Two of the studies conducted in an acute-care setting are relevant for long-term patient populations because, in both cases, the studies examined the effectiveness of dedicated geriatric beds.

The first question that arises is the extent to which functional status is a relevant outcome for nursing, as indicated by strong empirical evidence linking nursing variables to functional status outcomes. Ten randomized controlled trials examined a nursing intervention in which functional status was included as an outcome variable. McCusker, Verdon, Tousignant, de Courval, Dendukir, and Belzile (2001) evaluate the effect of a brief, standardized nursing assessment and referral to community services/follow-up for older people visiting the emergency department. They collected data on activities of daily living and instrumental activities of daily living using the Older American and Resources Services Scale.

Table 2.1. Studies Investigating the Relationship between Nursing Variables and Functional Status: Study Characteristics

Author/date	Design	Sample characteristics/ setting	Definition of the outcome concept	Intervention being evaluated/nursing variable being evaluated	Results	Limitations
Aiken et al. (1993)	Prospective cohort	Patient with HIV infection $N = 87$ ($RR = 84\%$); university outpatient setting (the NP group had more women).	Symptom occurrence & self-care management (author); functional status (Medical Outcome Study Short Form, SF-36).	Nurse practitioner-managed care vs. physician care.	NP patients reported significantly more symptoms (even after controlling for gender); NP patients reported poor health status; no significant difference between cohorts in the SF-36 subscales.	No information about the reliability and validity of the symptom and self-care instruments.
Alexy & Elnitsky (1998)	Case control pre-post test; baseline assessment and then 12–15 post-baseline assessment.	Recipients of mobile health unit ($n = 190$); project's home visit component ($n = 32$); $N = 222$.	Functional status (Katz, α .89); health status (two self-report questions); IOWA Self-Assessment Inventory [economic resources (α .90), anxiety/depression (α .84), physical health (α .68), alienation (α .83), mobility (α .83), cognitive status (α .79), social support (α .80)]; nutrition screening (α .40); Geriatric Depression Scale (Yesavage et al, 1983).	Community-based mobile health unit; clients participated in the project from 5–28 months (mean = 14.8) with a mean number of visits of 7.9; staffed by family nurse practitioner (FNP), MSCN nurse, and two FNP students.	There was a significant decline between the baseline and follow-up measures for the ADL scale (in the areas of continence and bathing) ($t = 2.83$, $p < .005$; mean 15.76 to 15.68 for community group; 12.75 to 11.21 for home group); there was a significant decline in the IADL scores (community 13 versus 12.70; home 7 versus 6.40; $t = 2.61$, $p < .01$).	Impossible to rule out a Hawthorne effect because of lack of a true control group; small number in the home visit sample.

Table 2.1 (continued)

Author/date	Design	Sample characteristics / setting	Definition of the outcome concept	Intervention being evaluated/nursing variable being evaluated	Results	Limitations
Barr Mazzuca et al. (1997)	RCT; prospective data collection over five times at 8-week intervals for 32 weeks.	Community setting; adults, insulin-dependent; $N = 22$ (RR not stated); age range 49–83.	Dietary adherence and weight; foot care (King, 1978); blood glucose monitoring; diabetes knowledge [Michigan Diabetes Research Training Center (MDRTC)]; self-care behaviors (The Self-Care Behaviors Questionnaire, Mendenhall, 1991); functional health status (SF-36; α .69 to .89).	Community health nursing by senior undergraduate nursing students.	No significant difference over time in the health status measures.	Small sample may have resulted in lack of power to test for significant change over time.
Boockvar et al. (2000)	Descriptive	409-bed nursing home; three floors; all daytime nursing assistants rated residents; all residents were observed ($n = 74$).	Illness Warning Instrument based on behavioral changes.	No intervention.	Primary outcome was acute illness (researcher went on rounds with nurses weekly to identify episodes of acute illness). Criteria for illness were limited to physical exam and lab tests. A resident for whom one or more of the five acute changes was endorsed was 4.1 times more likely to develop an illness within the next 7 days than a resident for whom no change was endorsed. The final instrument had a sensitivity of 53%, a positive predictive value of 17%, and a negative predictive value of 96%.	Testing limited to one setting.

Table 2.1 (continued)

Author/date	Design	Sample characteristics/ setting	Definition of the outcome concept	Intervention being evaluated/nursing variable being evaluated	Results	Limitations
Chan et al. (2000)	Pre-post test, RCT	Setting: Hong Kong; 80% diagnosis of schizophrenia; mean age = 39. N = 62; 31 in the experimental and control group, respectively.	Clinical and functional status: Brief Psychiatric Rating Scale (BPRS); Specific Level of Functioning Scale (SLOF, α reported .80); Risser Client Satisfaction.	Newly developed model for nurse case management vs. conventional care by case managers.	Clients in the experimental group showed more improvement on the BPRS in areas such as tension, suspiciousness, hallucinatory behavior and thought disturbance. Experimental group showed better improvement in SLOF personal care skills, interpersonal relationships, social acceptability, and community living skills. Significant difference between experimental and control subjects on the Risser scale for time to listen and talk to clients and feeling secure when being cared for by NCM.	Small sample
Cohen et al. (2000)	Prospective, single cohort design: 6-month and 1-year intervals.	Community setting; elderly clients receiving services from nurses; n = 68; mean age = 81.5; 79% women.	Functional status is defined as the ability to perform and adapt to the environment; Older Americans Resource & Services Tool (OARS).	Nurse-managed centers (NMC, neighborhood center & apartment building); services include assessment, medication review, safety counseling, symptom and illness management, personal care, etc.	There were no changes in scores among the total sample for any subscale of the OARS.	No control group
Dalton (2001)	Case study	Community clients receiving cardiac disease management; N = 51; sub-sample (n = 40) used to examine outcomes post-hospital discharge.	Functional status (OASIS).	Cardiac disease management home care program.	Improvement in the level of functioning was reflected in all of the functional status outcomes.	Small sample size; lack of a control group; no information about statistical significance provided.

Table 2.1 (continued)

Author/date	Design	Sample characteristics/ setting	Definition of the outcome concept	Intervention being evaluated/nursing variable being evaluated	Results	Limitations
Doran et al. (2002)	Longitudinal	Medical-surgical patients in 19 teaching hospitals; staff nurses ($n = 1085$, $RR = 97\%$); patients ($n = 835$, $RR = 87\%$); 74 units.	Ability to engage in activities of daily living and mobility assessed with Functional Independent Measure (FIM instrument; α .87 time 1, .88 time 2).	Nurse staff mix (proportion of RN/RPN staffing); nurse communication (Shortell et al., 1991).	The proportion of RN staffing, nurse experience, and effectiveness of nurses' communication had positive effects on patients' functional independence at discharge.	
Doran et al. (2002)	Cross-sectional	Medical-surgical patients in one teaching hospital; patients ($n = 372$, $RR = 73\%$); nurses ($n = 245$, $RR = 35\%$); 26 units.	Functional status: ability to resume usual activities of daily living; therapeutic self-care ability.	Educational preparation of nurses; staff mix; quality of nursing care (Shortell et al., 1991; α .94); quality of nurse communication (Shortell et al., 1991; α .85) and coordination of care (Shortell et al., 1991; α .77); nurse role tension (Lysons, α .78); and autonomy (Hackman & Oldhan, α .71).	Quality of nursing care was positively related to higher levels of therapeutic self-care and functional status at hospital discharge.	No control for admission level of functional status.
Fawcett & Tulman (1990)	Cross-sectional	Hospital and home setting; mothers of newborns.	Functional status defined as "the degree to which new role responsibilities and usual role activities are performed" [Inventory of Functional Status after Childbirth (IFSAC)].	No intervention.	Content validity of the IFSAC instrument established at 96.7%; construct validity supported by relative independence of the sub-scales with correlations ranging from 0.01 to 0.53.	

Table 2.1 (continued)

Author/date	Design	Sample characteristics/ setting	Definition of the outcome concept	Intervention being evaluated/nursing variable being evaluated	Results	Limitations
Gagnon et al. (1999)	RCT; baseline data; 10-month follow-up.	Frail elders; intervention ($n = 212$); control (usual care, $n = 215$); setting: university hospital and two community health centers.	Quality of life (SF-36); Client Satisfaction Questionnaire; ADL and IADL [Older Americans Resource & Services Multidimensional Functional Assessment (OARS)]; hospital admissions and emergency room visits.	Nurse case management providing in-hospital and out-patient services over a 10-month period.	There were no significant differences between elders in the interventions and control group in SF-36 physical functioning, role physical, bodily pain, general health, vitality, social functioning, role emotional, or mental health. No differences in OARS functional ability or satisfaction with care. Greater average number of ED visits in the NCM group.	None noted
Garrard et al. (1990)	Quasi-experimental; baseline, 3-, 6-, and 12-month assessments.	Nursing homes: five with NP and five without; two cohorts (long-stay, new admission); $N = 848$ (RR 43% by 12 months); 64% female; mean age = 80.24 in admission cohort, 82 in long-stay cohort.	Satisfaction (author developed); mental status (derived from Short Portable Mental Status Questionnaire); functional status (author developed).	Geriatric nurse practitioners.	For the new admission cohort, residents on non-geriatric NP units improved in functional status more than NP units. There was no significant change in functional status scores for the long-stay cohort, except for affect, with greater improvement in the non-NP units.	Differences between the nursing homes other than having NPs could have confounded the study results; limited psychometric testing of the functional status measure.
Griffiths (1996); Griffiths et al. (2000, 2001)	RCT; T1 = 24 h of referral and 48 h prior to discharge.	Hospital setting; inpatients; $N = 112$ ($RR = 84.2\%$); mean age = 77; 37% male.	Functional independence (Barthel Index); $N = 153$ ($RR = 76.62\%$).	Nurse-led intermediate care unit vs. usual care unit.	There were no statistically significant differences between the treatment and control groups in functional independence at discharge, although the difference was large and in favor of the nurse-led unit (73 compared with 53).	None noted

Table 2.1 (continued)

Author/date	Design	Sample characteristics/ setting	Definition of the outcome concept	Intervention being evaluated/nursing variable being evaluated	Results	Limitations
Hamilton & Lyon (1995)	Quasi-experimental; one-group pre-test/post-test.	Hospital setting; geriatric; N = 74; 54% women; mean age = 81.2.	Functional status was defined as the person's ability to carry out ADL (Modified Barthel Index); mental status defined as cognitive function in areas of orientation, attention, memory, and language (Mini-Mental State).	CNS-provided clinical support for nurses on a medical unit with six dedicated geriatric beds and where nurses practiced modular nursing.	There was a significant improvement in functional ability on all items of the Barthel Index between admission and discharge from the unit.	It is impossible to rule out the Hawthorne effect or other confounding variables, because of the absence of a control group. No information about the reliability of the modified Barthel Index in this study.
Harrell et al. (1989)	Cross-sectional	Hospital; two medical units; N = 150; age 65–93 (mean = 74).	Functional status (Katz Activities of Daily Living).	Nursing diagnoses gathered through retrospective chart review following discharge.	Those patients who improved in functional status from admission to discharge had the most number of nursing diagnoses. Predictors of functional status at discharge included Katz score at admission and nursing diagnosis of moving.	Small sample size; testing limited to one setting involving only two patient care units.
Heafey et al. (1994)	Descriptive, retrospective review of charts.	Hospital and home; subjects with lower extremity amputation (N = 96); 58.3% males; mean age for males = 60, for females = 68.	Safety awareness and functional ability [Safety Assessment and Functional Evaluation (SAFE) tool, developed in-hospital].	Rehabilitation following lower extremity amputation.	Patients demonstrated an improvement in functional status scores from the time of admission to discharge.	No information provided about the psychometric properties of the functional status instrument.

Table 2.1 (continued)

Author/date	Design	Sample characteristics/ setting	Definition of the outcome concept	Intervention being evaluated/nursing variable being evaluated	Results	Limitations
Helberg (1993)	Correlational	Home care patients ($N = 367$); primarily White; average age = 66.	Functional status (Older American Resources Survey, Pfeffer, 1975); Cronbach alpha .84.	Home care nursing.	Physical ADLs at admission correlated with independent discharge status ($r = .29$), institutionalized ($r = .19$) and died ($r = .27$); Instrumental IADLs correlated with independent at discharge ($r = 0.31$), need for family/community support ($r = 0.16$), and died ($r = -0.19$).	
Holzemer & Henry (1992)	Descriptive	Hospital; general medical-surgical units with AIDS patients; $N = 74$ male patients with HIV-related pneumocystis.	Functional status (measured with the Quality Audit Marker); internal consistency, total scale 0.90.	Use of a computer-generated vs. manually generated nursing care plan.	There were no significant differences in functional status, nutrition/elimination, and social isolation between those patients with the computer-supported care plans and those with the manually generated care plans.	Small sample size; non-random sampling procedure.
Howard & Reiley (1994)	Correlational	Patients admitted to a medical service of one hospital; $N = 87$; mean age = 65.	Functional status (not explicitly defined): Katz Index.	Nursing intensity system (author developed). Inter-rater reliability range from .82–99; Cronbach alpha in this study for Nursing Intensity (0.84).	Correlation between patient age and Katz ($r = .88$) and Nursing Intensity rating ($r = .81$). There were significant differences in functional status scores between patients admitted from home, versus those admitted from rehab, nursing homes, and other hospitals for the Katz instrument and the Nursing Intensity system.	Small sample size; no information about the psychometric properties of the Katz instrument in this study.

Table 2.1 (continued)

Author/date	Design	Sample characteristics/ setting	Definition of the outcome concept	Intervention being evaluated/nursing variable being evaluated	Results	Limitations
Irvine et al. (2000)	Correlational; prospective over two points in time.	Clients requiring community nursing; average age = 61; 60% female.	Functional health status (SF-36); reliability ranged from .76 to .94; quality of life [Quality of Life Profile: Seniors Version (QOLPSV, Raphael et al., 1995)]. Reliability ranged from .47 to .82.	Community nursing visits.	There was a significant improvement in health status scores for seven of the subscales of the SF-36 between Time 1 and Time 2. There was a significant improvement in four of the subscales of the QOLPSV over time. The proportion of visits made by a RN was significantly related to change in SF-36 subscales: bodily pain, vitality, and mental health.	Small sample size.
Johnson et al. (1997)	Quasi-experimental; control; pre-intervention; experimental: post-intervention; data collected prospectively over four points in time (pre-treatment to one month post-treatment).	Patients with breast or prostate cancer; N = 226 (RR = 77%).	Outcome expectancies [The Life Orientation Test (LOT)]; mood [Profile of Mood States (POMS)]; reliability ranged .77 to .83; reliability ranged .7 to .83; disruption in usual life activities [Sickness Impact Profile (SIP)]; SIP subscales had reliability of .66 to .88 except for the mobility subscale (α .43 to .54).	Nurses were trained to incorporate "self-regulation" theory into their practice.	The experimental group, as opposed to the control group, had a 31% reduction in disruption in home management at 4 weeks, and a 53% reduction at one month post-tx. In the experimental group, pessimistic patients were more positive than in the control group.	
Legge & Reilly (1980)	Pre-post test	Community setting; cancer patients in U.S.; N = 36; 50% female; 92% White.	Functional status (author developed); nurses assessed functional status and classified patients into four categories: dependent, needs assistance, needs supervision, and independent.	Home care nursing services.	The number of persons "dependent" rose over 36% between admission and discharge.	Instrument not well described; no psychometric information.

Table 2.1 (continued)

Author/date	Design	Sample characteristics/setting	Definition of the outcome concept	Intervention being evaluated/nursing variable being evaluated	Results	Limitations
Lush et al. (1997)	For the adult patients, the HSOD was completed at admission, at discharge, at admission and discharge from homecare, and 6 weeks post-hospital discharge. HSCODs were completed for pediatric patients at admission, and then in the medical office at monthly visits for 3 months.	Hospital setting; $N = 125$; adults with total joint replacement ($n = 57$); adults with acute congestive heart failure ($n = 37$); pediatric oncology patients receiving chemotherapy ($n = 31$); study conducted in four medical centers in California.	Health Status Outcome Dimensions (HSOD) instrument; dimensions include functional status (α .91), health care involvement (α .69), psychosocial well-being (α .77), caregiver status (α .67), and family status (α .83).	Change in functional status following health care; total patient care hours.	There was a significant change in functional status over time (FS scores lowest for joint replacement patients at discharge, lowest for CHF at hospital admission. No significant change for psychological status, family and caregiver status. There was a significant change over time for healthcare involvement. In the pediatric sample, child version ($n = 16$) the highest scores for all factors except functional status was at Time 3. There was a significant main effect of time on the caregiver factor and the family factor. In the toddler sample ($n = 9$), the only significant main effect of time was with the caregiver factor. For the total joint replacement sample, total patient care hours were negatively correlated with functional staus at hospital admission ($r = .39$) and discharge ($r = .42$), with healthcare involvement at discharge ($r = -.55$), and with psychological well-being at admission ($r = -.41$). Patient age correlated with functional status ($r = -.29$), health care involvement ($r = -.32$), and family status ($r = -.39$).	
McCusker et al. (2001)	RCT; T1 and T2 (1 month); T3 94-month follow-up); Intervention ($n = 178$; RR = 82.6%; 155 = 87.1% at T3); control ($n = 210$; 182 = 86.7% at T2).	Emergency department of four university affiliated hospitals in Montreal.	Functional status (Older American Resource & Services Scale); Geriatric Depression Scale; Caregiver health status (SF-36).	Intervention—brief standardized geriatric nursing assessment.	The intervention resulted in significantly reduced rate of functional decline at four months; no significant effect of the intervention on caregiver health status at four months.	

Table 2.1 (continued)

Author/date	Design	Sample characteristics/ setting	Definition of the outcome concept	Intervention being evaluated/nursing variable being evaluated	Results	Limitations
Meissner et al. (1989)	Descriptive comparative design.	Hospital setting; patients over 70 years old (N = 103); mean age = 81.	Functional status (Katz Activities of Daily Living); Instrumental Activities of Daily Living (Lawton & Brody, 1969).	Dedicated geriatric unit with a nurse specialist vs. similar medical unit.	Assess independence in six activities: bathing, dressing, toileting, transferring from bed to chair, continence, and feeding. Items rated on a 3-point scale.	
Milisen et al. (2001)	Cohort, prospective	Intervention (n = 60); nonintervention (n = 60); hospital setting in Belgium.	Functional status (Katz ADL).	Intervention to enhance the quality of nursing care focused on training in assessment and consultation with specialized nurses.	There was no statistically significant difference in functional status between the nonintervention and intervention cohorts.	
Mock et al. (1994)	RCT	Outpatient setting; women with breast cancer receiving chemotherapy (N = 14); mean age = 44; 93% White.	Performance status (Karnofsky Performance Status Scale); 12-Minute Walking Test.	Rehabilitation program: walking exercise.	Performance of physical activities.	

Table 2.1 (continued)

Author/date	Design	Sample characteristics/ setting	Definition of the outcome concept	Intervention being evaluated/nursing variable being evaluated	Results	Limitations
Mundinger et al. (2000)	RCT	Adult patients; $N = 1316$ ($RR = 66.4\%$); mean age = 45.9; 76.8% female; 90.3% Hispanic; community-based primary care clinics.	Functional health status (Medical Outcome Study Short-Form, SF-36).	Nurse practitioner vs. physician care.	No difference between NP and MD patients on any scale or summary score at 6 months; significant improvement in health status from baseline to 6-month follow-up for all sub-scales of the SF-36.	No data provided on the psychometric properties of the SF-36 for this particular sample.
Pettersson et al. (1999)	Prospective, single cohort design.	Swedish asthmatics; $N = 32$ ($RR = 53\%$); mean age = 43; 81% female; outpatient clinic.	Sickness Impact Profile (SIP).	Nurse-run asthma school.	Significant improvement in SIP physical health status sub-scale only.	No data on the psychometric properties of SIP in this sample; small sample size.
Pugh et al. (2001)	RCT	One community and one teaching hospital; $N = 58$, control ($n = 31$), intervention ($n = 27$).	Quality of life/functional status (SF-36) (all Cronbach alpha in this study greater than .50). Six-minute walking test.	Patient education and nurse case manager discharge planning and 6-month follow-up.	There was a trend to greater improvement in SF-36 physical functioning and mental health and 6-minute walking test for the intervention group, but none of the differences were statistically significant.	Small sample size and lack of control for patient risk profile.
Steiner et al. (2001)	RCT	Britain; 1 teaching and 9 community hospitals; $N = 238$ patients; nurse-led unit ($n = 119$) versus usual care. Six month follow-up.	Physical functioning (Barthel index).	Nurse-led unit.	No difference in functional status at discharge or at 6-month follow-up between intervention and nonintervention patients.	

Table 2.1 (continued)

Author/date	Design	Sample characteristics/ setting	Definition of the outcome concept	Intervention being evaluated/nursing variable being evaluated	Results	Limitations
Swan (1998)	Prospective, single cohort design.	Outpatient setting; ambulatory surgical patients ($N = 100$); attrition rate of 26%; mean age = 42.6 (SD = 12.83); 63% female; 72% White.	Symptom distress [General Symptom Distress Scale (GSDS, Lalonde, 1987)]; Functional Status Questionnaire [(FSQ) Jette et al., 1986].	Nurse caring behaviors: The Caring Behaviors Inventory (Wolf et al., 1994).	Post-operative nurse caring behaviours explained 7-day basic ADL, mental health, social activity, and 4-day postop social interaction.	
Walsh et al. (1999)	RCT; nurse-led inpatient care.	Hospital setting; post-acute medical patients.	Barthel Index.	Nurse-led inpatient care unit for post-acute medical patients.	There were no significant differences in the outcome measures, including Barthel scores between patients in the experimental and usual care groups.	No information on psychometric properties of Barthel in this study.
Wanich et al. (1992)	Quasi-experimental; intervention (one unit) vs. control group (two other inpatient units).	Patients aged 70 and over, admitted to urban teaching hospital ($N = 235$); mean age = 77.	Mini-Mental State Examination; Katz Index of Activities of Daily Living; diagnosis of delirium (psychiatrist).	Nursing intervention based on Orem's Self-Care Deficit Model.	More intervention group subjects improved in functional status in comparison to control subjects. Logistic regression indicated that subjects exposed to the intervention were three times as likely to improve in functional status in the hospital compared to subjects in the control group (OR 3.29).	Full version used in this study.

Note. RR = sample response rate; *RCT* = randomized control trial; *ADL* = activities of daily living; *IADL* = instrumental activities of daily living; *MD* = medical doctor; *MDS* = Minimum Data Set; *MDS-HC* = Minimum Data Set for Home Care.

Potential confounding variables were controlled for through initial screening and through statical analysis. McCusker et al. (2001) found a significant reduced rate of decline for the older people who received the nursing intervention at a four-month follow-up. When Chan, Mackenzie, Tin-Fu, and Leung (2000) evaluated a nurse case-management intervention, they found significant differences over time, and between the experimental and control groups, in outcomes measured by the Brief Psychiatric Rating Scale and the Specific Level of Functioning Scale. Barr Mazzuca, Farris, Mendenhall, and Stoupa (1997), who analyzed the effectiveness of community health nursing provided by senior undergraduate nursing students, found no significant difference in functional status scores over time, as measured by the Medical Outcome Study Short Form (SF-36). Gagnon, Schein, McVey, and Bergman (1999) examined a nurse case-management intervention and reported no significant differences in the SF-36 subscales over time and no differences in functional ability, as measured by the Older Americans Resource and Services Questionnaire. Likewise, Pugh, Havens, Xie, Robinson, and Blaha (2001) found no significant difference in SF-36 subscale scores six months after elderly persons with heart failure received a targeted educational and nurse case-management intervention compared with persons receiving usual care. When Mock et al. (1994) evaluated the effectiveness of a nurse-provided exercise program for women with breast cancer receiving chemotherapy, they found no differences between participants in the experimental and control groups on the Karnofsky Performance Status Scale.

A sub-set of studies sought to evaluate whether patients predominantly cared for by nurses achieved the same level of outcome as those receiving the usual level of medical care. For instance, Griffiths et al. (2000), who compared the functional status outcomes for patients admitted to a nurse-led intermediate care unit to those for patients admitted to a usual care unit, found no significant difference in functional status outcomes at discharge, as measured by the Barthel Index. Mundinger et al. (2000) reported no difference in SF-36 scores at a six-month follow-up between patients receiving care from primary care nurse practitioners and those receiving care from physicians. Steiner, Bronagh, Pickering, Wiles, Ward, and Brooking (2001) found no significant difference in the functional health outcomes for post-acute patients admitted to a nurse-led inpatient unit compared with patients admitted to usual care. In this study, the authors considered no difference a good outcome, because the purpose of the study was to assess whether similar health outcomes could be achieved for post-acute patients admitted to a unit where they did not receive the same level of medical coverage that was provided to patients on the conventional care units. Walsh, Pickering, and Brooking (1999) found no significant difference in scores on the Barthel Index between post-acute medical patients admitted to a nurse-led inpatient unit and similar patients admitted to a conventional medical unit. In summary, of the 10 randomized controlled trials reviewed, two found a significant impact of a nursing intervention on functional health outcomes and eight found no impact. However, in four of the studies finding no impact, negative findings were desirable. Negative findings demonstrated that the same level of functional health outcome was achieved for certain types of patients receiving care predominantly from nurses as that for patients receiving care from physicians.

Studies employing quasi-experimental designs were also reviewed in Table 2.1. Researchers in three of these found no significant effects for a nursing intervention/care on functional status outcomes, as measured by the SF-36 (Aiken et al., 1993), the Older Americans Resource and Services Questionnaire (Cohen, Gorenberg, & Schroeder, 2000), and the Quality Audit Marker (Holzemer & Henry, 1992). However, researchers in six other studies employing quasi-experimental designs reported significant findings based on a modified Barthel Index (Hamilton & Lyon, 1995), the Sickness Impact Profile (Johnson et al., 1997; Pettersson et al., 1999), the Katz Activities of Daily Living Scale (Meissner et al., 1989; Wanich et al., 1992), and the Jette et al. Functional Status Questionnaire (Swan, 1998).

Another set of studies reviewed in Table 2.1 did not evaluate a nursing intervention, but examined the relationship between functional status outcomes and nursing variables. Harrell, McConnell, Wildman, and Samsa (1989) reported a significant relationship between nursing diagnoses and Katz Activities of Daily Living scores. Patients who improved in functional status from admission to discharge from two medical units had the most number of nursing diagnoses recorded in the medical record when compared with patients who did not improve to the same extent. Howard and Reiley (1994) and Irvine et al. (2000) reported a significant relationship between nursing intensity and Katz scores and the SF-36 subscale scores, respectively. Irvine et al. also found that the proportion of visits made by a registered nurse was a significant predictor of improvements in SF-36 subscale scores for patients receiving home care nursing services. Lush, Henry, Foote, and Jones (1997) found a significant relationship between total patient care hours and functional status at hospital admission and discharge, as measured by the Health Status Outcomes Dimension. Doran, Sidani, Keatings, and Doidge (2002) noted that functional status scores of medical surgical patients at hospital discharge were significantly related to the quality of nursing care and the quality of nurse communication. Patients achieved better functional independence at hospital discharge on units where the quality of care was high and where communication among nurses and between nurses and physicians was accurate and timely. Doran et al. (2002) collected data on the functional status outcomes of 835 patients admitted to 19 teaching hospitals in Ontario. Functional status was assessed with the FIM instrument at the time of admission to the hospital, at discharge, and again at six weeks post-discharge. Patients achieved greater functional independence at hospital discharge on units where nurse communication was timely and accurate and where there was a high proportion of regulated staff (i.e., registered nurses and registered practical nurses).

In summary, a review of the empirical literature provides equivocal evidence concerning the impact of nursing variables on functional status outcomes. When the evidence from the most rigorous studies is considered, it does not appear that nursing interventions, such as case management, have an effect on patients' functional status outcomes. However, because the nursing interventions in these trials varied considerably in design, dose, setting, and patient populations, it is possible that the nursing intervention was not strong enough, or not properly designed and implemented, to test the impact of nursing on patients' functional health status. The conceptual and theoretical articles offer a rationale for including patients' functional status as an outcome of nursing care. The findings from the quasi-experimental studies and correlational studies offer evidence of a relationship between nursing variables and patients' functional health status. However, as compelling as this evidence is, it comes from studies of weaker research designs and does not corroborate the evidence from the clinical trials. Therefore, we recommend that more focused research be undertaken to establish the sensitivity of functional status outcomes to nursing interventions and care.

2.7 Evidence Concerning Approaches to Measurement

Only those functional status instruments that had been used in a study where the relationship between the instrument scores and nursing variables was examined were included in this review. Although many functional status instruments exist that may be relevant for assessing outcomes of nursing care, they require evaluation in studies where their sensitivity to nursing variables can be assessed. Thirteen instruments measuring functional status were identified in the empirical nursing literature. Their characteristics are summarized in Table 2.2. The name of the instrument and its author are identified. The domains of measurement, number of items, and response format are described. The method of administration is identified, and the evidence of reliability, validity, and sensitivity to nursing variables is summarized.

There are generally two different approaches to functional status assessment. One involves a trained clinician's assessment of clients/patients, based on chart abstraction, observation, and patient interview. This approach is favored by systems designed for outcome tracking and for collecting administrative data because it does not rely on self-report and, therefore, can be used to assess patients of varying levels of cognitive ability, severe limitation, and language competence. Other advantages to this approach include the fact that it is minimally intrusive for patients and family members, and can be completed by clinicians as part of the routine process of patient care and documentation.

Five instruments of this type were included in this review. The Nursing Outcomes Classification tool (NOC) (Johnson & Maas, 1997) was counted in this category. Indicators for the NOC are under development, with pilot testing

Table 2.2. Instruments Measuring Functional Status

Instrument (author)	Target population	Domains (number of items and response format)	Method of administration	Reliability	Validity	Sensitivity to nursing care
Barthel Index (Mahoney et al., 1958)	Chronic patients	Independence in personal care and mobility; two versions — original 10-item version and 15-item version.	Completed by health professional from the medical record and observation	Internal consistency 0.87 to 0.92 McDowell & Newell, 1996)	Concurrent validity, Construct validity (Wade & Hewer, 1987), Predictive validity (McDowell & Newell, 1996)	Griffiths et al. (2000) no effect; Hamilton & Lyon (1995) sensitivity to nursing; Walsh et al. (1999) no effect.
Functional Independence Measure (FIM) (Granger & Hamilton, 1993)	Patients of all ages and diagnoses	Domains include self-care, sphincter control, mobility, locomotion, communication, and social cognition. 18 items. Scores range from 1 to 7.	Completed by clinician based on observation of the patient	Inter-rater reliability 0.86 to 0.88 (Hamilton et al., 1987; Granger et al., 1990). Doran et al. (2002) reported an internal consistency reliability of 0.87 in a sample of medical-surgical patients.	Content validity, Construct validity (Granger et al., 1990)	Changes in the FIM instrument scores were significantly associated with the quality of nurse communication and nurse staff mix (Doran et al., 2002).
Functional Status Questionnaire (Jette et al., 1986)	Ambulatory patients	Ability to perform physical function, psychological function, work performance, social activity, social interaction; 34 items total 4–6-point rating scales.	Self-administered	Internal consistency of sub-scales ranges from 0.64 to 0.82 (Jette & Cleary, cited in McDowell & Newell, 1996)	Construct validity, Criterion validity, Predictive validity	Sensitivity to change shown with patients undergoing hip replacement (Katz et al., 1992).
Health Status Outcomes Dimension (HSOD) (Kaiser Permanente Northern California) (Lush & Jones, 1995; Lush et al., 1997).	Adult & pediatric vesions	Self-care ability/functional status; engagement in health care management; psychological distress; 14 items rated on 4-point scale.	Nurse based on patient observation and chart extraction; electronic documentation	No information available	Content validity	No information available

Table 2.2 (continued)

Instrument (author)	Target population	Domains (number of items and response format)	Method of administration	Reliability	Validity	Sensitivity to nursing care
Index of Independence in Activities of Daily Living (Katz & Akpom, 1959; revised 1976)	Elderly and chronically ill populations	Assess independence in six activities: bathing, dressing, toileting, transfer from bed to chair, continence, feeding. Items rated on a 3-point scale.	Nurse/therapist assesses based on observation	Alexy & Elnitsky (1998) reported internal consistency reliability of .89 in nursing study.	Predictive (Åsberg, 1987; Katz et al., 1970)	Association between Katz ADL scores and nursing diagnoses (Harrel et al., 1989); nursing intensity (Howard & Reiley, 1994); and dedicated geriatric nursing care (Meissner et al., 1989).
Inventory of Functional Status After Childbirth (Fawcett & Tulman, 1990; Fawcett et al., 1988)	Newborn mothers	Measures self-care, household, and infant care responsibilities; occupational, social, and community activities after childbirth. 36 items, rated on scale of 1 to 4.	Self-administered	Internal consistency reliability 0.76. Test-re-test reliability 0.86 (Fawcett & Tulman, 1990)	Content validity (Fawcett & Tulman, 1990), Construct validity (Fawcett & Tulman, 1990)	Sensitivity to change demonstrated in early post-partum period (Fawcett & Tulman, 1990).
Medical Outcome Study-Short Form (SF-36) (Stewart et al., 1988; Ware 1993)	Ambulatory	Physical function, mobility, social, mental, pain, general health (36-item and 12-item versions); Likert response format.	Self-administered or administered through interview	Internal consistency 0.76 and higher (Ware, 1993)	Construct validity, Criterion validity, Predictive validity	Irvine et al. (2000) found sensitivity to community nursing care; Barr Mazzuca et al. (1997); no effect Gagnon et al. (1999) found no effect.
Nursing Outcomes Classification Tool (NOC) Physical Function (Johnson & Maas, 1997)	All ages and practice settings	24 outcome category labels related to physical function, within which there are sub-category labels; 5-point scale; higher scores equal more independence	Nurse-assessed	No information available	Content validity	No information available

Table 2.2 (continued)

Instrument (author)	Target population	Domains (number of items and response format)	Method of administration	Reliability	Validity	Sensitivity to nursing care
Older American Resource and Services Questionnaire (OARS) (Fillenbaum, 1988)	Adults, particularly the elderly	Multidimensional functional and service assessment. Functional includes ADL, social, economic, mental and physical health. Functional assessment of 120 items.	Administered by trained interviewer	Inter-rater reliability and test-retest reliability (see McDowell & Newell, 1996)	Criterion validity (Fillenbaum & Smyer, 1981), Predictive validity (Fillenbaum, 1985)	Cohen et al. (2000) found no change in OARS scores over one year among elderly clients receiving services from nurse-managed community centers. Gagnon et al. (1999) reported no differences in ADL and IADL scores for clients receiving nurse case management and those with routine care.
Outcome Assessment Information Set (OASIS) (Shaughnessy et al., 1998)	Clients receiving home care services	General health, physical assessment, ADL, IADLs. Approximately 79 questions with sub-questions.	Completed by nurse/rater based on chart audit, client interview, nurse interview, observation	No published information found.	Content validity (Shaughnessy et al., 1998)	Dalton et al. (2001) described the use of OASIS for evaluating a cardiac disease management program and found OASIS data useful in the description of the patients, except that analysis of end-results outcomes proved to be the greatest challenge.
Quality Audit Marker (Holzemer et al., 1991; Holzemer & Henry, 1992)	Initial individuals with AIDS, although applicable to all populations	Three domains— functional status, nutrition/elimination, and social isolation. 17 items.	Completed on bases of chart audit, client interview, and observation	Cronbach alpha of 0.90 for total scale (Holzemer & Henry, 1992)	Construct validity through factor analysis (Holzemer & Henry, 1992)	No information found
Sickness Impact Profile (Bergner et al., 1976; revised 1981)	Adults experiencing an illness	Measures health status in 12 categories, including ambulation, mobility, body care and movement, social interaction, communication, alertness behavior, emotion, sleep and rest, eating, home management, recreation, work. 136 items.	Interview or self-administered	Test-retest reliability (DeBruin et al., 1992; McDowell & Newell, 1996). Internal consistency (0.84 to 0.91) (Bergner et al., 1981). Total alpha of 0.95 in a study of nursing home residents (Carter et al., 1976)	Extensive validity testing has been undertaken. Concurrent validity (Bergner et al., 1981), Criterion validity (DeBruin et al., 1992), Construct validity (Bergner et al., 1981)	Johnson et al. (1997) found change in the home maintenance subscale following a training program for nurses but no change in other sub-scales.

being conducted in a number of practice settings. There are 24 category labels related to physical function, within which there are sub-category labels. Although a significant amount of work has been done to establish the content validity of the NOC indicators (Johnson & Maas, 1997), no published information was found about the reliability and construct validity of the functional status sub-scales. The Health Status Outcomes Dimension (HSOD) (Lush et al., 1997; Lush & Jones, 1995) and the Quality Audit Marker (Holzemer et al., 1991) are two other outcome assessment tools that were specifically developed to evaluate the quality and outcomes of nursing care. The HSOD is designed to track outcomes across the continuum of care and includes a number of functional status indicators. The functional status indicators have demonstrated sensitivity to change over time in adult medical and surgical patients and in pediatric patients. The Quality Audit Marker was originally designed for use with an AIDS population but is applicable to other patient populations. Both tools have had limited testing in different practice settings, and there is no published information about their sensitivity to changes in patients' functional health outcomes following nursing interventions. The Outcome Assessment Set (Shaughnessy et al., 1998) was developed to assess service needs and the outcomes of clients receiving home care services. It has good evidence of reliability and validity; however, the evidence is limited concerning its sensitivity to change in outcomes following nursing intervention (Dalton, 2001). Hamilton, Granger, Sherwin, Zielezny, and Tashman (1987) developed the Functional Independence Measurement (FIM instrument) to assess functional health outcomes for patients of all ages and diagnoses. It has been used extensively in rehabilitation populations with good evidence of reliability, validity, and sensitivity to change (McDowell & Newell, 1996). Doran et al. (2002) used the FIM instrument to assess functional health outcomes of medical and surgical patients admitted to 19 acute-care teaching hospitals in Ontario. They found the FIM instrument sensitive to several nursing variables, including variation in nursing staff mix across the hospital units and variations in the quality of nursing care (Doran et al., 2002). The Resident Assessment Instrument (RAI) is a series of instruments that involves person-specific assessment in which data are recorded on a Minimum Data Set (MDS) form (Hawes et al., 1997; Hirdes et al., 1999). The MDS functional status indicators include cognitive items, activities of daily living, and instrumental activities of daily living. The RAI series of instruments have been developed for nursing homes and home care settings (Hirdes et al., 1999). An acute-care, mental health, and post-acute-care series are under development and/or have undergone initial psychometric testing (Hirdes et al., 1999). The reliability and validity of the MDS long-term care version has been confirmed in multiple studies (Casten et al., 1998; Frederiksen et al., 1996; Hartmaier et al., 1995; Hawes et al., 1995; Hirdes et al., 1999).

The other approach to assessing functional status is the use of a self-report questionnaire, which is completed by the patient or through an interview guide.

This approach is evidently favored in the research literature, since the majority of empirical studies reviewed here that investigated functional status in relationship to nursing care utilized a structured instrument, based on patients' self-report, to measure functional status outcomes: (a) six used the SF-36 (Aiken et al., 1993; Barr Mazzuca et al., 1997; Gagnon et al., 1999; Irvine et al., 2000; Mundinger et al., 2000; Pugh et al., 2001); (b) six used the Katz Activities of Daily Living Scale (Alexy & Elnitsky, 1998; Harrell et al., 1989; Howard & Reiley, 1994; Meissner et al., 1989; Milisen et al., 2001; Wanich et al., 1992); (c) four used the Older Americans Resource and Services Questionnaire (Cohen et al., 2000; Gagnon et al., 1999; Helberg, 1993; McCusker et al., 2001); (d) four used the Barthel Index (Griffiths et al., 2000; Hamilton & Lyon, 1995; Steiner et al., 2001; Walsh et al., 1999); (e) two used the Sickness Impact Profile (Johnson et al., 1997; Pettersson et al., 1999); (f) one used the Inventory of Functional Status After Child Birth (Fawcett & Tulman, 1990); and (g) one used the Jette Functional Status Questionnaire (Swan, 1998). Commenting on a measure's sensitivity is difficult when evidence is derived from only one or two studies. Therefore, the review is limited to those instruments that were used in multiple studies.

Of the studies employing the SF-36, only one found a significant relationship between the SF-36 and nursing variables (Irvine et al., 2000). Five of the six studies that used the Katz Activities of Daily Living scale found sensitivity to nursing practice variables. Only one of the studies using the Older Americans Resource and Services Questionnaire demonstrated sensitivity to nursing variables (McCusker et al., 2001), and only one of the studies using the Barthel Index (Hamilton & Lyon, 1995) demonstrated sensitivity to nursing care. Based on this empirical evidence, it appears that the most compelling evidence of sensitivity to nursing variables is in favor of the Katz Activities of Daily Living Scale.

The Katz Activities of Daily Living Scale is an older instrument that was first introduced in 1959 and revised in 1976 (McDowell & Newell, 1996). When reviewing the instrument, McDowell and Newell concluded that there was surprisingly little published evidence on the tool's reliability and validity. It is important to consider the types of items that comprise the Katz Activities of Daily Living Scale because this may reveal why the tool was found to be sensitive to nursing variables. The items comprising the Katz Activities of Daily Living Scale are focused on patients' self-care activities in relation to personal care (e.g., bathing, toileting, dressing) and on mobility (e.g., moving in bed, sitting transfer, standing transfer). These very specific activities of daily living reflect the foci of nursing care. For many patient populations, it is possible to see changes in these activities within a relatively short period. Think, for example, about the course of clinical and functional recovery for a patient undergoing an uncomplicated surgical intervention, such as a total knee replacement. In the immediate 24-hour postoperative period, the nurse helps the patient to sit in bed and transfer from the bed to chair. By the next day, the nurse may be assisting the patient to ambulate from the bed to a bathroom or along the hospital corridor. In addition, the nurse reinforces the physiotherapist's instructions and supervises range of motion exercises. The nurse begins to gage nursing care to promote graduated recovery of personal self-care activities so that, at the time of hospital discharge to home/community or to a rehabilitation setting, the patient may have made significant progress towards functional independence. The nurse's effective management of postoperative pain will also have an important effect on the patient's clinical and functional recovery.

This brief clinical example illustrates the applicability of the kinds of items that comprise the Katz Activities of Daily Living Scale to nursing practice. Since its introduction, other instruments have been developed that assess similar activities of daily living and that should be considered for nursing outcomes measurement research. Some of these were reviewed in this chapter, such as the FIM instrument, the HSOD, and the MSD functional status scales. For this reason, we conclude that there is good evidence (a) that items measuring activities of daily living, such as the Katz instrument, are sensitive to nursing, and (b) that the Katz Activities of Daily Living Scale has demonstrated sensitivity to nursing variables, but (c) that there may yet be other instruments measuring similar items that could be considered for nursing outcomes measurement.

2.8   Recommendations Necessary for Future Research

Improvement in functional status outcomes is often identified as an intended goal of nursing care. Indeed, much of nursing practice is devoted to the promotion and restoration of healthy functioning, as evidenced by such grand nursing theories as Orem's Self-Care Deficit Theory (Orem, 1980) and Roy's Adaptation Theory (Roy & Roberts, 1981). However, the strong theoretical rationale for identifying functional status as a nursing-sensitive patient outcome is not matched by comparable strong empirical evidence linking functional status outcomes to nursing practice variables. The weight of the evidence from the randomized controlled trials is negative.

Despite this lack of evidence, we do not believe that nursing should dismiss functional status as a relevant outcome of our practice. We have based our assertion on several reasons. The studies testing the effect of nursing interventions on functional status outcomes have differed in the types of interventions tested, the patient populations targeted, the outcome assessment tools employed, and the timing of measurement. A problem with the design or implementation of the nursing intervention may have led to non-significant findings. Alternatively, problems with the validity of the outcome assessment tool for the population studied may have resulted in non-significant findings. Problems may have arisen with the timing of assessment. Changes in functional status indicators related to activities of daily living, such as bathing and dressing, would occur over a short period of time for medical surgical patients following an uneventful hospital stay, and would probably plateau soon after hospital discharge. But changes in instrumental activities of daily living and social functioning would occur only after hospital discharge, once individuals were home and interacting with their family and social network. Measurement of change in ADLs and IADLs would have to be timed to capture the expected clinical and functional course of recovery. For these reasons, we suggest that further research is needed to evaluate the sensitivity of functional status as an outcome of nursing care. This research must be undertaken in a variety of practice settings, such as acute care, home care, and long-term care.

Two approaches to measuring functional status warrant evaluation: one based on a trained clinician's assessment and the other on patient self-report. Yet evidence suggests that the two approaches may not yield comparable results with regard to patients' actual level of functioning (Reiley et al., 1996; Rubenstein et al., 1984). Therefore, research is needed to evaluate the approaches to measurement for different patient populations and practice settings.

A systematic review of the nursing studies indicated that functional status as measured by activities of daily living appears sensitive to nursing care and that the Katz Activities of Daily Living Scale has shown promise as an instrument for use in nursing studies, but that other instruments measuring similar items should be evaluated. The evidence of sensitivity of instruments measuring the broader domains of functional status, such as social and work role activities, is less conclusive. Further research is needed to evaluate the reliability, validity, and sensitivity of functional status instruments measuring the broader domains of human functioning in different practice settings. For example, there is reason to expect that indicators measuring the domains that reflect instrumental activities of daily living would be more sensitive to nursing in community settings (Irvine et al., 2000) than in institutional settings.

References

Aiken, L. H., Lake, E. T., Semaan, S., Lehman, H. P., O'Hare, P. A., Cole, C. S., Dunbar, D., & Frank, I. (1993). Nurse practitioner managed care for persons with HIV infection. *Image: Journal of Nursing Scholarship, 25*, 172–177.

Alexy, B. B., & Elnitsky, C. (1998). Rural mobile health unit: Outcomes. *Public Health Nursing, 15*, 3–11.

Asberg, K. H. (1987). Disability as a predictor of outcome for the elderly in a department of internal medicine. *Scandinavian Journal of Social Medicine, 15*, 261–265.

Aydelotte, M. (1962). The use of patient welfare as a criterion measure. *Nursing Research, 11*, 10–14.

Barr Mazzuca, K., Farris, N. A., Mendenhall, J., & Stoupa, R. A. (1997). Demonstrating the added value of community nursing for clients with insulin-dependent diabetes. *Journal of Community Health Nursing, 14*, 211–224.

Bergner, M., Bobbitt, R. A., Carter, W. B., & Gilson, B. S. (1981). The Sickness Impact Profile: Development and final revision of a health status measure. *Medical Care, 21*, 787–805.

Bergner, M., Bobbitt, R. A., Kressel, S., Pollard, W. E., Gilson, B. S., & Morris, J. R. (1976). The Sickness Impact Profile: Conceptual formulation and methodology for the development of a health status measure. *International Journal of Health Services, 6*, 393–415.

Bergner, M., Bobbitt, R. A., Pollard, W. E., Martin, D. P., & Gilson, B. S. (1976). The Sickness Impact Profile: Validation of a health status measure. *Medical Care, 14*, 57–67.

Boockvar, K., Brodie, H. D., & Lachs, M. (2000). Nursing assistants detect behavioral changes in nursing home residents that precede acute illness: Development and validation of an illness warning instrument. *Journal of the American Geriatric Society, 48*, 1086–1091.

Bourret, E.M., Bernick, L.G., Cott, C.A., & Kontos, P.C. (2002). The meaning of mobility for residents and staff in long-term care facilities. *Journal of Advanced Nursing, 37*, 338–345.

Brown, S. A., & Grimes, D. E. (1995). A meta-analysis of nurse practitioners and nurse midwives in primary care. *Nursing Research, 44*(6), 332–339.

Burns, R. B., Moskowitz, M. A., Ash, A., Kane, R. L., Finch, M. D., & Bak, S. M. (1992). Self-report versus medical record functional status. *Medical Care, 30*(Suppl.), MS85–MS95.

Carter, W. B., Bobbitt, R. A., Bergner, M., & Gilson, B. S. (1976). The validation of an interval scaling: The Sickness Impact Profile. *Health Services Research, 11*, 516–528.

Casten, R., Powell-Lawton, M., Parmelee, P. A., & Kleban, M. H. (1998). Psychometric characteristics of the Minimum Data Set I: Confirmatory factor analysis. *Journal of the American Geriatrics Society, 46*, 726–735.

Chan, S., Mackenzie, A., Tin-Fu, D., & Leung, J. K. (2000). An evaluation of the implementation of case management in the community psychiatric nursing service. *Journal of Advanced Nursing, 31*, 144–156.

Cohen, J., Gorenberg, B., & Schroeder, B. (2000). A study of functional status among elders at two academic nursing centers. *Home Care Provider, 5*, 108–112.

Cooley, M. E. (1998). Quality of life in persons with non-small cell lung cancer: A concept analysis. *Cancer Nursing, 21*, 151–161.

Dalton, J. M. (2001). Using OASIS patient outcomes to evaluate a cardiac disease management program: A case study. *Outcomes Management for Nursing Practice, 5*, 167–172.

Davids, D., & Verderber, A. (1995). Functional outcomes of cardiac surgery for the elderly. *Journal of Cardiovascular Nursing, 9*, 96–101.

DeBruin, A. F., De Witte, L. P., Stevens, F., & Diederiks, J. P. (1992). Sickness Impact Profile: The state of the art of a generic functional status measure. *Social Science & Medicine, 35*, 1003–1014.

Ditmyer, S., Koepsell, B., Branum, V., Davis, P., & Lush, M. T. (1998). Developing a nursing outcomes measurement tool. *Journal of Nursing Administration, 28*, 10–16.

Doran, D. M., McGillis Hall, L., Sidani, S., O'Brien-Pallas, L., Donner, G., Baker, G. R., et al. (2002). Nursing staff mix and patient outcome achievement: The mediating role of nurse communication. *The Journal of International Nursing Perspectives, 1*, 74–83.

Doran, D. M., Sidani, S., Keatings, M., & Doidge, D. (2002). An empirical test of the Nursing Role Effectiveness Model. *Journal of Advanced Nursing, 38*, 29–39.

Fawcett, J., & Tulman, L. (1990). Building a programme of research from the Roy Adaptation Model of Nursing. *Journal of Advanced Nursing, 15*, 720–725.

Fawcett, J., Tulman, L., & Samarel, N. (1995). Enhancing function in life transitions and serious illness. *Advanced Practice Nursing Quarterly, 1*(3), 50–57.

Fawcett, J., Tulman, L., & Taylor Myers, S. (1988). Development of the inventory of functional status after childbirth. *Journal of Nurse-Midwifery, 33*, 252–260.

Fillenbaum, G. G. (1988). *Multidimensional functional assessment of older adults: The Duke Older Americans Resources and Services procedures.* Hillsdale, NJ: Lawrence Erlbaum Associates.

Fillenbaum, G. G. (1985). Screening the elderly: A brief instrumental activities of daily living measure. *Journal of the American Geriatric Society, 33*, 698–706.

Fillenbaum, G. G., & Smyer, M. A. (1981). The development, validity, and reliability of the OARS Multidimensional Functional Assessment Questionnaire. *Journal of Gerontology, 36*, 428–434.

Frederiksen, K., Tariot, P., & Jonghe, E. D. (1996). Minimum data set plus (MDS+) scores from five rating scales. *Journal of the American Geriatrics Society, 44*, 305–309.

Gagnon, A. J., Schein, C., McVey, L., & Bergman, H. (1999). Randomized controlled trial of nurse case management of frail older people. *Journal of the American Geriatrics Society, 47*, 1118–1124.

Gant, M. J. (1996). Comparison of nurses' and patients' perceptions about patients' functional levels after discharge. *Perspectives in Respiratory Nursing, 7*(4), 7,10.

Garrard, J., Kane, R. L., Radosevich, D. M., Skay, C. L., Arnold, S., Kepferle, L., McDermott, S., & Buckanan, J. L. (1990). Impact of geriatric nurse practitioners on nursing-home residents' functional status, satisfaction, and discharge outcomes. *Medical Care, 28*, 271–283.

Gillette, B., & Jenko, M. (1991). Major clinical functions: A unifying framework for measuring outcomes. *Journal of Nursing Care Quality, 6*, 20–24.

Granger, C. V., Cotter, A. C., Hamilton, B. B., Fiedler, R. C., & Hens, M. M. (1990). Functional assessment scales: A study of persons with multiple sclerosis. *Archives of Physical Medicine and Rehabilitation, 71*, 870–875.

Granger, C. V., & Hamilton, B. B. (1993). The Uniform Data System for Medical Rehabilitation report of first admissions for 1991. *American Journal of Physical Medical Rehabilitation, 72*, 33–38.

Granger, C.V., Hamilton, B.B., Keith, R.A., Zielezny, M., & Sherwin, F. S. (1986). Advances in functional assessment for medical rehabilitation. *Topics in Geriatric Rehabilitation, 1*(3), 59–74.

Griffiths, P. (1996). Clinical outcomes for nurse-led in-patient care. *Nursing Times, 92*(9), 40–43.

Griffiths, P., Harris, R., Richardson, G., Hallett, N., Heard, S., & Wilson-Barnett, J. (2001). Substitution of a nursing-led inpatient unit for acute services: Randomized control trial of outcomes and cost of nursing-led intermediate care. *Age and Aging, 30*, 483–488.

Griffiths, P., Wilson-Barnett, J., Richardson, G., Spilsbury, K., Miller, F., & Harris, R. (2000). The effectiveness of intermediate care in a nursing-led in-patient unit. *International Journal of Nursing Studies, 37*, 153–161.

Hackman, J. R., & Oldham, G. R. (1980). *Work redesign*. Reading, MA: Addison-Wesley.

Hamilton, B. B., Granger, C. V., Sherwin, F. S., Zielezny, M., & Tashman, J. S. (1987). A uniform national data system for medical rehabilitation. In M. J. Fuhrer (Ed.), *Rehabilitation outcomes: Analysis and measurement* (pp. 135–147). Baltimore: Paul H. Brooks.

Hamilton, L., & Lyon, P. S. (1995). A nursing-driven program to preserve and restore functional ability in hospitalized elderly patients. *Journal of Nursing Administration, 25*, 30–37.

Harrell, J. S., McConnell, E. S., Wildman, D. S., & Samsa, G. P. (1989). Do nursing diagnoses affect functional status? *Journal of Gerontological Nursing, 15*(10), 13–19.

Hartmaier, S. L., Sloane, P. D., Guess, H. A., Koch, G. G., Mitchell, M., & Phillips, C. D. (1995). Validation of the minimum data set cognitive performance scale: Agreement with the mini-mental state examination. *Journal of Gerontology, 50A* (2), M128–133.

Hawes, C., Morris, J. N., Phillips, C. D., Mor, V., Fries, B. E., & Nonemaker, S. (1995). Reliability estimates for the minimum data set for nursing home resident assessment and care screening. *The Gerontologist, 35*, 172–178.

Hawes, C., Morris, J. N., Phillips, C. D., Fries, B. E., Murphy, K., & Mor, V. (1997). Development of the nursing home resident assessment instrument in the USA. *Age and Aging, 26* (S2), 19–25.

Heafey, M. L., Golden-Baker, S. B., & Mahoney, D. W. (1994). Using nursing diagnoses and interventions in an inpatient amputee program. *Rehabilitation Nursing, 19*, 163–168.

Helberg, J. L. (1993). Patients' status at home care discharge. *Image: Journal of Nursing Scholarship, 25*, 93–99.

Hirdes, J. P., & Carpenter, G. I. (1997). Health outcomes among the frail elderly in communities and institutions: Use of the minimum data set (MDS) to create effective linkages between research and policy. *Canadian Journal on Aging*, Supplement, 53–69.

Hirdes, J. P., Fries, B. E., Morris, J. N., Steel, K., Mor, V., Frijters, D., LaBine, S., Schalm, C., Stones, M. J., Teare, G., Smith,T., Marhaba, M., Perez, E., & Jonsson, P. (1999). Integrated health information systems based on the RAI/MDS series of instruments. *Healthcare Management Forum, 12*(4), 30–40.

Holzemer, W. L., & Henry, S. (1992). Computer-supported versus manually-generated nursing care plans: A comparison of patient problems, nursing interventions, and AIDS patient outcomes. *Computers in Nursing, 10*, 19–24.

Holzemer, W. L., Henry, S. B., Stewart, A., & Janson-Bjerklie, S. (1993). The HIV Quality Audit Marker (HIV-QAM): An outcome measure for hospitalized AIDS patients. *Quality of Life Research, 7,* 99–107.

Holzemer, W. L., Janson-Bjerklie, S., Brown, D. S., & Henry, S. B. (1991). The Quality Marker: A measure of outcomes of nursing care. *Communicating Nursing Research, 24,* 201.

Howard, E., & Reiley, P. (1994). Use of a nursing intensity system as a measure of patient function. *Applied Nursing Research, 7,* 178–182.

Irvine, D. M., O'Brien-Pallas, L., Murray, M., Cockerill, R., Sidani, S., Laurie-Shaw, B., et al. (2000). The reliability and validity of two health status measures for evaluating outcomes of home care nursing. *Research in Nursing & Health, 23,* 43–54.

Jette, A. M., Davies, A. R., Cleary, P. D., Calkins, D. R., Rubenstein, L. V., Finke, A., et al. (1986). The functional status questionnaire: Reliability and validity when used in primary care. *Journal of General Internal Medicine, 1,* 143–149.

Johnson, J. E., Fieler, V. K., Saidel Wlasowicz, G., Mitchell, M. L., & Jones, L. S. (1997). The effects of nursing care guided by self-regulation theory on coping with radiation therapy. *Oncology Nursing Forum, 24,* 1041–1050.

Johnson, M., & Maas, M. (Eds.). (1997). *Nursing outcome classification (NOC).* St. Louis, MO: Mosby.

Johnson, S. J., Brady-Schluttner, K., Ellenbecker, S., Johnson, M., Lassegard, E., Maas, M., et al. (1996). Evaluating physical functional outcomes: One category of the NOC system. *MEDSURG Nursing, 5,* 157–162.

Katz, J. N., Larson, M. G., Phillips, C. B., Fossel, A. H., & Liang, M. H. (1992). Comparative measurement sensitivity of short and longer status instruments. *Medical Care, 30,* 917–925.

Katz, S., & Akpom, C. A. (1976). Index of ADL. *Medical Care, 14,* 116–118.

Katz, S., Downs, T., Cash, H., & Grotz, R. (1970). Progress in development of the index of ADL. *The Gerontologist, 10,* 20–30.

Katz, S., Ford, A. B., Moskowitz, R. W., Jackson, B. A., & Jaffe, M. W. (1963). Studies of illness of the aged. *Journal of the American Medical Association, 185,* 94–99.

Kaufert, J. M. (1983). Functional ability indices: Measurement problems in assessing their validity. *Archives of Physical Medicine and Rehabilitation, 64,* 260–267.

Kline Leidy, N. (1994). Functional status and the forward progress of merry-go-rounds: Toward a coherent analytic framework. *Nursing Research, 43,* 196–202.

Knight, M. M. (2000). Cognitive ability and functional status. *Journal of Advanced Nursing, 31,* 1459–1468.

Lalonde, B. (1987). The general symptom distress scale: A home care outcome measure. *Quality Review Bulletin, 7,* 243–250.

Lang, N. M., & Clinton, J. F. (1984). Assessment of quality of nursing care. *Annual Review of Nursing Research, 2,* 135–163.

Lang, N. M., & Marek, K. D. (1990). The classification of patient outcomes. *Journal of Professional Nursing, 6,* 153–163.

Lawton, M. P., & Brody, E. M. (1969). Assessment of older people: Self-maintaining and instrumental activities of daily living. *The Gerontologist, 9,* 179–186.

Legge, J. S., & Reilly, B. J. (1980). Assessing the outcomes of cancer patients in a home nursing program. *Cancer Nursing, 3,* 357–363.

Lush, M. T., Henry, S. B., Foote, K., & Jones, D. L. (1997). Developing a generic health status measure for use in a computer-based outcomes infrastructure. In U. Gerdin, M. Tallberg, & P. Wainwright (Eds.), *Nursing informatics* (pp. 229–234). Amsterdam: IOS Press.

Lush, M. T., & Jones, D. L. (1995). Developing an outcome infrastructure for nursing. In *JAMIA Symposium Supplement, SCAMC Proceeding* (pp. 625–629). American Medical Informatics Association. Philadelphia: Hanley & Belfus.

Lyons, T. F. (1971). Role clarity, need for clarity, satisfaction, tension, and withdrawal. *Organizational Behavior and Human Performance, 6,* 99–100.

Mahoney, F. L., Wood, O. H., & Barthel, D. W. (1958). Rehabilitation of chronically ill patients: the influence of complications on the final goal. *Southern Medical Journal, 51,* 605–609.

McCorkle, R., Benoliel, J. Q., Donaldson, G., Georgiadou, F., Moinpour, C., & Goodell, B. (1989). A randomized clinical trial of home nursing care for lung cancer patients. *Cancer, 64,* 1375–1382.

McCormich, K. (1991). Future data needs for quality care monitoring, DRG considerations, reimbursement and outcome measurement. *Image: Journal of Nursing Scholarship, 23*(1), 29–32.

McCusker, J. M., Verdon, J., Yousignant, P., de Courval, L.P., Dendukuri, N., & Belzile, E. (2001). Rapid emergency department intervention for older people reduces risk of functional decline: Results of a multicenter randomized trial. *Journal of the American Geriatric Society, 49,* 1272–1281.

McDowell, I., & Newell, C. (1996). *Measuring health: A guide to rating scales and questionnaires* (2nd ed.). New York: Oxford University Press.

Meissner, P., Andolsek, K., Mears, P. A., & Fletcher, B. (1989). Maximizing the functional status of geriatric patients in an acute community hospital setting. *The Gerontologist, 29,* 524–528.

Mendenhall, J. (1991). Diabetes self-care behaviors assessment. (Unpublished tool).

Middleton, S., & Lumby, J. (1998). Exploring the precursors of outcome evaluation in Australia: Linking structure, process and outcome by peer review. *International Journal of Nursing Practice, 4,* 151–155.

Milisen, K., Foreman, M. D., Abraham, I. L., De Geest, S., Godderis, J., Vandermeulen, E., Fischler, B., Delooz, H. H., Spiessen, B., & Broos, P. L. (2001). A nurse-led interdisciplinary intervention program for delirium in elderly hip-fracture patients. *Journal of the American Geriatrics Society, 49,* 523–532.

Mill Barrell, L., Irving Merwin, E., & Poster, E. C. (1997). Patient outcomes used by advanced practice psychiatric nurses to evaluate effectiveness of practice. *Archives of Psychiatric Nursing, 11,* 184–197.

Mock, V., Barton Burke, M., Sheehan, P., Creaton, E. M., Winningham, M. L., McKenney-Tedder, S., et al. (1994). A nursing rehabilitation program for women with breast cancer receiving adjuvant chemotherapy. *Oncology Nursing Forum, 21,* 899–907.

Moinpour, C. M., McCorkle, R., & Saunders, J. (1988). *Measuring functional status.* In M. Frank-Storomberg (Ed.), *Instruments for Clinical Nursing Research.* Connecticut: Appleton & Lang.

Morris, J. N., Fries, B. E., Steel, K., Ikegami, N., Bernabei, R., Carpenter, G. I., et al. (1997). Comprehensive clinical assessment in community setting: Applicability of the MDS-HC. *Journal of the American Geriatrics Society, 45,* 1017–1024.

Mundinger, M. O., Kane, R. L., Lenz, E. R., Totten, A. M., Tsai, W. Y., Cleary, P. D., et al. (2000). Primary care outcomes in patients treated by nurse practitioners or physicians. *Journal of the American Medical Association, 283,* 59–68.

Naylor, M. D. (1990). Comprehensive discharge planning for the elderly. *Research in Nursing & Health, 13,* 327–347.

Naylor, M. D., Munro, B. H., & Brooten, D. A. (1991). Measuring the effectiveness of nursing practice. *Clinical Nurse Specialist, 5,* 210–215.

Nikolaus, T., Bach, M., Oster, P., & Schlierf, G. (1996). Prospective value of self-report and performance-based tests of functional status for 18-month outcomes in elderly patients. *Aging Clinical Experimental Research, 8,* 271–276.

Olson, R. S. (2001). Community re-entry after critical illness. *Critical Care Nursing Clinics of North America, 13,* 449–461.

Orem, D. E. (1980). *Nursing: Concepts of practice* (2nd ed.). New York: McGraw-Hill.

Ouellet, L. L., & Rush, K. L. (1996). A study of nurses' perception of client mobility. *Western Journal of Nursing Research, 18,* 565–579.

Pettersson, E., Gardulf, A., Nordström, G., Svanberg-Johnsson, C., & Bylin, G. (1999). Evaluation of a nurse-run asthma school. *International Journal of Nursing Studies, 36,* 145–151.

Pfieffer, E. (Ed). (1975). *Multidimensional functional assessment: The OARS methodology.* Durham, NC: Center for the Study of Aging and Human Development.

Pugh, L. C., Haven, D. S., Xie, S., Robinson, J. M., & Blaha, C. (2001). Case management for elderly persons with health failure: The quality of life and cost outcomes. *MEDSURG Nursing, 10,* 71–78.

Ramler, C. L., Kraus, V. L., Pringle Specht, J., & Titler, M. G. (1996). MOS SF-36: Clinical and administrative implications for nurses. In K. Kelly & M. Maas (Eds.), *Outcomes of effective management practice* (pp. 71–93). Thousand Oaks, CA: Sage.

Raphael, D., Smith, T., Brown, I., & Renwick, R. (1995). Development and properties of the short and brief version of the quality of life profile: Senior version. *International Journal of Health Sciences, 6,* 161–168.

Reiley, P., Lezzoni, L. I., Phillips, R., Davis, R. B., Tuchin, L. I., & Calkins, D. (1996). Discharge planning: Comparison of patients' and nurses' perception of patients following hospital discharge. *Image: Journal of Nursing Scholarship, 28,* 143–147.

Richmond, T., McCorkle, R., Tulman, L., & Fawcett, J. (1997). *Measuring function.* In M. Frank-Stromborg & S. J. Olsen (Eds.), *Instruments for clinical health-care research* (2nd ed., pp. 75–85). Boston: Jones and Bartlett.

Roy, C., & Roberts, S. L. (1981). *Theory construction in nursing: An adaptation model.* Englewood Cliffs, NJ: Prentice-Hall.

Rubenstein, L. Z., Schairer, C., Wieland, G. D., & Kane, R. (1984). Systematic biases in functional status assessment of elderly adults: Effects of different data sources. *Journal of Gerontology, 39,* 686–691.

Shah, S., Vanclay, F., & Cooper, B. (1989). Improving the sensitivity of the Barthel Index for stroke rehabilitation. *Journal of Clinical Epidemiology, 42,* 703–709.

Shaughnessy, P. W., Crisler, K. S., & Schlenker, R. E. (1998). Outcome-based quality improvement in home health care: The OASIS indicators. *Home Health Care Management & Practice, 10* (2), 11–19.

Shortell, S. M., Rousseau, D. M., Gilles, R. R., Devers, K. J., & Simon, T. L. (1991). Organizational assessment in intensive care units (ICUs): Construct development, reliability, and validity of the ICU nurse-physician questionnaire. *Medical Care, 29,* 709–726.

Steiner, A., Bronagh, W., Pickering, R. M., Wiles, R., Ward, J., & Brooking, J. I. (2001). Therapeutic nursing or unblocking beds? A randomized controlled trial of a post-acute intermediate care unit. *British Medical Journal, 322,* 453–459.

Stewart, A. L., Hays, R. D., & Ware, J. E., Jr. (1988). The MOS Short Form General Health Survey: Reliability and validity in a patient population. *Medical Care, 26,* 724–735.

Swan, B. A. (1998). Postoperative nursing care contributions to symptom distress and functional status after ambulatory surgery. *MEDSURG Nursing, 7,* 148–158.

Tulman, L., & Fawcett, J. (1990). Functional status during pregnancy and the postpartum: A framework for research. *Image: Journal of Nursing Scholarship, 22,* 191–194.

van Bennekom, C. A. M., Jelles, F., Lankhorst, G. J., & Bouter, L. M. (1996). Responsiveness of the Rehabilitation Activities Profile and the Barthel Index. *Journal of Clinical Epidemiology, 49,* 39–44.

Wade, D. T., & Hewer, R. L. (1987). Functional abilities after stroke: Measurement, natural history and prognosis. *Journal of Neurology, Neurosurgery, and Psychiatry, 50,* 177–182.

Walsh, B., Pickering, R. M., & Brooking, J. I. (1999). A randomized controlled trial of nurse-led inpatient care for post-acute medical patients: A pilot study. *Clinical Effectiveness in Nursing, 3,* 88–90.

Waltz, C. F., & Strickland, O. L. (1988). *Measurement of nursing outcomes, Volume 1: Measuring client outcomes.* New York: Springer Publ.

Wanich, C. K., Sullivan-Marx, E. M., Gottlieb, G. L., & Johnson, J. C. (1992). Functional status outcomes of a nursing intervention in hospitalized elderly. *Image: Journal of Nursing Scholarship, 24,* 201–207.

Ware, J. E. (1993). *SF-36 Health Survey: Manual and interpretation guide.* Boston: New England Medical Center, The Health Institute.

Wolf, Z., Giardino, E., Osbourne, P., & Ambrose, M. (1994). Dimensions of nurse caring. *Image: Journal of Nursing Scholarship, 26,* 107–111.

Zemore, R., & Shepel, L. (1989). Effects of breast cancer and mastectomy on emotional support and adjustment. *Social Science and Medicine, 28,* 19–27.

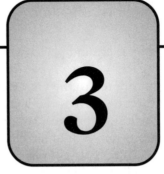

3

Self-Care

Souraya Sidani, RN, PhD

3.1 Introduction

Self-care is the key dimension of health care (Nelson McDermott, 1993; Slusher, 1999) and is viewed as a philosophical orientation that underlies nursing and distinguishes it from other disciplines (Bennett, 1980; Orem, 1991). It is regarded as a framework that underpins the design of health-promoting interventions and guides practice across the continuum of care, which includes primary care, acute care, home care, long-term care, and rehabilitation settings. Self-care is the focus and the goal of nursing care aimed at improving the health status, coping, and functioning of clients (Dodd & Miaskowski, 2000; Gantz, 1990; Henry & Holzemer, 1997; Keller et al., 1989; McCaleb & Edgil, 1994). Furthermore, self-care represents the theoretical foundation for psychoeducational, cognitive, behavioral, and symptom management interventions. These interventions involve informing clients about their condition and its treatment, and instructing them in (a) self-monitoring, perceiving, and identifying changes in functioning; (b) judging the meaning and severity of these changes; (c) assessing options for actions to manage these changes; and (d) selecting and performing appropriate actions. Self-care also is viewed as an outcome of nursing care (Gillette & Jenko, 1991; Irvine et al., 1998; Johnson & Maas, 1997; Mitchell et al., 1998), where clients are expected to select and perform actions to maintain life, healthy functioning, and well being.

Several factors have contributed to the importance of self-care as an outcome desired for clients seen in settings across the healthcare continuum: (a) shifting patterns of disease (from acute to chronic); (b) an ideological shift from a cure to a care orientation; (c) healthcare economics characterized by limited resources and funds and by an emphasis on cost containment, which lead to shorter hospital lengths of stay and to delivery of care on an outpatient basis; and (d) a consumer movement in which patients are more knowledgeable about health issues, demand increased control of their health care and increased involvement in health-related decisions and care, and demonstrate a desire and motivation to improve their health, functioning, and well-being (Anastasio et al., 1995; Bennett, 1980; Craddock et al., 1999; Dodd & Miaskowski, 2000; McCaleb & Edgil, 1994; Padula, 1992; van Agthoven & Plomp, 1989).

As a result of these changes, self-care has been identified as critical for effective health promotion in the general population (Moore, 1995) and in older adults (Nicholas, 1993), and for successful home health care of acute and chronic conditions (Jopp et al., 1993; Rice, 1998). Self-care has gained most attention in the management of chronic illness, which places many demands on patients as well as on the healthcare system. Chronic illnesses, such as cancer, asthma, chronic obstructive pulmonary disease, diabetes, and end-stage renal disease, impose multiple and new demands on the affected persons. These are associated with the physical symptoms characterizing the illness and its treatment, the emotional stresses of coping with and adjusting to the chronic condition, and the changes in interpersonal relationships and physical and social functioning (Burks, 1999; Richardson, 1991). Much of the required treatment and care for these conditions is provided in outpatient settings. Consequently, patients must assume primary responsibility for addressing these demands, carrying out the therapeutic regimen on a long-term basis, and identifying and successfully managing any changes in their condition (Craddock et al., 1999; Nail et al., 1991).

Self-care is considered an integral component both of managing these demands and of preserving an acceptable level of healthy functioning (Anastasio et al., 1995). Self-care enables patients to observe themselves, recognize symptoms, determine the severity of symptoms, and choose appropriate strategies for treating the symptoms. The goals are to minimize the symptoms and maximize health (Baker, 1999; Coates & Boore, 1995). In chronic illness, self-care is thus considered an important aspect of health and nursing care, as well as an instrumental outcome of care.

Although self-care is recognized as an outcome of nursing care and has been discussed in a large number of publications, studies that have investigated self-care are scarce (Rice, 1998; van Agthoven & Plomp, 1989). Research on self-care has been hampered by a lack of consistent conceptualization of its dimensions, which has resulted in variability in its operationalization and in a lack of well-established, reliable, and valid instruments to measure self-care accurately and comprehensively (Padula, 1992).

This chapter reviews the available literature on self-care. The first section provides a conceptual definition of self-care based on a concept analysis that clarifies the concept at the theoretical and operational levels. The second section identifies factors that have been found to influence self-care and that need to be taken into account when evaluating the effectiveness of nursing care in promoting the achievement of self-care. The third section summarizes the empirical evidence linking self-care to nursing. The purpose of this literature review is to determine the extent to which self-care is an outcome that is sensitive to nursing. The fourth section identifies instruments measuring self-care that demonstrated reliability, validity, and sensitivity to change. The last section discusses issues in the measurement of self-care that should be taken into consideration when this outcome is assessed in research or in everyday practice.

3.2 Self-Care: A Concept Analysis and Definition

Self-care is a term that appeared in health-related literature in the 1970s (e.g., Levin, 1976). In nursing, Orem (1971, 1985, 1991) developed and refined a model of self-care that served as the basis for deriving middle-range theories of self-care. These theories formed the frame of reference for multiple studies that described the self-care practices of various patient populations, explored factors influencing self-care, and investigated the effects of nursing interventions on self-care.

In Orem's (1985, 1991) conceptualization, self-care is represented by two distinct yet interrelated concepts: self-care agency and self-care behavior. The first refers to the capacity of an individual to engage in self-care behaviors. It denotes the *ability* to initiate and perform actions directed toward the care of oneself by oneself. Self-care agency involves several domains, including (1) the cognitive domain, that is, knowledge of the health condition and of the skills necessary to fulfill the self-management action, as well as decision-making and judgment ability; (2) the physical domain, that is, the physical ability to carry out the self-management action; (3) the emotional or psychosocial domain, that is, attitude, values, desire, and motivation, as well as perceived competence in performing the self-management action; and (4) the behavioral domain, which refers to having the necessary skills for performing the self-care behaviors (Burks, 1999; Joseph, 1980; Lantz et al., 1995; Orem, 1991).

Self-care behavior refers to the *practice* of activities that maturing and mature persons initiate and perform, within time frames, on their own behalf in the interests of maintaining life, healthy functioning, continuing personal development, and well-being (Orem, 1991). The domains comprising self-care behavior are defined in relation to the universal, developmental, and health-deviation requisites. Universal requisites are concerned with basic life processes, such as maintaining an adequate intake of air, and a balance between activity and rest. Developmental requisites focus on the life cycle changes. Health-deviation requisites are related to appropriate health care, such as health monitoring, seeking health care as needed, participating in treatment, and living with illness (Orem, 1991).

Orem characterized self-care behavior as being performed by oneself for oneself (i.e., controlled by the individual) and consisting of deliberate, patterned, sequential, and purposeful activities. These behaviors could be performed continuously and voluntarily on the individual's own behalf, could be learned, and are goal-oriented (i.e., to improve, maintain, or restore health). Other nursing scholars have advanced the following definitions of self-care:

- The process that permits people and families to take initiative and responsibility, and to function effectively in developing their potential for health (Norris, 1979).

- The process of taking responsibility for developing one's own health potential (Spradley, 1981).

- The level of direct action behaviors for prevention or attenuation of treatment side effects or of preventable complications of illness (Braden, 1993).

- The performance of preventive or therapeutic healthcare activities that promote optimum participation in normal activities (Anderson, 1990).

- The set of activities in which one engages throughout life on a daily basis (Hartweg, 1990).

- Self-care in health refers to the activities that individuals, families, and communities undertake with the intention of enhancing health, preventing disease, limiting illness, and restoring health. These activities are derived from technical knowledge and skills from the pool of both professional and lay experience. They are undertaken by lay people on their own behalf, either separately or in participative collaboration with professionals (Ad Hoc Work Group on self-care education, as cited in Lenihan, 1988).

Three qualitative studies that were conducted to investigate the patients' perception of self-care provided the perspective of those involved in self-care, which complemented the scholars' conceptualization. Patients with chronic illness described self-care as taking care, not harming self, and listening to the body (Leenerts & Megilvy, 2000). Others defined it as a focused set of actions that participants used to enhance their mental and physical health. It entailed a process involving five dimensions: cognitive (i.e., normalizing), attitudinal (i.e., focusing on living), behavioral (i.e., taking care of oneself), interpersonal (i.e., being in relation to others), and existential (i.e., triumphing) (Barroso, 1995). Elderly persons living at home viewed self-care as involving caring for health and illnesses and carrying out activities of daily living. They identified four categories or levels of self-care performance, which they labeled as responsible, formally guided, independent, and abandoned. Responsible self-care implied activity and responsibility in all activities of daily living. Formally guided self-care consisted of regular but uncritical observance of medical instructions and routine performance of daily tasks. Independent self-care was based on the person's desire to listen to his or her internal voice. Helplessness and lack of responsibility characterized abandoned self-care (Backman & Hentinen, 1999).

3.2.1 Essential Attributes of Self-Care

These definitions provide a rather consistent conceptualization of self-care. It is viewed as the ability to perform, and the actual involvement in, actions aimed at promoting, enhancing, or maintaining health. The activities are selected and enacted by the individuals on their own behalf, independently or in collaboration with health care professionals.

Self-care has been operationalized as the perceived ability and/or actual performance of the actions or behaviors related to health maintenance and promotion, disease prevention, and self-treatment. The specific actions reflective of self-care vary based on the purpose for which they are carried out (e.g., health promotion, disease prevention), the target population (e.g., healthy children, clients with chronic illness), and the setting of healthcare delivery (e.g., community at large, home health, long-term care).

3.2.2 Antecedents of Self-Care

The actual performance of self-care behavior is posited as being directly influenced by the person's perceived self-care agency, that is, the person's ability and willingness to engage in self-care activities (Gantz, 1990; Orem, 1991). In addition, researchers have proposed a variety of factors that affect the exercise of self-care agency and/or performance of self-care behavior. The factors are classified into five categories: cognitive, psychosocial, physical, demographic, and socio-cultural. The first includes learning skills, memory, problem-solving skills, organizational skills, and knowledge, as well as the perception that the action/behavior or treatment to be carried out is efficacious (Harper, 1984; Jaarsma et al., 1998). Psychosocial factors comprising the second category include self-concept, self-esteem, self-discipline, personality traits, perceived self-competence, and motivation (Gantz, 1990; Harper, 1984; Horsburgh et al., 2000; Joseph, 1980; Whetstone & Hansson, 1989). The third category entails physical factors such as dexterity, psychomotor skills, activity or movement level, health functional state, and disability or injury (Gaffney & Moore, 1996; Harper, 1984; Joseph, 1980). Demographic factors such as age or maturity, gender, education, socioeconomic status, and living arrangement (Gaffney & Moore, 1996; Hanucharurnkul, 1989; Joseph, 1980) form the fourth category of factors affecting self-care. The last category includes sociocultural factors such as family system, cultural practices and beliefs, health values and beliefs, social support, and availability of resources (Gaffney & Moore, 1996; Gantz, 1990; Hanucharurnkul, 1989; Joseph, 1980). Backman and Hentinen (1999) identified the following factors as contributing to the performance of self-care in elderly persons living at home: (a) external factors, such as living condition and social support; and (b) internal factors, including health and functional state, individual thoughts concerning health, and attitude toward health and self-care.

Several studies examined the effects of selected factors on self-care. The results are summarized in relation to the self-care concept (i.e., self-care agency or behavior) investigated.

Gender, age, perceived health status, health locus of control, perceived self-efficacy, learned helplessness, personality traits, and marital status were found to influence self-care agency in healthy and ill adults. Women reported higher levels of self-care agency than men in a sample of healthy adults (Whetstone & Hansson, 1989) and in patients with end-stage renal disease on dialysis (Horsburgh, 1999). Older persons reported higher levels of self-care agency than younger ones in a sample of healthy adults (Whetstone & Hansson, 1989) and in patients with end-stage renal disease on dialysis (Horsburgh, 1999). Perceived health status was positively correlated to self-care agency in older patients with end-stage renal disease (Horsburgh et al., 2000). Perceived health locus of control and perceived self-efficacy were positively related to the exercise of self-care agency in patients with hypertension; that is, patients who perceived more control over their health and had higher self-efficacy had higher scores on self-care agency (Chen, 1999). Learned helplessness was negatively related to self-care agency in healthy adults (Nelson McDermott, 1993). Various personality traits were associated with self-care agency in patients with end-stage renal disease. Patients reporting higher levels of consciousness, openness, and extroversion had higher self-care agency scores (Horsburgh, 1999; Horsburgh et al., 2000). Married adults, whether healthy or with end-stage renal disease, had higher self-care agency scores (Horsburgh, 1999).

Multiple factors influenced performance of self-care behaviors in children and adolescents. Although gender differences in self-care behavior performance were reported, the direction of the difference varied with the nature of the specific behaviors (McCaleb & Cull, 2000). Older adolescents tended to engage less in self-care practices (McCaleb & Cull, 2000; Moore & Mosher, 1997). Those who reported experiencing some health problems tended to engage less in self-care practices (McCaleb & Cull, 2000). Lower socioeconomic status, indicated by participation in a paid lunch program, was associated with increased self-care practices (McCaleb & Edgil, 1994). Church attendance had a positive influence on self-care; that is, healthy adolescents who attended church tended to practice self-care (McCaleb & Cull, 2000; McCaleb & Edgil, 1994). Ethnicity was also related to self-care behaviors; being White was associated with increased self-care behavior performance by healthy adolescents (Gaffney & Moore, 1996; McCaleb & Edgil, 1994; Moore & Mosher, 1997). Self-concept and self-care agency were positively correlated with performance of self-care behavior in healthy adolescents (McCaleb & Edgil, 1994; Slusher, 1999).

Similar factors were reported to affect self-care behavior in adults. Women engaged in self-care activities more than men in samples of patients with first time myocardial infarction (Rodeman et al., 1995). Older patients with chronic illness tended to report minimal engagement in self-care behaviors (Carroll, 1995; Wang & Lee, 1999). Increased socioeconomic status was consistently associated with increased performance of self-care behaviors in patients with cancer receiving radiation therapy (Hanucharurnkul, 1989), in elderly women living in rural areas (Wang & Lee, 1999), and in healthy older adults (Nicholas, 1993). Social support was positively correlated with self-care behavior performance. This finding was consistent across samples of patients with first time myocardial infarction (MI), patients receiving radiation therapy, and elderly women living in rural areas, despite differences in the operationalization of social support measured with established questionnaires (Hanucharurnkul, 1989; Rodeman et al., 1995). Living with others was also associated with increased self-care behavior performance in healthy older adults (Nicholas, 1993). Being married was related to increased adherence to self-care recommendations in patients with congestive heart failure (Ni et al., 1999).

Individuals' health status had an effect on self-care behavior performance, but the effect's direction was inconsistent, due to variability in the operationalization of health status across studies. When health status was measured with general perceived health scales, the relationship with self-care behavior was positive; when health status was measured as perceived disability, the relation was negative. Perception of high level of health correlated positively with perceived effectiveness of self-care behaviors undertaken to manage the side effects of chemotherapy (Dodd et al., 1991), and with performance of self-care by elderly women living in rural areas (Wang & Lee, 1999) and by healthy adults (Nicholas, 1993). In contrast, when health state was measured with perceived disability (LeFort, 2000) or with stage of cancer (Hanucharurnkul, 1989), it was associated with decreased self-care behavior performance. A high level of perceived self-care efficacy was consistently related to increased self-care practices, despite variability in the measurement of these two variables and variability in the target populations, including patients on hemodialysis (Lev & Owen, 1998), patients recovering from cardiovascular surgery (Carroll, 1995), patients with idiographic pain (LeFort, 2000), and patients with congestive heart failure (Ni et al., 1999). Resourcefulness was also associated with increased engagement in self-help behaviors in patients with idiographic pain (LeFort, 2000). Having high levels of perceived self-care agency had a significant positive influence on self-care behaviors performance, as reported by pregnant women (Hart, 1995), older patients with end-stage renal disease (Horsburgh et al., 2000), and patients with advanced heart failure (Jaarsma et al., 2000). In elderly patients on hemodialysis, Badzek and colleagues (1998) found a significant positive correlation between the patients' educational level and length of time on hemodialysis, and knowledge of self-care activities related to food and fluid restrictions. Similarly, Ni et al. (1999) found a positive relationship between knowledge of, and adherence to, self-care recommendations in patients with congestive heart failure.

The results of these studies provide evidence supporting the influence of antecedent factors on self-care. Briefly, these factors could be viewed as determinants or risk factors of self-care, and should be taken into consideration when evaluating self-care as an outcome of nursing care. Therefore, it is recommended that nurses:

- Assess these factors when planning care aimed at enhancing self-care in clients seen in everyday practice.

- Design the care to fit the demographic, sociocultural, physical, psychosocial, and cognitive characteristics of individual patients (i.e., individualize care).

- Account for these factors when monitoring clients'/patients' self-care practices, and when evaluating outcomes of care in practice.

- Examine or control for the influence of these factors on the self-care outcomes expected of nursing care/interventions in research.

3.2.3 Consequences of Self-Care

The performance of self-care behavior is considered beneficial to the individual patient and to the healthcare system. The following were mentioned as favorable consequences of self-care behavior:

- Achievement of desired outcomes (Badzek et al., 1998).

- Decreased risk for complications (Badzek et al., 1998; Hanucharurnkul & Vinya-nguag, 1991; Kimberly, 1997; Nail et al., 1991).

- Decreased rate of re-admission (Dunbar, Jacobson, & Deaton, 1998).

- Increased patient satisfaction (Hanucharurnkul & Vinya-nguag, 1991; Slusher, 1999).

- Decreased healthcare costs (Leveille et al., 1998; Slusher, 1999).

- Increased sense of responsibility, control, independence, and autonomy (Skoner, 1994; Slusher, 1999).

- Enhanced coping with or adjustment to illness (Slusher, 1999) and decreased burden of chronic illness (Leveille et al., 1998).

- Improved sense of well-being, functioning, and quality of life (Slusher, 1999).

- Decreased health services utilization (Leveille et al., 1998).

- Enhanced recovery from surgery or illness (Hanucharurnkul & Vinya-nguag, 1991).

- Symptom control (Dodd et al., 1991; Richardson, 1991).

No studies were located that investigated the effects of self-care on the proposed consequences. In the future, researchers need to examine the relationship of self-care agency and behavior with these variables, with the aim of demonstrating the instrumental role of self-care in achieving desired patient outcomes.

In summary, self-care is considered an outcome that is sensitive to nursing care. As an outcome, self-care refers to the clients' perceived ability to engage in self-care behaviors, as well as the clients' performance of actions or behaviors that aim at promoting and maintaining health, preventing disease, and managing or treating illness or changes in body function. Clients initiate these actions independently or in collaboration with health care professionals. The specific actions in which clients engage vary under different circumstances. Several factors have been identified as potentially influencing self-care. These should be accounted for when providing nursing care and then evaluating its effects on self-care.

3.3 Empirical Evidence Linking Self-Care to Nursing

Self-care is the fundamental principle underlying many nursing interventions. It is considered the primary concern and goal of educational, psychoeducational, cognitive, behavioral, and symptom management interventions. These interventions focus on teaching individuals self-care related knowledge, and on instructing them in the skills necessary to perform self-care. Examples include the Pro-Self Program (Dodd & Miaskowski, 2000), the Self-Help Intervention (Braden et al., 1993), psychoeducational programs for managing chronic pain (LeFort et al., 1998), and the Arthritis Self-Management Program (Lorig et al., 1987). Although self-care is a theoretically anticipated outcome of these interventions, few studies have evaluated their effectiveness in achieving self-care.

A total of 23 studies were analyzed for this review. Almost all evaluated the effectiveness of educational or psychoeducational interventions that nurses provided. Table 3.1 summarizes information pertinent to the studies' design, sample, outcome and measures, intervention, and results.

Table 3.1. Studies Investigating the Relationships between Nursing Interventions and Self-Care

Author	Design	Sample size and characteristics	Interventions and outcomes	Major results	Limitations
Gregory (2000)	Quasi-experimental (one group)	$N = 150$. Grade 3–5 students with asthma.	Education by school nurse. Strategies for managing asthma signs and symptoms.	Attendance at the educational sessions increased adequacy in describing reactions to asthma, recognizing signs and symptoms, and managing signs and symptoms through medical or non-medical strategies.	Outcome measures not validated; no monitoring of treatment implementation; experimenter expectancy.
Hagopian (1996)	Experimental with post-test only	$N = 31$ in control and 38 in experimental groups. Patients being treated with radiation therapy; mean age = 53; majority White, female.	Listening to audiotapes that discussed side effects and suggested SC[1] activities. Radiation side effects experienced and use and effectiveness of SC measures.	Experimental group reported greater use of SC measures and a higher level of perceived effectiveness of SC measures used.	Lack of pre-testing; outcome measure not validated.
Blair et al. (1996)	Repeated measures with three groups exposed to different conditions	$N = 15$. Residents in nursing home; mean age = 78; mean residency period = 18 months; mean MMSE[2] = 25.	Group 1: operant behavior management; group 2: mutual goal-setting; group 3: usual care. SC behavior (e.g., bathing, dressing, feeding self).	Patients in group 1 performed SC behaviors more frequently than those in the other two groups.	Very small sample size; experimenter expectancy; no monitoring of treatment implementation; Hawthorne effects.
Blair (1995)	Quasi-experimental with three groups	$N = 37$ in group 1, 16 in group 2, 26 in group 3. Residents in nursing homes; females; mean age 80; mean residency period = 2 years.	Group 1: behavioral management of dependent behaviors; group 2: goal attainment preparation; group 3: control. Attainment of goal and frequency of performance of ADLs[3].	Patients in group 1 showed significant improvement in performance of ADLs.	Possible placebo effect; experimenter expectancy.

Table 3.1 (continued)

Author	Design	Sample size and characteristics	Interventions and outcomes	Major results	Limitations
Watson et al. (1997)	Experimental	$N = 27$ in control and 29 in treatment groups. Patients with COPD[4]; smoking history of 10 years; mean age = 67; more males.	Patient education about self-medication. Use of medications, respiratory status.	Patients in the experimental group showed improvement in self-medication adjustment.	Possible dissemination of the intervention; selection bias.
Gallefoss & Bakke (1999)	Experimental	$N = 140$. Patients with asthma or COPD; majority women.	Patient education on self-management of medications. Compliance with medications.	The odds ratio for having a compliance rate greater than 75% were 2.8 in the education group.	Outcome measures not validated.
Turner et al. (1998)	Experimental with two experimental groups	$N = 117$. Patients with asthma; 53% women.	Group 1: patient education; group 2: self-management plans. Medications usage and symptom control.	Significant decrease in signs and symptoms scores in both groups; improvement in medications usage as prescribed in both groups.	21% of patients were non-compliant with treatment plan.
Blair (1999)	Quasi-experimental with repeated measures	$N = 20$. Residents in nursing homes; more females; mean age = 78; mean duration of residency 19 months; mean MMSE score = 25.	Combination of educative-supportive system of care and operant behavior management. Performance of morning SC and ADLs.	Patients in experimental groups showed greater engagement in SC activities of daily living than those in the control group did.	Small sample size; possible experimenter expectancy.
Hanucharurnkul & Vinya-nguag (1991)	Experimental with blocking on age	$N = 40$, 20 in each group. Patients who underwent pyelo- or nephrolithotomy.	Patient education. Pain and ambulation.	Experimental group reported less pain severity and distress and greater ambulation than the control group did.	Small sample size; possible dissemination of treatment.

Table 3.1 (continued)

Author	Design	Sample size and characteristics	Interventions and outcomes	Major results	Limitations
Williams et al. (1988)	Quasi-experimental with repeated measures post-test only	N = 60. Mastectomy or hysterectomy; 72% less than 50 years old; 65% married; had stage 1 or 2 cancer.	Patient education pre- and post-op with a focus on SC activities. SC behavior performance.	Patients in the experimental group performed the SC behaviors earlier and more appropriately than those in the control group.	High drop-out rate; small sample size; possible Hawthorne effect with observation of SC behavior performance.
Dodd (1983)	Experimental with four groups	N = 48, 12 in each group. Patients with cancer receiving chemotherapy.	Group 1: drug info; group 2: informational package for symptom management; group 3: combination; group 4: control. SC behavior.	Significant difference among groups on the number of SC behaviors performed (highest mean for patients who received the informational package).	Heterogeneous sample on diagnostic categories and chemotherapy protocols; small sample size; recall bias.
Jaarsma et al. (2000)	Experimental with repeated measures	N = 132. Patients with advanced heart failure; mean age = 72; 60% men.	Patient education. SC agency; SC behaviors.	No difference in SC agency; significant difference in SC behaviors at post-test and follow-up.	Differential attrition rates (higher in experimental group); significant difference between dropouts and participant completers in stage of heart disease; SC measures lack sensitivity to change.
Aish (1996)	Experimental	N = 104. Patients hospitalized for MI[5]; 60% men.	Home visit and instructions on diet management. Food habits; SC agency.	Experimental group showed significant decrease in fat intake and increase in healthy food habits.	Pre-existing differences in the groups not controlled for; treatment implementation not monitored.
LeFort et al. (1998)	Experimental with block on gender	N = 110, 57 in treatment and 53 in control groups. Patients with idiographic, chronic pain; more women; middle age; mean pain duration 6 years; taking medications.	Psychoeducational program. Pain, performance of self-help activities.	Patients in experimental group reported less pain and more involvement in valued adult role activities.	Dropouts had too much pain.

Table 3.1 (continued)

Author	Design	Sample size and characteristics	Interventions and outcomes	Major results	Limitations
Hart & Foster (1998)	Secondary data analysis	$N = 246$. Pregnant women enrolled in prenatal care, or in childbirth education classes.	Patient education. SC agency.	Women who had childbirth education, and were primiparous and college-educated had higher scores on SC agency.	None.
Harper (1984)	Experimental with repeated measures	$N = 60$, 30 in each group. Women with essential hypertension; mean age = 66; widowed; had other diseases.	Patient education about medications. Knowledge of medications; SC behaviors.	Patients in the experimental group had a significant increase in knowledge and SC behavior.	Outcome measures not validated.
Craddock et al. (1999)	Quasi-experimental	$N = 48$, 26 in experimental group and 22 in control group. Women with breast cancer receiving chemotherapy; stage 1 or 2; well-educated; mean age = 49; 65% married.	Patient education and phone follow-up on side effects. SC agency; effectiveness of SC.	No significant difference between groups on effectiveness of SC measures and SC agency.	Small sample size; treatment and response burden were reasons for refusal to participate; treatment implementation not monitored.
Albrecht et al. (1993)	Correlational	$N = 154$. Patients with arthritis; mean age = 56; 85% women; 73% White; 55% marrried.	Patient education at home. SC behaviors.	No effect on SC behavior performance reported; however, sex (B = .20), age (.23), and number of lessons (.18) affected satisfaction with intervention.	Outcome measure not validated; self-selection bias.
Folden (1993)	Quasi-experimental	$N = 34$ in control group, 34 in experimental group. Patients with stroke; mean age = 75; 74% married; 56% men.	Guided decision-making. SC agency; performance of ADLs.	Patients in the experimental group increased SC agency scores and performance of ADLs.	High attrition; initial difference between groups not accounted for.

Table 3.1 (continued)

Author	Design	Sample size and characteristics	Interventions and outcomes	Major results	Limitations
LeFort (2000)	Experimental	N = 102. Pregnant women; 75% White; mean age = 40; mean pain duration 6 years.	Psychoeducation. SC behaviors.	Psychoeducation associated with self-efficacy (.27), resourcefulness (.21), disability (−.40).	None.
Goeppinger et al. (1995)	Quasi-experimental with one group	N = 154. Patients with arthritis at home.	Patient education. SC behaviors.	Patients showed improvement in SC behavior performance.	Outcome measures not validated; treatment implementation not monitored.

[1] SC = Self-Care
[2] MMSE = Mini-Mental State Exam
[3] ADLs = Activities of Daily Living
[4] COPD = Chronic Obstructive Pulmonary Disease
[5] MI = Myocardial Infarction

In several studies, the intervention was based on Orem's model of self-care, in which the nurses' role in promoting self-care is described as supportive-educative. The nurses' functions involved providing patients with the information and resources needed to perform self-care, and assisting them in incorporating the self-care behaviors in their everyday lives. The outcome of self-care was operationalized as the engagement in, or the performance of, self-care actions. The specific actions measured varied across the studies, depending on the focus of the intervention and on the target population. The specific actions represented were (1) adherence to prescribed drug regimen or self-care recommendations such as diet, exercise, and stress management; (2) engagement in self- or healthcare providers' prescribed strategies for managing symptoms; (3) performance of activities of daily living; (4) performance of valued adult role activities such as work and recreation; and (5) knowledge or perceived ability to perform self-care behaviors.

The target populations included children with asthma, patients who were recovering from CABG, patients with cancer receiving adjuvant therapy, residents in nursing homes, adult patients with COPD or asthma, patients who had surgery, patients with advanced heart failure or with MI, patients with idiopathic pain, pregnant women, patients with hypertension, patients with arthritis, and patients with stroke.

The research designs were experimental or quasi-experimental, which is appropriate to address the study purpose. However, only a few studies included one or two follow-up post-test measurements. Most did not include any at all. Yet follow-ups are useful for examining changes in behaviors, which are known to require some time to take place.

The sample sizes ranged from 15 to 246. The smallest one involved nursing home residents. In 10 studies (48% of studies reviewed), the sample size was greater than 100. The rather small sample size observed in these studies is characteristic of experimental design. Nonetheless, none was based on a power analysis. The demographic characteristics of the participants varied, but were consistent with those of the target population. For instance, most nursing home residents were older women, whereas most patients with heart disease were middle-aged men.

The instruments used to measure self-care differed. Most were developed for the study and addressed the specific self-care behaviors of concern. In few studies, self-care agency was measured in addition to or instead of actual performance of self-care behaviors. Most measures were not well validated. In one study, knowledge of self-care strategies was measured as the outcome. The variability observed in these studies limited the ability to synthesize the results. Therefore, they are summarized in point form here:

- Children with asthma who attended educational sessions provided by school nurses were able to adequately describe physical reactions to asthma, recognize symptoms, and manage the symptoms by properly using medications and applying non-medical strategies such as trying to calm down, resting or slowing down, and taking deep breaths, more so than children in the control group (Gregory, 2000).

- No significant difference in knowledge of self-care strategies was found among three groups of patients recovering from cardiovascular surgery. The three groups received education in three different formats: (a) inpatient individual sessions, (b) inpatient individual sessions with follow-up phone call after discharge, and (c) group session held after discharge. Patients in all groups demonstrated increased self-care knowledge at posttest (Barnason & Zimmerman, 1995).

- Patients receiving radiation therapy for cancer who listened to audiotapes instructing them in self-care activities to manage the side effects of treatment reported more use of self-care measures and a higher level of perceived effectiveness of the self-care measures used than patients in the control group did (Hagopian, 1996).

- Residents in nursing homes who were supported and encouraged by nursing staff to engage in morning care (i.e., bathing, grooming, dressing, feeding self) showed significant improvement in performing these activities of daily living independently and more frequently than those who received usual care (Blair, 1995, 1999; Blair et al., 1996).

- Patients with COPD who were instructed by nurses on when and how to adjust their medications showed more appropriate self-medication adjustment than those in the control group (Watson et al., 1997). Similar improvement in medication self-management was observed in patients with asthma (Gallefoss & Bakke, 1999; Turner et al., 1998) and in patients with hypertension (Harper, 1984).

- Surgical patients instructed in the performance of postoperative exercises and ambulation engaged in these activities earlier and performed them more appropriately than those who received usual care (Hanucharurnkul & Vinya-nguag, 1991; Williams et al., 1988).

- Patients with cancer who were receiving chemotherapy and who also received drug information and an informational package for symptom management performed more self-care behaviors than those who received (a) the drug information only, (b) the informational package only, or (c) no information (Dodd, 1983). In contrast, patient education with a follow-up contact to reinforce self-management did not influence performance or perceived effectiveness of self-care measures to manage the side effects of chemotherapy in patients with breast cancer (Craddock et al., 1999).

- Patient education had a significant impact on self-care (i.e., increased engagement in self-care behaviors) in patients with advanced heart failure; however, it did not affect self-care agency (Jaarsma et al., 2000). A similar effect was reported in patients with MI (Aish, 1996) who altered their dietary intake in accordance with given recommendations. In contrast, patient education did not affect self-care behaviors or self-care agency in patients with heart failure, despite the observed increased engagement in self-care activities in both groups over time (Jaarsma et al., 1999).

- Patients with idiographic pain and with breast cancer reported increased involvement in valued adult role activities after attending a psychoeducational program, more so than patients in the control group did (Braden et al., 1993; LeFort et al., 1998).

- The results of a secondary data analysis indicated that pregnant women who attended childbirth education classes had higher level of self-care agency than those who did not (Hart & Foster, 1998).

- The effects of patient education on self-care behaviors in patients with arthritis were inconsistent. Although Goeppinger, Macnee, Anderson, Boutaugh, & Stewart (1995) found a significant improvement in self-care behaviors performance, Albrecht et al. (1993) did not.

- Patients with stroke who were provided with guided decision-making showed increased performance of activities of daily living (e.g., walking) compared to those in the control group (Folden, 1993).

Several threats to the validity of the studies' conclusions were identified. Those commonly found across the studies were: (1) inadequate validation of the outcome measures, (2) possible low power to detect significant effects with a small sample size (i.e., small number of cases per group), and (3) possible experimenter expectancy bias since the outcome measurement was not blinded.

When only methodologically sound studies were reviewed (i.e., no or limited threats to validity), the results indicated that educational/psychoeducational interventions are effective in improving individuals' performance of self-care activities. This conclusion was supported by the results of meta-analyses. Psychoeducational interventions demonstrated the following effects:

- Strong positive effect on adherence to treatment (effect size = .78), use of PRN medications (effect size = .62), and psychomotor skills (i.e., use of inhaler, effect size = 1.02) in adults with asthma (Devine, 1996).

- Increased practice of desired behaviors (e.g., exercise, relaxation, and joint protection) in patients with arthritis. This favorable effect was reported in 77% to 91% of the studies reviewed by Hirano, Laurent, and Lorig (1994) and Lorig et al. (1987), respectively.

- Favorable influence on behavioral change related to smoking or alcohol, nutrition and weight control, and breast self-examination in the general population (Mullen et al., 1997).

- Low to moderate effect on self-care behaviors, operationalized in terms of loss of weight, in patients with diabetes of different age groups (Brown, 1992).

- Strong positive effect on medication compliance (effect size = .74) in patients with hypertension (Devine & Reifschneider, 1995).

- Moderate positive effect on self-care behaviors (effect size = .55) in patients with various conditions (McCain & Lynn, 1990).

The empirical evidence presented supports the conclusion that patient education provided by nurses with a focus on self-care is effective in improving performance of specific self-care behaviors, particularly those targeted by the educational intervention. Self-care can, in turn, yield favorable patient outcomes. Consequently, self-care is sensitive to nursing care, and is instrumental for achieving desired patient outcomes in different patient populations cared for across healthcare settings.

3.4 Instruments Measuring Self-Care

Self-care is represented by two concepts: self-care agency (i.e., the perceived ability of an individual to engage in self-care behaviors) and self-care behavior (i.e., the individual's practice or performance of self-care actions). Several instruments have been developed to measure each of these concepts. Tables 3.2 and 3.3 present information on the domains captured by the instruments measuring self-care agency and self-care behavior, respectively, and summarize the evidence supporting their reliability, validity, and sensitivity to change.

3.4.1 Measures of Self-Care Agency

Five instruments were used to measure the concept of self-care agency (see Table 3.2). They were all based on Orem's conceptualization of self-care. Since self-care agency refers to the person's capability or perceived ability to perform self-care behaviors, clients or patients themselves would be the best persons to judge or rate the self-care agency. This point implies that measures of this concept should be self-administered, which was the case for four of the instruments reviewed. The ASA Scale has two versions: one is self-administered and one is completed by a caregiver. The reported discrepancies between the patient's and the nurse's scores on this scale (Halfens et al., 1998) renders the nurse's assessment of the patient's self-care agency of limited clinical utility, and confines it to specific conditions in which the patient is unable to self-report.

Table 3.2. Instruments Measuring Self-Care Agency

Instrument (author)	Target population	Domains; number of items; response format	Method of administration	Reliability	Validity	Sensitivity to change and nursing care
Denyes Self-Care Agency Questionnaire (Denyes, 1980; as cited in Lantz et al., 1995)	Children and adolescents	Ability to meet universal self-care requisites; 34 items for adolescent's version, 25 for children's version; 5-point Likert-type.	Self-administered	ICR: split-half r of .80 to .83 in healthy children (Moore, 1995); α of .81 and .90 in healthy adolescents (Slusher, 1999). TRR: no data available.	Content: no data available. Construct: positive r with SC practice and with health status in children (Moore, 1995; Slusher, 1999).	Sensitivity to change: no data available. Sensitivity to nursing: no data available.
Exercise of Self-Care Agency Scale (Kearny & Fleischer, 1979)	Adults	Personal motivation, knowledge base and information seeking, active versus passive response to situations, self-concept or sense of self-worth; 43 items in original version, 35 in adapted version for patients with CABG (Carroll, 1995; Chen, 1999); 5-point Likert-type.	Self-administered	ICR: split-half r of .77 to .81 in healthy adults; α of .77 and .87 in healthy adults, elderly women, patients with hypertension, and patients recovering from CABG (Carroll, 1995; Chen, 1999; Kearny & Fleischer, 1979; Wang & Lee, 1999). TRR: r of .77 in healthy adolescents (Moore, 1995); .79 to .94 in chronically ill patients and healthy adults (Folden, 1993).	Content: established by five experts in SC. Factorial structure: four factors consistent with domains (Chen, 1999; Whetstone & Hansson, 1989). Construct: positive r with self-confidence in adolescents (Moore, 1995).	Sensitivity to change: change in scores observed following surgery (Folden, 1993). Sensitivity to nursing: change in scores observed following a supportive-educative intervention (Carroll, 1995).

Table 3.2 (continued)

Instrument (author)	Target population	Domains; number of items; response format	Method of administration	Reliability	Validity	Sensitivity to change and nursing care
Appraisal of Self-Care Agency Scale (ASA) (Evers et al., 1986 as cited in Hart & Foster, 1998).	Adults	Ability to perform the SC behaviors related to eight universal SC requisites; 24 items; 5-point Likert-type.	2 versions: one self-administered (ASA-A) and the other completed by the individuals' significant other or caregiver, such as nurse (ASA-B)	ICR: for ASA-A version, α of .76 to .77 for pregnant women (Hart, 1995; Hart & Foster, 1998); .80 to .87 for patients with cardiac disease (Jaarsma et al., 1999); .84 for adults awaiting renal transplant (Horsburgh et al., 2000); for the ASA-B version α of .77 to .87 for nurses (Soderhamn et al., 1996). TRR: r of .72 in elderly patients who underwent cardiac surgery (Aish, 1996). IRR: .64 to .71 for ASA-B version for nurses caring for patients (van Achterberg et al., 1991).	Content: considered relevant by Orem and eight experts in the theory of SC. Construct: positive r with performance of SC behaviors in pregnant women (Hart, 1995) and in cardiac patients (Jaarsma et al., 2000); convergence of the ASA-A and ASA-B scores. (van Achterberg et al., 1991).	Sensitivity to change: no change in scores following cardiac surgery (Jaarsma et al., 2000). Sensitivity to nursing: no data available.
Perception of Self-Care Agency Questionnaire (Hanson, 1981, as cited in Nelson McDermott, 1993)	Adults	Orem's 10 power components; 53 items; 5-point Likert-type.	Self-administered	ICR: α of .92 to .96 for healthy adults (Nelson McDermott, 1993). TRR: No data available.	Content: validated by a panel of experts. Factorial Structure: five factors; factorial invariance was not maintained (Nelson McDermott, 1993).	Sensitivity to change: no data available. Sensitivity to nursing: no data available.

Table 3.2 (continued)

Instrument (author)	Target population	Domains; number of items; response format	Method of administration	Reliability	Validity	Sensitivity to change and nursing care
Self-Care Agency Inventory (Lantz et al., 1995)	Adults	Person's SC knowledge and actions (enabling perceptual elements of motivation, responsibility, and decision making; enactment of self-care; and self-care factors); 40 items; multiple-choice.	Self-administered	ICR: α of .65 in patients and staff in family practice physician offices (Lantz et al., 1995). TRR: r of .83 for adults (Lantz et al., 1995).	Content: established by two panels of professionals with expertise in the area of SC (CVI .95). Construct: no clear evidence (Lantz et al., 1995).	Sensitivity to change: no data available. Sensitivity to nursing: no data available.

r = correlation coefficient

α = Cronbach's alpha coefficient

ICR = Internal Consistency Reliability

TRR = Test Re-test Reliability

IRR = Inter-Rater Reliability

SC = Self-Care

CABG = Coronary Artery Bypass Graft surgery

CVI = Content Validity Index

The capabilities captured in the scale varied across the instruments. The Denyes Self-Care Agency Questionnaire (Denyes, 1980, as cited in Lantz et al., 1995) and the ASA Scale measure the person's ability to perform self-care behaviors related to universal needs and demands. The other three scales capture the domains of self-care agency, including the cognitive, physical, emotional, and behavioral abilities needed to perform self-care behaviors. The operationalization of self-care agency in terms of the cognitive, physical, emotional, and behavioral elements is consistent with the conceptualization of self-care agency advanced earlier. It is encompassing because it is applicable to various situations and conditions of health and illness, as well as to the self-care behaviors to be performed.

Two instruments, the Perception of Self-Care Agency and the Self-Care Agency Inventory, were each discussed in one study (Hanson, 1981, as cited in Nelson McDermot, 1993; Lantz et al., 1995). The study was methodological in nature and aimed at assessing the instruments' psychometric properties. The Perception of Self-Care Agency demonstrated acceptable reliability and validity. The Self-Care Agency Inventory had high test-retest reliability but rather low internal consistency reliability; it had acceptable content and concurrent validity. These two measures are newly developed and require further testing before they can be recommended for practice.

The Denyes Self-Care Questionnaire was used in two studies, one involving children (Moore, 1995) and the other adolescents (Slusher, 1999). It demonstrated acceptable reliability and validity. However, the number of items comprising it, as described in Table 3.2, may require these populations to spend some effort and time to complete it.

The Exercise of Self-Care Agency was used in seven studies involving various client populations, including healthy adolescents, adults, and older adults, as well as patients with chronic illnesses. The reported results provide adequate evidence supporting its reliability and initial evidence for its validity and sensitivity to change. Its factorial structure seems to be consistent or invariant across samples of individuals residing in North America only (Chen, 1999); differences in factorial structure were reported for individuals residing in Northern Europe (Whetstone & Hanson, 1989). The shorter version, comprised of 35 items, requires a short time to complete.

The ASA Scale was used in 10 studies; it was self-administered in nine studies to healthy persons and to patients with chronic illnesses. The reported reliability coefficients tended to be slightly lower than those reported for the Exercise of Self-Care Agency Scale, but were still supportive of its consistency in measuring the concept. The evidence for its validity is contradictory. Although results provided adequate support for its content, convergent, and construct validity, some findings pointed to the possibility of response bias (i.e., acquiescence and social desirability) by patients (Halfens et al., 1998; Horsburgh et al., 2000). Its sensitivity to change was not demonstrated. Its short length (only 24 items) and its translated versions in four languages other than English render it useful in clinical settings serving persons with different cultural backgrounds.

The empirical evidence on the psychometric properties of self-care agency measures is rather limited. Consequently, it is difficult to make any recommendations about which are the most reliable, valid, sensitive to change, and clinically useful measures of self-care agency. All instruments need further testing.

3.4.2 Measures of Self-Care Behavior

A total of 32 instruments have been used to measure the concept of self-care behavior (see Table 3.3). The development of the instruments was guided, to various extents, by Orem's model of self-care. Some were designed to measure the universal self-care demands only, whereas others incorporated elements of developmental and/or health deviations demands in addition to universal demands (e.g., Denyes Self-Care Practice Instrument, Children Self-Care Performance Questionnaire). Other instruments did not accurately reflect the different self-care demands that Orem identified. They were rather heuristic, developed to capture the specific self-care behaviors that the target population was expected to perform. Vrijhoef, Diederiks, & Spreeuwenberg (2000) reached similar conclusions in the literature review they conducted to examine the contribution of advanced practice nurses on quality of care outcomes. Although they reported that implementation of this role component was associated with improved self-care, they found that validated instruments were not always used to assess self-care. Self-care was assessed in different ways, depending on the activities involved.

The literature reviewed and clinical experience suggest that the expected self-care behaviors vary across client populations and across healthcare settings. This variability accounts for the large number of pertinent instruments found. Investigators interested in assessing self-care behaviors in a particular situation seemed to have either (a) developed a new instrument to measure those self-care behaviors of primary concern in the study, as was the case for most of the studies reviewed (e.g., Dellasega & Clark, 1995; Harper, 1984) or (b) adapted previously developed instruments in an attempt to enhance the relevance of their content to the target population and setting involved in the study. The adaptation often consisted of generating additional items related to new/different behaviors expected of clients/patients, as illustrated by the work of Moore (1995), Gaffney and Moore (1996), and Moore and Mosher (1997). These authors adapted the original scale to measure self-care behaviors in various groups encompassing healthy children and adolescents and their parents, and children with cancer and their parents.

The variability in the self-care behaviors expected of various populations in different healthcare settings appears to be associated with variability in the operationalization of the concept. The following patterns were observed:

- Some researchers operationalized self-care behaviors as the performance

Table 3.3. Instruments Measuring Self-Care Behavior

Instrument (author)	Target population	Domains; number of items; response format	Method of administration	Reliability	Validity	Sensitivity to change and nursing care
Denyes Self-Care Practice Instrument (Denyes, 1980, as cited in Lantz et al., 1995)	Healthy adolescents	SC actions performed in meeting the universal SC requisites and general SC actions; 17 items; numeric rating scale.	Self-administered	ICR: α of .84 in adolescents (McCaleb & Edgil, 1994); .82 to .89 for healthy adolescents (McCaleb & Cull, 2000; Slusher, 1999). TRR: r of .84 in healthy adolescents (McCaleb & Edgil, 1994).	Content: established. Construct: positive r with SC agency in healthy adolescents (Slusher, 1999).	Sensitivity to change: no data available. Sensitivity to nursing: no data available.
Children and Adolescent Self-Care Practice Questionnaire (Moore, 1995)	Children 9–18 years old	Activities that children perform to meet their developmental and universal needs as identified (Orem, 1991); 35 items; 5-point Likert-type.	Self-administered	ICR: α of .83 in healthy children (Moore, 1995). TRR: no data available.	Content: rated as valid by a panel of seven experts. Factorial Structure: 10 factors representing the developmental and universal SC requisites. Construct: positive r with SC agency in children (Moore, 1995).	Sensitivity to change: no data available. Sensitivity to nursing: no data available.
Children Self-Care Performance Questionnaire (Moore, 1995; Moore & Mosher, 1997)	Children with cancer	Developmental, universal, and health-deviation SC requisites; 51 items; 5-point Likert-type.	Self-administered	ICR: α of .83 for children with cancer (Moore & Mosher, 1997). TRR: no data available.	Content: rated as valid by pediatric oncology nurses. Construct: performance of SC behaviors decreased with increasing age (Moore & Mosher, 1997).	Sensitivity to change: no data available. Sensitivity to nursing: no data available.

Table 3.3 (continued)

Instrument (author)	Target population	Domains; number of items; response format	Method of administration	Reliability	Validity	Sensitivity to change and nursing care
Dependent Care Agent Performance Questionnaire (Moore & Gaffney, 1989)	Caregivers of children, primarily mothers (parents of children with cancer and parents of healthy children).	SC activities directed toward meeting children's universal, development, and health-deviation needs; 39 items in healthy version, and 55 in children with cancer version; 5-point Likert-type.	Self-administered	ICR: α of .99 for healthy caregivers (Gaffney & Moore, 1996); .91 to .93 for mothers of children with cancer (Moore & Mosher, 1997). TRR: no data available.	Content: established by panels of experts. Construct: for healthy version: low r with social desirability; negative r with desirability; negative r with child's age (Gaffney & Moore, 1996). For children with cancer version: positive r with children's performance of SC activity (Moore & Mosher, 1997).	Sensitivity to change: no data available. Sensitivity to nursing: no data available.
Personal Life Style Questionnaire (Muhlenkamp & Brown, 1983, as cited in Nicholas, 1993)	Healthy older adults	Engagement in health promotion or SC activities; 24 items; 4-point rating scale.	Self-administered	ICR: α of .74 to .76 for healthy adults (Nicholas, 1993). TRR: r of .78 and .88 (Nicholas, 1993).	Content: no data available. Construct: positive r with perceived health status in healthy older adults (Nicholas, 1993).	Sensitivity to change: no data available. Sensitivity to nursing: no data available.
Self-Care Behaviors Inventory (Goeppinger et al., 1995)	Patients with arthritis	Performance of 16 SC activities; 16 items; report number of times each activity was performed in the last 7 days.	Self-administered	ICR: α of .75 for patients with arthritis (Goeppinger et al., 1995). TRR: no data available.	Content: no data available. Construct: no data available.	Sensitivity to change and to nursing: significant increase observed following a psychoeducational intervention.

Table 3.3 (continued)

Instrument (author)	Target population	Domains; number of items; response format	Method of administration	Reliability	Validity	Sensitivity to change and nursing care
Self-Care Diary (Nail et al., 1991)	Patients with cancer receiving chemotherapy	Incidence and severity of side effects experienced by patient receiving chemotherapy, and use and perceived effectiveness of SC activities to manage the side effects (Craddock et al., 1999; Nail et al., 1991); 18 items; 6-point rating scale to indicate use and effectiveness of SC activities.	Self-administered	ICR: Not applicable. TRR: r of .80 in patients with cancer receiving chemotherapy (Nail et al., 1991).	Content: reviewed by patients, oncology clinical nurse specialists, and physicians (Craddock et al., 1999; Nail et al., 1991). Construct: positive r between use of SC activities and SC agency in patients with breast cancer (Craddock et al., 1999).	Sensitivity to change: no data available. Sensitivity to nursing: no data available.
Hart Prenatal Care Actions Scale (Hart, 1995)	Pregnant women	Areas of prenatal health activities (health supervision, nutrition maintenance, balancing activity and rest, maintenance of social interaction, abstinence from hazards, and knowledge acquisition); 41 items; 5-point Likert-type.	Self-administered	ICR: α of .80 (Hart, 1995). TRR: no data available.	Content: established by SC theory experts, childbirth educators, nurses, and pregnant women. Factorial structure: 8 factors. Construct: positive r with SC agency (Hart, 1995).	Sensitivity to change: no data available. Sensitivity to nursing: no data available.

Table 3.3 (continued)

Instrument (author)	Target population	Domains; number of items; response format	Method of administration	Reliability	Validity	Sensitivity to change and nursing care
Inventory of Adult Role Behaviors (Braden, 1990a, 1990b)	Adults	Ability to perform adult role responsibilities (e.g., involvement in family roles, leisure and recreation, household duties, and SC activities); 16 items; VAS.	Self-administered	ICR: α > .80 in patients with arthritis, breast cancer, and chronic pain (Braden, 1990a; 1990b; Braden et al., 1993; LeFort, 2000). TRR: no data available.	Content: reviewed by experts in the field of SC (Braden, 1990a). Construct: *r* with theoretically relevant concepts (e.g., disability, sense of well-being, and affect) (Braden, 1990a, 1990b; LeFort, 2000; Sidani, 1994).	Sensitivity to change and to nursing: increase in scores following a psychoeducational intervention in patients with breast cancer (Sidani, 1994) and in patients with pain (LeFort, 2000).
Items (unnamed) developed to measure SC behavior (Jopp et al., 1993)	Older adults after rehabilitation	Performance of ADLs; one item; 3-point rating scale.	Not clear	ICR: not applicable. TRR: no data available.	Content: no data available. Construct: no data available.	Sensitivity to change: no data available. Sensitivity to nursing: no data available.
Jenkins Activity Checklist (Jenkins, 1985, as cited in Carroll, 1995)	Adults	Five categories of ADLs representing SC behaviors (i.e., walking, climbing stairs, roles, and relationships); 51 items; three response options (No, Yes, Not applicable).	Self-administered	ICR: α of .53 to .92 for the five subscales, in elderly patients recovering from CABG (Carroll, 1995). TRR: no data available.	Content: no data available. Construct: no data available.	Sensitivity to change: scores increased following cardiac surgery (Carroll, 1995). Sensitivity to nursing: no data available.

Table 3.3 (continued)

Instrument (author)	Target population	Domains; number of items; response format	Method of administration	Reliability	Validity	Sensitivity to change and nursing care
Self-Care Behavior Inventory (Albrecht et al., 1993)	Patients with arthritis	No domain specified; 17 items; no clearly defined response format.	Self-administered	ICR: α of .75 in patients with arthritis (Albrecht et al., 1993) TRR: no data available.	Content: no data available. Construct: no data available.	Sensitivity to change: no data available. Sensitivity to nursing: no data available.
Universal Self-Care Inventory (Gazda, 1986, as cited in Horsburgh et al., 2000)	Adults	SC behaviors undertaken in response to universal self-care requisites; 10 items; 6-point Likert-type.	Self-administered	ICR: α of .78 to .88 in various patient populations (Horsburgh et al., 2000; Horsburgh, 1999). TRR: no data available.	Content: reported to be supported. Construct: reported to be supported.	Sensitivity to change: no data available. Sensitivity to nursing: no data available.
Heart Failure Self-Care Behavior Scale (Jaarsma et al., 1999)	Patients with heart failure	SC activities that are essential parts of the therapeutic regimen, to be performed (e.g., managing dyspnea and restricting sodium intake); 19 items; Yes-No response format.	Self-administered	ICR: α of .62 to .68 in patients with heart failure (Jaarsma et al., 1999; 2000). TRR: No data available.	Content: established by a panel of experts in cardiac care (Jaarsma et al., 1999). Construct: No data available.	Sensitivity to change: no data available. Sensitivity to nursing: increase in scores in patients with heart failure following an educational intervention (Jaarsma et al., 1999, 2000).
Items (unnamed) developed to measure SC behavior (Ni et al., 1999)	Patients with heart failure	Adherence to therapeutic regimen (e.g., medication, sodium intake, and weight monitoring); 8 items; response reflected frequency of peformance of SC behaviors.	Self-administered	ICR: not applicable. TRR: no data available.	Content: no data available. Construct: positive *r* with knowledge of therapeutic regimen (Ni et al., 1999).	Sensitivity to change: no data available. Sensitivity to nursing: no data available.

Table 3.3 (continued)

Instrument (author)	Target population	Domains; number of items; response format	Method of administration	Reliability	Validity	Sensitivity to change and nursing care
Self-Care Behavioral Rating Scale (Harper, 1984)	Patients with hypertension	SC behaviors related to safe self-medication; 12 items; 5-point rating scale.	Administered by trained observers	ICR: inter-item r of .73 to .74 for the subscales in patients with hypertension (Harper, 1984). TRR: r of .94 in patients with hypertension (Harper, 1984). IRR: ICC of .88 to 1.00 (Harper, 1984).	Content: established by expert nurses. Construct: no data available.	Sensitivity to change and to nursing: increase in scores observed in patients with hypertension, following an educational intervention (Harper, 1984).
Self-Care Burden Scale (Oberst et al., 1991)	Adults	Illness and universal SC demands and behaviors; 16 items; 5-point rating scale.	Self-administered	ICR: α of .79 to .90 in various patient populations. TRR: no data available.	Content: reported to be established. Construct: Reported to be established.	Sensitivity to change: no data available. Sensitivity to nursing: no data available.
Self-Care Assessment Tool (SCAT) (Boss et al., 1996)	Patients with spinal cord injury	Eight areas of SC (bathing, nutritional management, medications, mobility, skin management, bladder and bowel management, and dressing); 8 items; Yes-No response format.	Administered by a nurse observer	ICR: no data available. TRR: r of .06 to .86 (Boss et al., 1996). IRR: agreement 94%–100%; r of .69–.94 (Boss et al., 1996).	Content: validated by a panel of 10 clinical nurse specialists (CVI .90) (Boss et al., 1996). Construct: discharge scores accounted for 82% of the variance in scores obtained at six months post discharge (Boss et al., 1996).	Sensitivity to change: no data available. Sensitivity to nursing: no data available.

Table 3.3 (continued)

Instrument (author)	Target population	Domains; number of items; response format	Method of administration	Reliability	Validity	Sensitivity to change and nursing care
Strategies Used by Patients to Promote Health (Lev & Owen, 1996)	Adults	Self-confidence to perform strategies to promote health; 29 items; 5-point scale.	Self-administered	ICR: α of .94–.96 in patients with renal failure on hemodialysis (Lev & Owen, 1998). TRR: no data available.	Content: no data available. Factorial structure: four factors (Lev & Owen, 1996). Construct: no data available.	Sensitivity to change: increase in the scores was observed over time (Lev & Owen, 1998). Sensitivity to nursing: no data available.
High Intensity Self-Care Needs and Interventions Survey (Robinson & Posner, 1992)	Patients with cancer receiving biologic response modifier therapy	SC interventions performed to manage the side effects of biologic response modifier therapy; unknown number of items; open-ended questions.	May be self-administered or administered by health care providers	ICR: not applicable. TRR: not applicable.	Content: no data available. Construct: no data available.	Sensitivity to change: no data available. Sensitivity to nursing: no data available.
Self-Care Behavior Log (Dodd, 1982b)	Patients with cancer receiving chemotherapy	Initiation of SC behaviors and perception of the effectiveness of the behaviors used to manage the side effects of chemotherapy; no pre-set number of items: patients asked to identify symptoms and strategies used to manage each symptom; 5-point rating scale to rate effectiveness of SC behaviors.	Self-administered	ICR: not applicable. TRR: reported to be established.	Content: established by two groups of oncologists and four nurse clinical oncology specialists (Dodd, 1982). Construct: no data available.	Sensitivity to change and to nursing: increase in scores following an educational intervention (Dodd, 1983).

95

Table 3.3 (continued)

Instrument (author)	Target population	Domains; number of items; response format	Method of administration	Reliability	Validity	Sensitivity to change and nursing care
Self-Care Rating Scale (Williams et al., 1988)	Post-surgical patients who underwent either mastectomy or hysterectomy	Performance of SC behaviors to be carried out by patients at home following mastectomy or hysterectomy; 20 items for the mastectomy version and 12 items for the hysterectomy version; 4-point rating scale.	Either self-administerd or administered by the nurse	ICR: not applicable. TRR: no data available.	Content: two versions developed in consultation with physicians and nurses. Construct: no data available.	Sensitivity to change and to nursing: increase in scores following an educational intervention Williams et al., 1988).
Self-Care Behavior Questionnaire (Hanucharurnkul, 1989)	Patients with cancer	SC performed by patients with cancer receiving radiation therapy; 41 items; 5-point Likert-type.	Self-administered	ICR: α of .87 in patients with head/neck cancer; .86 in patients with cervical cancer. TRR: r of .90.	Content: judged as valid by two groups of experts. Construct: positive r with life satisfaction ($r = .63$) in patients with cancer (Hanucharurnkul, 1989).	Sensitivity to change: no data available. Sensitivity to nursing: no data available.
Self-Care Assessment Tool (Johannsen, 1992)	Cardiac patients	Ability to seek medical assistance, attend to the effects of the illness, carry out the therapeutic regimen, regulate the deleterious effects of the therapeutic regimen, live with the illness, and modify self-concept (for each domain, the tool assesses the patient's knowledge base, decision, and action); 86 items; checklist format.	Administered by the nurse	ICR: no data available. TRR: no data available.	Content: domains reflective of Orem's six health-deviation self-care requisites. Construct: no data available.	Sensitivity to change: no data available. Sensitivity to nursing: no data available.

Table 3.3 (continued)

Instrument (author)	Target population	Domains; number of items; response format	Method of administration	Reliability	Validity	Sensitivity to change and nursing care
Self-Care Assessment Tool (SCAT) (McFarland et al., 1992)	Patients with spinal cord injury	Two domains of SC: cognitive skills (e.g., selecting appropriate action) and functional skills (e.g., bathing, nutritional management, taking medications, mobility); 81 items; three response options (No, Yes, and Not Applicable).	Administered by the nurse	ICR: no data available. TRR: r of .47 to .80 for the cognitive subscale; –.06 to .86 for the functional subscale; and .45 to .69 for the total scale (McFarland et al., 1992). IRR: r of .69 to .94 for the cognitive subscale; .74 to .92 for the functional subscale; and .74 to .94 for the total scale.	Content: reviewed by a panel of 10 clinical nurse specialists in spinal cord injury or neuroscience nursing (McFarland et al., 1992). Construct: predictive reported to be supported (.61 for cognitive subscale, .90 for functional subscale, and .82 for total scale) (McFarland et al., 1992).	Sensitivity to change: no data available. Sensitivity to nursing: no data available.
Measure (unnamed) developed by (Lenihan, 1988)	Elderly residents living in non-institutional settings in the community	Universal SC demands, health deviation SC demands, and medically derived self-care demands; 123 items; response format unclear.	No data available	ICR: no data available. TRR: no data available.	Content: developed in consultation with experts in the areas of gerontology and geriatrics, health promotion, and self-care. Construct: no data available.	Sensitivity to change: no data available. Sensitivity to nursing: no data available.
Health Behavior Scale (Miller et al., 1982)	Adults with cardiac disease	Performance of recommended SC behaviors (e.g., diet, medication and exercise, smoking cessation, and stress management); 20 items; 5-point Likert-type.	Self-administered	ICR: α of .82 and .95. TRR: no data available.	Content: no data available. Construct: no data available.	Sensitivity to change: no data available. Sensitivity to nursing: no data available.

Table 3.3 (continued)

Instrument (author)	Target population	Domains; number of items; response format	Method of administration	Reliability	Validity	Sensitivity to change and nursing care
Self-Care of Older Persons Evaluation (SCOPE) (Dellasega & Clark, 1995)	Older adults in rehabilitation	Universal SC domains (e.g., food, elimination processes, activity and rest, bathing, prevention of hazards, and social interaction); 13 items; 6-point Likert-type.	Administered by observer/health care provider	ICR: α of .89 in patients with rehabilitation needs. TRR: no data available. IRR: complete agreement was accomplished during the training session (Dellasega & Clark, 1995).	Content: established by a panel of 30 experts. Factorial structure: three factors. Construct: no data available.	Sensitivity to change: no data available. Sensitivity to nursing: no data available.
Interstitial Cystitis-Self-Care Responses (Webster & Brennan, 1998)	Women with interstitial cystitis	SC related to universal, developmental, and health deviations demands (e.g., hygiene, diet, and use of medications); about 300 items; rating scale from 0 to 3 (to rate frequency of using and effectiveness of SC strategies).	Self-administered	ICR: no data available. TRR: no data available.	Content: developed based on the responses of women with interstitial cystitis to open-ended questions. Construct: positive r with adjustment to the illness (Webster & Brennan, 1998).	Sensitivity to change: no data available. Sensitivity to nursing: no data available.
Epilepsy Self-Management Scale (DiIorio & Henry, 1995)	Patients with epilepsy	Performance of tasks that are helpful in managing seizures (e.g., medication, self-monitoring, stress management, hypnosis, and biofeedback); 26 items; 5-point scale.	Self-administered	ICR: α of .81 to .86 in persons with epilepsy (DiIorio & Henry, 1995). TRR: No data.	Content: derived from the literature; CVI 93%. Construct: no data available.	Sensitivity to change: no data available. Sensitivity to nursing: no data available.

Table 3.3 (continued)

Instrument (author)	Target population	Domains; number of items; response format	Method of administration	Reliability	Validity	Sensitivity to change and nursing care
Therapeutic Self-Care (Sidani & Irvine, 1999)	Adult patients in acute care settings	Taking medications, recognizing and managing symptoms, carrying out ADLs, and managing changes in health condition; 13 items; 5-point numeric rating scale.	Self-administered	ICR: α of .62 to .85 for the subscales; .89 for total scale in patients admitted to cardiac and general medical and surgical units (Sidani & Irvine, 1999; Sidani et al., 2002). TRR: No data available.	Content: maintained by generating items based on literature review. Factorial structure: four factors, as hypothesized. Construct: negative r with age, affect, number of symptoms experienced; positive r with functional status and perceived health (Sidani & Irvine, 1999; Sidani et al., 2002).	Sensitivity to change: no data available. Sensitivity to nursing: correlated with patient education given by nurses in the hospital (Sidani & Irvine, 1999).
Health Promoting Lifestyle Profile (Walker, Sechrist & Pender, 1995, as cited in Acton & Malathum, 2000)	Adults	Actions that maintain or enhance wellness (e.g., physical activity, nutrition, interpersonal relations, stress management); 52 items; 4-point rating scale.	Self-administered	ICR: α of .83 to .90 for the subscales; .90 for total scale (Acton & Malathum, 2000). TRR: no data available.	Content: no data available. Construct: no data available.	Sensitivity to change: no data available. Sensitivity to nursing: no data available.

r = correlation coefficient
α = Cronbach's alpha coefficient
ICR = Internal Consistency Reliability
TRR = Test Re-test Reliability
IRR = Inter-Rater Reliability
SC = Self-Care
CABG = Coronary Artery Bypass Graft surgery

CVI = Content Validity Index
VAS = Visual Analogue Scale
ICC = Intra-Class Correlation Coefficient

of usual activities, that is, activities of daily living, instrumental activities of daily living, and adult role behaviors such as involvement in family, recreational, social, and work-related activities. These activities were measured with various instruments, including the following: items developed by Jopp et al. (1993); the Jenkins Activity Checklist used by Carroll (1995); and the Inventory of Adult Behavior developed by Braden (1990b) and used by LeFort (2000). The activities were investigated in community-dwelling adults with chronic illnesses who were recovering from an acute episode or who required long-term management.

• Some investigators operationalized self-care behaviors in terms of activities performed to meet universal self-care demands. These demands encompassed (a) air, food, and water; (b) elimination processes (bladder and bowel); (c) activity and rest; (d) normalcy (i.e., bathing and grooming); (e) prevention of hazards; and (f) solitude and social interactions. The scales used to measure these behaviors were (a) the Denyes Self-Care Practice Instrument used by McCaleb and Edgil (1994), Slusher (1999), and McCaleb and Cull (2000); (b) the Children and Adolescent Self-Care Practice Questionnaire and the Dependent Care Agent Questionnaire used by Moore (1995) and Gaffney and Moore (1996); (c) the Universal Self-Care Inventory used by Horsburgh (1999) and Horsburgh et al. (2000); and (d) the Self-Care of Older Persons Evaluation developed by Dellasega and Clark (1995). These instruments have been used in studies involving healthy adolescents and their parents, healthy children, elderly patients with rehabilitation needs, and patients with end-stage renal disease who were on dialysis, respectively.

• Other investigators operationalized self-care behaviors in terms of engagement in health-promotion activities such as nutrition, exercise, and relaxation. The instruments used in these situations were (a) the Personal Lifestyle Questionnaire used by Nicholas (1993) with healthy older adults; (b) the Hart Prenatal Care Actions Scale used by Hart (1995) with pregnant women; and (c) Strategies Used by Patients to Promote Health used by Lev and Owen (1996) with patients with renal failure who were on hemodialysis. All client/patient populations were community-dwelling adults.

• Most investigators operationalized self-care as the performance of activities aimed at maintaining health and managing the presenting problem(s) related to illness. That is, the measures included various combinations of (a) health maintenance activities such as exercising, nutrition, sleep, and relaxation; (b) activities associated with implementation of the prescribed therapeutic regimen (e.g., taking medications, adhering to dietary or fluid restriction recommendations, skin management, and appointment keeping); and (c) strategies, whether self-initiated or suggested by health care providers, for recognizing and monitoring symptoms or alterations in body functions and for relieving the symptoms.

Most instruments reviewed could be classified in this last category. They have been used with patients with chronic illnesses, such as patients with cancer who are receiving therapy; patients with arthritis, cardiac diseases, and hypertension; patients with injuries requiring long-term rehabilitation (i.e., spinal cord injury); and patients with acute conditions (i.e., admitted for acute medical problems or for surgery). Measurement of self-care behaviors took place in a few instances when the patient was institutionalized, but was conducted primarily after discharge or on an outpatient basis (either in a clinic or at home).

The specific self-care behaviors for managing the presenting problem that were measured varied across populations. For instance, those measured for patients with cancer receiving adjuvant therapy related to using strategies for managing the symptoms or side effects of cancer treatment that patients commonly experience (e.g., Dodd et al., 1991; Nail et al., 1991). The self-care behaviors focused on diet modification, weight reduction, exercise, smoking cessation, and stress management for patients with cardiac disease (e.g., Jaarsma et al., 1999; Ni et al., 1999; Rodeman et al., 1995). For patients with hypertension, the self-care behaviors measured related to taking medications as prescribed and communicating concerns about medications to health care providers (Harper, 1984). The relevant self-care behaviors for patients with arthritis concerned exercise, saving energy, rest, medication taking, and using community resources. For patients with acute conditions, the self-care behaviors related to medication taking, recognizing and managing symptoms or changes in condition, and following prescribed instructions (like post-surgery exercises). Through qualitative interviews with patients and nurses, van Agthoven and Plomp (1989) identified two categories of self-care activities required by patients receiving home health care. The first included practical or physical self-care activities related to (a) general care (like washing, dressing, eating/drinking, and bladder/bowel management); (b) nursing activities associated with therapeutic regimen (e.g., injections); (c) mobility and exercises (e.g., walking, getting in/out of bed); and (d) household duties. The second category referred to psychosocial self-care activities related to accepting illness and managing psychological, family, and/or marital problems.

The observed pattern underscores the importance of assessing self-care behaviors comprehensively but differently, based on the target population. To be consistent with the conceptualization of self-care behaviors presented in the theoretical background section of this review, nurses should address the following domains of self-care behaviors: health promotion/maintenance, recognizing and monitoring changes in functioning, selecting and applying appropriate strategies for managing these changes, and coping with/adjusting to long-term changes. The domains to be assessed could vary with the patient population. For instance, the assessment of self-care behaviors could be confined to those reflective of health promotion/maintenance for healthy persons. All these domains could be assessed in patients presenting with an illness, whether chronic or acute. Although none of the reviewed instruments adequately reflect all these domains, those classified under category four (i.e., those measuring health maintenance and managing the presenting problems) seem to fit for ill individuals. For example, the Therapeutic Self-Care Scale focuses on activities associated with monitoring symptoms and changes in body function, managing these symptoms, and implementing the prescribed therapeutic regimen. The items' content is stated in general terms. It is relevant to patients admitted to various clinical areas, and seems appropriate for assessing self-care behaviors in patients with acute and chronic conditions. It demonstrated acceptable validity and sensitivity to nursing care. Specifically, it was correlated with the receipt of education that nurses provided in the hospital (Sidani & Irvine, 1999; Sidani et al., 2002). Therefore, the Therapeutic Self-Care Scale is a promising measure of this instrumental outcome.

The reviewed instruments have been used in a rather small number of studies. Dodd's Self-Care Behavior Log, Nail and colleagues' Self-Care Diary, the Denyes Self-Care Practice instrument, and the Therapeutic Self-Care Scale were used in more than two studies. Each of the other measures has been either developed and tested in one study, or has been used in one study included in the review, as Vrijhoef et al. (2000) also explained. This state of affairs precludes accumulating sound and adequate evidence to support their psychometric properties. Nonetheless, the available results indicate that all instruments are consistent in measuring self-care behaviors, with minimal error. The reliability coefficients, which were lower than the criterion of .70 value, do not detract from the measures' internal consistency and stability over time. This is because the observed low values of the Cronbach's alpha coefficients could be explained with minimal variability in the scores, which is anticipated in homogenous groups, and with the nature of the responses, in which the performance of one specific self-care behavior does not necessarily imply performance of another. The observed low values of the test-retest correlation coefficients could be explained by the changes in self-care behavior performance over time and, therefore, could be indicative of the instruments' sensitivity to change.

The content validity for most instruments was established, as reported by the tool developers or by investigators who used the measure. However, the evidence supporting the construct validity of the measures is limited. Similarly, few instruments demonstrated changes in their respective scores, which provides initial evidence of their sensitivity to change.

This review indicates that the 32 instruments seem promising in assessing different domains of self-care behaviors expected of various client/patient populations. They require further testing to establish their reliability, validity, and sensitivity to change.

3.5   Issues in the Measurement of Self-Care

This review of the literature on self-care raised some issues about measurement of self-care as an outcome that is sensitive to nursing care. The first issue relates to the content of self-care instruments, and more specifically to whether to use global or specific measures of self-care. Global measures capture domains and behaviors of self-care that are relevant to various client populations seen in various practice settings. This general applicability makes global measures standard criteria that are useful for evaluating nursing care. Specific measures, in contrast, are adapted to particular clients or conditions. They tend to be responsive to particular interventions and sensitive to the context and condition of the particular clients receiving the interventions. Using specific measures, however, limits the ability to compare the effectiveness of different interventions delivered to address the same problem in different client populations (Guyatt et al., 1993). Therefore, a combination of global and specific measures is most effective for conducting a comprehensive assessment of self-care (Sidani & Braden, 1998). Except for the Therapeutic Self-Care Scale, the instruments reviewed previously were categorized as specific measures of self-care because they captured different domains and specific behaviors that were of interest and relevant to the particular situation, target population, and intervention of interest. Developing a global measure is necessary, but it requires clarifying domains and behaviors expected of different client populations seen across the healthcare continuum.

The second issue concerns the operationalization of self-care. The more specific questions are whether to measure self-care agency or self-care behavior, and under what condition to measure each. Self-care agency and behavior, although viewed as distinct concepts, are interrelated. Although assessing both concepts is highly recommended, administering relevant measures may increase response burden, especially in acutely ill and frail elderly clients. The selection of either as an outcome of nursing care and interventions should be guided by an understanding of the components comprising nursing practice in various settings, and by the theory underlying the interventions (Sidani & Braden, 1998). It may be meaningful to assess the clients' perceived ability to engage in self-care behaviors when institutionalized, and their actual performance of these behaviors in outpatient settings. Institutionalization, especially in acute-care settings, may preclude clients from initiating and/or actively undertaking some self-care actions, such as taking medications as prescribed. Furthermore, most nursing interventions are delivered to enhance the clients' ability for self-care. After discharge, clients are expected to assume the responsibility of taking care of themselves; it is therefore logical to inquire about their actual performance of self-care behaviors.

The third issue relates to the method of assessing self-care. Self-care agency, as the person's capability or perceived ability to perform self-care behaviors, is a subjective phenomenon. Consequently, clients themselves would be the best persons to judge or rate self-care agency. This observation implies that measures of this concept should be self-administered, as was the case for the instruments reviewed earlier. When clients are not able to self-report (e.g., children), a caregiver or health care professional may be needed to assess self-care agency. The results of such assessments should be viewed with caution, due to reported discrepancies between the clients' and others' perceptions. Self-care behavior refers to a person's practice or performance of self-care actions. Although clients can report about engaging in these behaviors, the accuracy of their responses may be questionable in light of response bias (Horsburgh, 1999). Having the clients' significant others report on the clients' performance of self-care behaviors provides another source of information to validate the clients' self-report. This strategy is recommended to enhance validity of outcome measurement. However, no instrument that measures self-care behavior and that is completed by the adult clients' significant other was found.

3.6 Conclusions and Recommendations for Practice and Research

Self-care is an instrumental outcome that is consistent with nursing and is sensitive to nursing interventions and care. The main points of this chapter are summarized as follows:

- Self-care is operationalized as the clients' perceived ability and actual practice of behaviors aimed at promoting and maintaining health, preventing disease, and managing or treating illness or changes in body function.

- Self-care is a critical concept in the current healthcare system, where much of the required treatment and care is provided in outpatient settings. Self-care enables patients, particularly those with chronic illnesses, to observe themselves, recognize symptoms or changes in functioning, and choose and implement appropriate strategies for managing these changes or symptoms.

- The performance of self-care behaviors is influenced by cognitive, psychological, physical, demographic, and sociocultural factors. Engagement in self-care is considered beneficial to the patient and the healthcare system. Self-care is believed to reduce the risk of complications; to enhance adjustment to illness, symptom control, and functioning; and, consequently, to improve quality of life and reduce health services utilization.

- Self-care formed the framework guiding the design of educational and psychoeducational nursing interventions for various client populations. These interventions focused on teaching individuals self-care-related knowledge and on instructing them in the skills necessary to perform self-care. Although the actual performance of self-care behaviors was not measured as an outcome expected of these interventions, educational or psychoeducational interventions were effective in improving the participants' self-care-related knowledge and their physical and psychological functioning, and in reducing health services utilization. The evidence supporting the beneficial effects of these interventions was obtained from rigorous primary studies and from several meta-analytic studies.

- The evidence reviewed provides support for the benefits of nursing educational or psychoeducational interventions in enhancing engagement in or enactment of self-care behaviors. Self-care is considered an outcome that is sensitive to nursing care and that is instrumental for achieving other patient outcomes, such as symptom control, improved functioning, and sense of well-being.

- Self-care is relevant to clients seen across the healthcare continuum (i.e., primary, acute, home, rehabilitation, and long-term care). However, the expected self-care behaviors vary across client populations and health care settings. This variability in the expected self-care behaviors accounts for the large number of pertinent measures found and poses some challenges in its clinical assessment.

- A large number of instruments that measured self-care behaviors was found. Most assess a combination of health maintenance activities and activities associated with implementing the therapeutic regimen or with strategies for recognizing, monitoring, and managing symptoms. They captured various domains and behaviors of self-care that are relevant to different client populations in different practice settings. The instruments demonstrated acceptable reliability; however, the evidence supporting their validity is limited.

These points lead to three main recommendations. First, the measurement of self-care should be further refined. Generic measures of self-care that are relevant and applicable to different client populations are needed. Generic measures are useful for evaluating the impact of nursing care in general, for comparing the effectiveness of different nursing interventions, and for developing a database. Such generic measures should be complemented with specific ones so that comprehensive assessments of self-care can be conducted for clients seen across healthcare settings. Refinement of self-care measures is a prerequisite for investigating the outcome's sensitivity to nursing care. The second recommendation concerns the cognitive, physical, demographic, and sociocultural factors that influence perceived ability and the performance of self-care. These factors should be taken into consideration when researchers or health care professionals design interventions aimed at promoting self-care, and when they evaluate the effects of nursing care on this outcome. Finally, additional studies that evaluate the impact of nursing input and care on self-care are needed to strengthen the empirical evidence supporting the sensitivity of self-care to nursing, as well as the benefits of promoting self-care for patients.

References

Acton, G. J., & Malathum, P. (2000). Basic need status and health-promoting self-care behavior in adults. *Western Journal of Nursing Research, 22,* 796–811.

Aish, A. (1996). A comparison of female and male cardiac patients' responses to nursing care promoting nutritional self-care. *Canadian Journal of Cardiovascular Nursing, 7*(3), 4–13.

Albrecht, M., Goeppinger, J., Anderson, M. K., Boutaugh, M., Macnee, C., & Stewart, K. (1993). The Albrecht nursing model for home healthcare: Predictors of satisfaction with a self-care intervention program. *Journal of Nursing Administration,* (1), 51–54.

Anastasio, C., McMahan, T., Daniels, A., Nicholas, P. K., & Paul-Simon, A. (1995). Self-care burden in women with human immunodeficiency virus. *Journal of the Association of Nurses in AIDS Care, 6*(3), 31–42.

Anderson, J. (1990). Home care management in chronic illness and the self-care movement. *Advances in Nursing Science, 12,* 71–83.

Backman, K., & Hentinen, M. (1999). Model for the self-care of home-dwelling elderly. *Journal of Advanced Nursing, 30,* 564–572.

Badzek, L., Hines, S. C., & Moss, A. H. (1998). Inadequate self-care knowledge among elderly hemodialysis patients: Assessing its prevalence and potential causes. *ANNA Journal, 25,* 293–300.

Baker, C. (1999). From chaos to order: A nursing-based psycho-education program for parents of children with attention-deficit hyperactivity disorder. *Canadian Journal of Nursing Research, 31*(2), 71–75.

Barnason, S., & Zimmerman, L. (1995). A comparison of patient teaching outcomes among postoperative coronary artery bypass graft (CABG) patients. *Progress in Cardiovascular Nursing, 10*(4), 11–20.

Barroso, J. (1995). Self-care activities of long-term survivors of acquired immunodeficiency syndrome. *Holistic Nursing Practice, 10*(1), 44–53.

Bennett, J. G. (1980). Symposium on the self-care concept of nursing. Foreword. *Nursing Clinics of North America, 15*(1), 129–130.

Blair, C. E. (1995). Combining behavior management and mutual goal setting to reduce physical dependency in nursing home residents. *Nursing Research, 44,* 160–165.

Blair, C. E. (1999). Effect of self-care ADLs on self-esteem of intact nursing home residents. *Issues in Mental Health Nursing, 20,* 559–570.

Blair, C. E., Lewis, R., Wieweg, V., & Tucker, R. (1996). Group and single-subject evaluation of a programme to promote self-care in elderly nursing home residents. *Journal of Advanced Nursing, 24,* 1207–1213.

Boehm, S., Schlenk, E. A., Raleigh, E., & Ronis, D. (1993). Behavioral analysis and behavioral strategies to improve self-management of type II diabetes. *Clinical Nursing Research, 2*, 327–344.

Boss, B. J., Barlow, D., McFarland, S. M., & Sasser, L. (1996). A self-care assessment tool (SCAT) for persons with a spinal cord injury: An expanded abstract. *Axon, 17*, 66–67.

Braden, C. J. (1990a). Learned self-help response to chronic illness experience: A test of three alternative learning theories. *Scholarly Inquiry for Nursing Practice, 1*(1), 23–41.

Braden, C. J. (1990b). A test of the self-help model: Learned response to chronic illness experience. *Nursing Research, 39*, 42–47.

Braden, C. J. (1993). Research program on learned response to chronic illness experience: Self-help model. *Holistic Nursing Practice, 8*(1), 38–44.

Braden, C. J., Mishel, M. H., Longman, A., & Burns, L. R. (1993). Nurse interventions promoting self-help response to breast cancer (Grant No. NCI 1R01 CA48450-01 A1). Washington, DC: National Cancer Institute.

Brown, S. A. (1992). Meta-analysis of diabetes patient education research: Variations in intervention effects across studies. *Research in Nursing & Health, 15*, 409–419.

Burks, K. J. (1999). A nursing practice model for chronic illness. *Rehabilitation Nursing, 24*, 197–200.

Carroll, D. L. (1995). The importance of self-efficacy expectations in elderly patients recovering from coronary artery bypass surgery. *Heart & Lung, 24*, 50–59.

Chang, B. L., Uman, G. C., & Hirsch, M. (1998). Predictive power of clinical indicators for self-care deficit. *Nursing Diagnosis, 9*(2), 71–82.

Chen, Y. M. (1999). Relationships among health locus of control, self-efficacy, and self-care of the elderly with hypertension. *Nursing Research, 7*, 504–516.

Classon, B. L., Mattingly, L. J., Finne, K. M., & Larson, J. A. (1994). Telephone follow-up program evaluation: Application of Orem's self-care model. *Rehabilitation Nursing, 19*, 287–292.

Coates, V. E., & Boore, J. R. P. (1995). Self-management of chronic illness: Implications for nursing. *International Journal of Nursing Studies, 32*, 628–640.

Craddock, R. B., Adams, P. F., Usui, W. M., & Mitchell, L. (1999). An intervention to increase use and effectiveness of self-care measures for breast cancer chemotherapy patients. *Cancer Nursing, 22*, 312–319.

Dellasega, C., & Clark, D. (1995). SCOPE: A practical method for assessing the self-care status of elderly persons. *Rehabilitation Nursing Research, 4*, 128–135.

Devine, E. C. (1996). Meta-analysis of the effects of psychoeducational care in adults with asthma. *Research in Nursing & Health, 19*, 367–376.

Devine, E. C., & Cook, T. D. (1983). A meta-analytic analysis of effects of psychoeducational interventions on length of postsurgical hospital stay. *Nursing Research, 32*, 267–274.

Devine, E. C., & Cook, T. D. (1986). Clinical and cost-saving effects of psychoeducational interventions with surgical patients: A meta-analysis. *Research in Nursing & Health, 9*, 89–105.

Devine, E. C., & Reifschneider, E. (1995). A meta-analysis of the effects of psycho-educational care in adults with hypertension. *Nursing Research, 44*, 237–245.

DiIorio, C., & Henry, M. (1995). Self-management in persons with epilepsy. *Journal of Neuroscience Nursing, 27*, 338–343.

Dodd, M. J. (1982a). Assessing patient self-care for side effects of cancer chemotherapy. *Cancer Nursing, 5*, 447–451.

Dodd, M. J. (1982b). Chemotherapy knowledge in patients with cancer: Assessment and informational interventions. *Oncology Nursing Forum, 9*(3), 39–44.

Dodd, M. J. (1983). Self-care for side effects in cancer chemotherapy: An assessment of nursing interventions. Part II. *Cancer Nursing, 6*, 63–67.

Dodd, M. J. (1988). Patterns of self-care in patients with breast cancer. *Western Journal of Nursing Research, 10*, 7–14.

Dodd, M. J., & Miaskowski, C. (2000). The Pro-Self Program: A self-care intervention program for patients receiving cancer treatment. *Seminars in Oncology Nursing, 16*, 300–308.

Dodd, M. J., Thomas, M. L., & Dibble, S. L. (1991). Self-care for patients experiencing cancer chemotherapy side effects: A concern for home care nurses. *Home Healthcare Nurse, 9*(6), 21–26.

Dunbar, S. B., Jacobson, L. H., & Deaton, C. (1998). Heart failure: Strategies to enhance patient self-management. *AACN Clinical Issues, 9*, 244–256.

Easton, K. L. (1993). Defining the concept of self-care. *Rehabilitation Nursing, 18*, 384–387.

Ekman, I., Anderson, B., Ehnfors, M., Makjkat, G., Person, B., & Fagerberg, B. (1998). Feasibility of a nurse-monitored, outpatient-care programme for elderly patients with moderate-to-severe, chronic heart failure. *European Heart Journal, 19*, 1254–1260.

Folden, S. L. (1993). Effect of a supportive-educative nursing intervention on older adults' perceptions of self-care after a stroke. *Rehabilitation Nursing, 18*, 162–167.

Foltz, A. T., Gaines, G., & Gullatte, M. (1996). Recalled side effects and self-care actions of patients receiving inpatient chemotherapy. *Oncology Nursing Forum, 23*, 679–683.

Gaffney, K. F., & Moore, J. B. (1996). Testing Orem's theory of self-care deficit: Dependent care agent performance for children. *Nursing Science Quarterly, 9*, 160–164.

Gallefoss, F., & Bakke, P. S. (1999). How does patient education and self-management among asthmatics and patients with chronic obstructive pulmonary disease affect medication? *American Journal of Respiratory and Critical Care Medicine, 160*, 2000–2005.

Gantz, S. B. (1990). Self-care: Perspectives from six disciplines. *Holistic Nursing Practice, 4*(2), 1–12.

Gillette, B., & Jenko, M. (1991). Major clinical functions: A unifying framework for measuring outcomes. *Journal of Nursing Care Quality, 6*, 20–24.

Goeppinger, J., Macnee, C., Anderson, M. K., Boutaugh, M., & Stewart, K. (1995). From research to practice: The effects of the jointly sponsored dissemination of an arthritis self-care nursing intervention. *Applied Nursing Research, 8*, 106–113.

Gregory, E. K. (2000). Empowering students on medication for asthma to be active participants in their care: An exploratory study. *Journal of School Nursing, 16*(1), 20–27.

Guyatt, G. H., Feeny, D. H., & Patrick, D. L. (1993). Measuring health-related quality of life. *Annals of Internal Medicine, 118,* 622–629.

Hagopian, G. A. (1996). The effects of informational audiotapes on knowledge and self-care behaviors of patients undergoing radiation therapy. *Oncology Nursing Forum, 23,* 697–700.

Halfens, R. J. G., van Alphen, A., Hasman, A., & Philipsen, H. (1998). The effect of item observability, clarity and wording on patient/nurse ratings when using the ASA scale. *Scandinavian Journal of Caring Science, 13,* 159–164.

Hanson, B. R., & Bickel, L. (1985). Development and testing of the questionnaire on perception of self-care agency. In Riehl-Sisca (Ed.), *The science and art of self-care.* Norwalk, CT: Appleton-Century-Crofts.

Hanucharurnkul, S. (1989). Predictors of self-care in cancer patients receiving radiation therapy. *Cancer Nursing, 12,* 21–27.

Hanucharurnkul, S. & Vinya-nguag, P. (1991). Effects of promoting patients' participation in self-care on postoperative recovery and satisfaction with care. *Nursing Science Quarterly, 4,* 14–20.

Harper, D. C. (1984). Application of Orem's theoretical constructs to self-care medication behaviors in the elderly. *Advances in Nursing Science, 6*(3), 29–46.

Hart, M. A. (1995). Orem's self-care deficit theory: Research with pregnant women. *Nursing Science Quarterly, 8,* 120–126.

Hart, M. A., & Foster, S. N. (1998). Self-care agency in two groups of pregnant women. *Nursing Science Quarterly, 11,* 167–171.

Hartweg, D. L. (1990). Health promotion self-care within Orem's general theory of nursing. *Journal of Advanced Nursing, 15,* 35–41.

Hathaway, D. (1986). Effect of preoperative instruction on postoperative outcomes: A meta-analysis. *Nursing Research, 35,* 269–275.

Henry, S. B., & Holzemer, W. L. (1997). Achievement of appropriate self-care. Does care delivery system make a difference? *Medical Care, 35,* NS33–NS40.

Hibbard, J. H., Greenlick, M., Jimison, H., Kunkel, L., & Tusler, M. (1999). Prevalence and predictors of the use of self-care resources. *Evaluation & the Health Professions, 22* (1), 107–122.

Hickey, T. (1981). *Health and aging.* Monterey, CA: Brooks/Cole.

Hirano, P. C., Laurent, D. D., & Lorig, K. (1994). Arthritis patient education studies, 1987–1991: A review of the literature. *Patient Education & Counseling, 24,* 9–54.

Hogan, L., Morin, D., & Lepine, R. (2000). Evaluation of telenursing outcomes: Satisfaction, self-care practice, and cost savings. *Public Health Nursing, 17,* 305–313.

Holoday, B., Turner-Henson, A., Harkins, A., & Swan, J. (1993). Chronically ill children in self-care: Issues for pediatric nurses. *Journal of Pediatric Health Care, 7,* 256–263.

Horsburgh, M. E. (1999). Self-care of well adult Canadians and adult Canadians with end stage renal disease. *International Journal of Nursing Studies, 36,* 443–453.

Horsburgh, M. E., Beanlands, H., Looking-Cusolito, H., Howe, A., & Watson, D. (2000). Personality traits and self-care in adults awaiting renal transplant. *Western Journal of Nursing Research, 22*, 407–437.

Irvine, D., Sidani, S., & McGillis Hall, L. (1998). Linking outcomes to nurses' roles in health care. *Nursing Economics, 16*, 58–64.

Jaarsma, T., Halfens, R., Abu-Saad, H. H., Dracup, K., Gorgels, T., van Ree, J., et al. (1999). Effects of education and support on self-care and resource utilization in patients with heart failure. *European Heart Journal, 20*, 673–682.

Jaarsma, T., Halfens, R., Senten, M., Abu-Saad, H. H., & Dracup, K. (1998). Developing a supportive-educative program for patients with advanced heart failure within Orem's general theory of nursing. *Nursing Science Quarterly, 11*, 79–85.

Jaarsma, T., Halfens, R., Tan, F., Abu-Saad, H. S., Dracup, K., & Diederiks, J. (2000). Self-care and quality of life in patients with advanced heart failure: The effect of a supportive educational intervention. *Heart & Lung, 29*, 319–330.

Johannsen, J. M. (1992). Self-care assessment: Key to teaching and discharge planning. *Dimensions of Critical Care Nursing, 11*, 48–56.

Johnson, M., & Maas, M. (Eds). (1997). *Nursing Outcome Classification* (NOC). St. Louis, MO: Mosby.

Jopp, M., Carroll, M. C., & Waters, L. (1993). Using self-care theory to guide nursing management of the older adult after hospitalization. *Rehabilitation Nursing, 18*, 91–94.

Joseph, L. S. (1980). Self-care and the nursing process. *Nursing Clinics of North America, 15*(1), 131–143.

Kearney, B., & Fleischer, B. (1979). Development and testing of an instrument to measure exercise of self-care agency. *Research in Nursing & Health, 2*, 25–34.

Keller, M. L., Ward, S., & Baumann, L. J. (1989). Processes of self-care: Monitoring sensations and symptoms. *Advances in Nursing Science, 12*(1), 54–66.

Kemper, D. (1980). Medical self-care: A stop on the road to high level wellness. *Health Values, 4*(2), 63–68.

Kimberly, O. (1997). Home-taught pediatric asthma program improves outcomes, cuts hospital, physician visits. *Health Care Cost Reengineering Report, 2*(3), 40–43.

Lachman, V. S. (1996). Stress and self-care revisited: A literature review. *Holistic Nursing Practice, 10*(2), 1–12.

Lang, N. M., & Marek, K. D. (1990). The classification of patient outcomes. *Journal of Professional Nursing, 6*, 158–163.

Lantz, J. M., Fullerton, J., & Quayhagen, M. P. (1995). Perceptual and enactment measurement of self-care. *Advanced Practice Nursing Quarterly, 1*, 29–33.

Larson, P. J., Miaskowski, C., MacPhail, L., Dodd, M. J., Greenspan, D., Dibble, S. L., et al. (1998). The PRO-SELF mouth aware program: An effective approach for reducing chemotherapy-induced mucosistis. *Cancer Nursing, 21*, 263–268.

Leenerts, M. H., & Megilvy, J. K. (2000). Investing in self-care: A midrange theory of self-care grounded in the lived experience of low-income HIV-positive White women. *Advances in Nursing Science, 22*(3), 58–75.

LeFort, S. M. (2000). A test of Braden's self-help model in adults with chronic pain. *Journal of Nursing Scholarship, 32,* 153–160.

LeFort, S. M., Gray-Donald, K., Rowat, K. M., & Jeans, M. E. (1998). Randomized controlled trial of a community-based psychoeducation program for the self-management of chronic pain. *Pain, 74,* 297–306.

Lenihan, A. A. (1988). Identification of self-care behaviors in the elderly: A nursing assessment tool. *Journal of Professional Nursing, 4,* 285–288.

Lev, E. L. (1997). Bandura's theory of self-efficacy: Applications to oncology. *Scholarly Inquiry for Nursing Practice: An International Journal, 11*(1), 21–37.

Lev, E. L., & Owen, S. V. (1996). A measure of self-care self-efficacy. *Research in Nursing & Health, 19,* 421–429.

Lev, E. L., & Owen, S. V. (1998). A prospective study of adjustment to hemodialysis. *ANNA Journal, 25,* 495–506.

Leveille, S. G., Wagner, E. H., Davis, C., Grothaus, L., Wallace, J., LoGerfo, M., et al. (1998). Preventing disability and managing chronic illness in frail older adults: A randomized trial of a community-based partnership with primary care. *Journal of the American Geriatrics Society, 46,* 1191–1198.

Levin, L. S. (1976). The layperson as primary care provider. *Public Health Report, 91,* 206–210.

Levin, L. S., Katz, A. H., & Holst, E. (1979). *Self-care: Lay initiatives in health.* New York: Prodist.

Lipsey, M. W. (1990). *Design sensitivity: Statistical power for experimental research.* Newbury Park, CA: Sage.

Lorig, K., Konkol, L., & Gonzalez, V. (1987). Arthritis patient education: A review of the literature. *Patient Education & Counseling, 10,* 207–252.

McCain, N. L., & Lynn, M. R. (1990). Meta-analysis of a narrative review. Studies evaluating patient teaching. *Western Journal of Nursing Research, 12,* 347–358.

McCaleb, A., & Cull, V. V. (2000). Sociocultural influences and self-care practices of middle adolescents. *Journal of Pediatric Nursing, 15,* 30–35.

McCaleb, A. & Edgil, A. (1994). Self-concept and self-care practices of healthy adolescents. *Journal of Pediatric Nursing, 9,* 233–238.

McFarland, S. M., Sasser, L., Boss, B. J., Dickerson, J. L., & Stelling, J. D. (1992). Self-care assessment tool for spinal cord injured persons. *Science Nursing, 9*(4), 111–116.

McKinney, B. (1995). Under new management: Asthma and the elderly. *Journal of Gerontological Nursing, 21*(11), 39–45.

Miller, P., Wikoff, R., & McMahon, A. (1982). Development of a health attitude scale. *Nursing Research, 31,* 132–135.

Mitchell, P. H., Ferketich, S., & Jennings, B. M. (1998). Quality health outcomes model. *Image: Journal of Nursing Scholarship, 30,* 43–46.

Moore, J. B. (1995). Measuring the self-care practice of children and adolescents: Instrument development. *Maternal-Child Nursing Journal, 23*(3), 101–108.

Moore, J. B., & Gaffney, K. G. (1989). Development of an instrument to measure mothers' performance of self-care activities for children. *Advances in Nursing Science, 12,* 76–83.

Moore, J. B., & Mosher, R. B. (1997). Adjustment responses of children and their mothers to cancer: Self-care and anxiety. *Oncology Nursing Forum, 24,* 519–525.

Mullen, P. D., Green, L. W., & Persinger, G. S. (1985). Clinical trials of patient education for chronic conditions: A comparative meta-analysis of intervention types. *Preventive Medicine, 14,* 753–781.

Mullen, P. D., Simons-Morton, D. G., Ramirez, G., Frankowski, R. F., Green, L. W., & Mains, D. A. (1997). A meta-analysis of trials evaluating patient education and counseling for three groups of preventive health behaviors. *Patient Education & Counseling, 32,* 157–173.

Nail, L. M., Jones, L. S., Greene, D., Schipper, D. L., & Jensen, R. (1991). Use and perceived efficacy of self-care activities in patients receiving chemotherapy. *Oncology Nursing Forum, 18,* 883–887.

Nelson McDermott, M. A. (1993). Learned helplessness as an interacting variable with self-care agency: Testing a theoretical model. *Nursing Science Quarterly, 6,* 28–38.

Ni, H., Nauman, D., Burgess, D., Wise, K., Crispell, K., & Hershberger, R. E. (1999). Factors influencing knowledge of and adherence to self-care among patients with heart failure. *Archives of Internal Medicine, 159,* 1613–1619.

Nicholas, P. K. (1993). Hardiness, self-care practice, and perceived health status in older adults. *Journal of Advanced Nursing, 18,* 1085–1094.

Norris, C. M. (1979). Self-care. *American Journal of Nursing, 3,* 486–489.

Novak, M. M. (1988). Innovations in family and community health. *Family and Community Health, 11*(1), 76–81.

Oberst, M., Hughes, S., Chang, A., & McCubbin, M. (1991). Self-care burden, stress appraisal, and mood among persons receiving radiotherapy. *Cancer Nursing, 14,* 71–78.

Orem, D. E. (1971). *Nursing: Concepts of practice.* New York: McGraw Hill.

Orem, D. E. (1985). *Nursing: Concepts of practice* (3rd ed.). New York: McGraw Hill.

Orem, D. E. (1991). *Nursing: Concepts of practice* (5th ed.). St. Louis, MO: Mosby.

Padula, C. A. (1992). Self-care and the elderly: Review and implications. *Public Health Nursing, 9*(1), 22–28.

Page, P., Lengacher, C., Holsonback, C., Himmelgreen, D., Pappalardo, L. J., Lipana, M. J., et al. (1999). Quality of care-risk adjustment outcomes model: Testing the effects of a community-based educational self-management program for children with asthma. *Nursing Connections, 12*(3), 47–58.

Parcel, G. S., Nade, P. R., & Tiernan, K. (1980). A health education program for children with asthma. *Journal of Developmental and Behavioral Pediatrics, 1,* 128–132.

Persaud, D. I., Barnett, S. E., Weller, S. C., Baldwin, C. D., Niebuhr, V., & McCormick, D. (1996). An asthma self-management program for children, including instruction in peak flow monitoring by school nurses. *Journal of Asthma, 33*(1), 37–43.

Rice, R. (1998). Key concepts of self-care in the home: Implications for home care nurses. *Geriatric Nursing, 19*(1), 52–54.

Richardson, A. (1991). Theories of self-care: Their relevance to chemotherapy-induced nausea and vomiting. *Journal of Advanced Nursing, 16,* 671–676.

Robinson, K. D., & Posner, J. D. (1992). Patterns of self-care needs and interventions related to biologic modifier therapy: Fatigue as a model. *Seminars in Oncology Nursing, 18*(4), 17–22.

Rodeman, B. J., Conn, V. S., & Rose, S. (1995). Myocardial infarction survivors: Social support and self-care behaviors. *Rehabilitation Nursing Research, 4*, 58–63, 71.

Ruland, C. M. (1999). Decision support for patient preference-based care planning: Effects on nursing care and patient outcomes. *Journal of the American Medical Informatics Association, 6*, 304–312.

Sidani, S. (1994). *Empirical testing of a conceptual model to evaluate psychoeducational interventions.* Unpublished doctoral dissertation, University of Arizona, Tucson.

Sidani, S., & Braden, C. J. (1998). *Evaluating nursing interventions: A theory-driven approach.* Thousand Oaks, CA: Sage.

Sidani, S., & Irvine, D. (1999). *Evaluation of the care delivery model and staff mix redesign initiative: The collaborative care study.* Unpublished report.

Sidani, S., Irvine, D., Porter, H., LeFort, S., O'Brien-Pallas, L. L., & Zahn, C. (2002). *Evaluating the impact of nurse practitioners in acute care settings.* Final Report, submitted to Canadian Institutes of Health Research.

Singleton, J. K. (2000). Nurses' perspectives of encouraging clients' care-of-self in a short-term rehabilitation unit within a long-term care facility. *Rehabilitation Nursing, 25*, 23–30.

Skoner, M. M. (1994). Self-management of urinary incontinence among women 31 to 50 years of age. *Rehabilitation Nursing, 19*, 339–347.

Slusher, I. L. (1999). Self-care agency and self-care practice of adolescents. *Issues in Comprehensive Pediatric Nursing, 22*, 49–58.

Soderhamn, O., Evers, G., & Hamrin, E. (1996). A Swedish version of the Appraisal of Self-Care Agency (ASA) Scale. *Scandinavian Journal of Caring Science, 10*, 3–9.

Spradley, B. W. (1981). *Community health nursing: Concepts and practice.* Boston: Little Brown.

Thomas, V., & Riegel, B. (1999). A computerized method of identifying potentially preventable heart failure admissions. *Journal of Nursing Care Quality, 13*(5), 1–10.

Turner, M. O., Taylor, D., Bennett, R., & Fitzgerald, J. M. (1998). A randomized trial comparing peak expiratory flow and symptom self-management plans for patients with asthma attending a primary care clinic. *American Journal of Respiratory and Critical Care Medicine, 157*, 540–546.

van Achterberg, T., Lorensen, M., Isneberg, M. A., Evers, G. C. M., Levin, E., & Philipsen, H. (1991). The Norwegian, Danish & Dutch version of the Appraisal of Self-Care Agency Scale: Comparing reliability aspects. *Scandinavian Journal of Caring Science, 5*, 101–108.

van Agthoven, W. M., & Plomp, H. N. (1989). The interpretation of self-care: A difference in outlook between clients and home-nurses. *Social Science & Medicine, 29*, 245–252.

Vickery, D. (1986). Medical self-care: A review of the concept and program models. *American Journal of Health Promotion, 1*(3), 23–28.

Vrijhoef, H. J. M., Diederiks, J. P. M., & Spreeuwenberg, C. (2000). Effects on quality of care for patients with NIDDM or COPD when the specialized nurse has a central role: A literature review. *Patient Education & Counseling, 41*, 243–250.

Wang, H. H., & Lee, I. (1999). A path analysis of self-care of elderly women in a rural area of Southern Taiwan. *Kaohsiung Journal of Medical Science, 15*, 94–103.

Watson, P. B., Town, G. I., Holbrook, N., Dwan, C., Toop, L. J., & Drennan, C. J. (1997). Evaluation of a self-management plan for chronic obstructive pulmonary disease. *The European Respiratory Journal, 10*, 1267–1271.

Webster, D. C., & Brennan, T. (1998). Self-care effectiveness and health outcomes in women with interstitial cystitis: Implications for mental health clinicians. *Issues in Mental Health Nursing, 19*, 495–519.

Whetstone, W. R., & Hansson, A. M. O. (1989). Perceptions of self-care in Sweden: A cross-cultural replication. *Journal of Advanced Nursing, 14*, 962–969.

Williams, P. D., Valderrama, D. M., Gloria, M. D., Pascoguin, L. G., Saaveda, L. D., De La Roma, D. T., et al. (1988). Effects of preparation for mastectomy/ hysterectomy on women's post-operative self-care behaviors. *International Journal of Nursing Studies, 25*, 191–206.

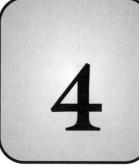

4

Symptom Management

Souraya Sidani, RN, PhD

4.1 Introduction

Symptoms play an important role in the health-illness experience. They signal a change in functioning and represent the reason for seeking health care (Dodd et al., 2001; O'Neill & Morrow, 2001; University of California, San Fransisco (UCSF), School of Nursing Symptom Management Faculty Group, 1994). Experienced by clients with various acute and chronic conditions, symptoms are the primary concern of patients and health care providers. Effective symptom management, which is viewed as an essential component of nursing practice (Johnson, 1993), has taken precedence in the care of patients with chronic illness.

Effective symptom management or symptom control (the two terms are used interchangeably) is considered an outcome of nursing practice (Irvine et al., 1998; Lang & Marek, 1991; Mitchell et al., 1998). It begins with a comprehensive and accurate assessment of the client's symptom experience. Assessment is followed by selecting appropriate strategies to prevent or relieve the symptoms, implementing the strategies, and evaluating their effectiveness in controlling the symptoms (Dodd et al., 2001; Haworth & Dluhy, 2001). Symptom assessment, therefore, forms the foundation for effective management.

This chapter presents an overview of how symptom experience is conceptualized. A clear understanding of the symptom experience is necessary for accurate management. Issues in symptom measurement are discussed and instruments for assessing general symptoms are briefly reviewed. These instruments contain lists of symptoms commonly experienced by clients with a particular condition; they can be used to conduct comprehensive symptom assessment in the respective client population. Finally, the conceptualization, measurement, and sensitivity to nursing care of the following three symptoms are discussed: fatigue, nausea and vomiting, and dyspnea. They were selected based on their reported frequency of occurrence and impact on daily functioning in different patient populations across healthcare settings.

4.2 Symptom Experience: Conceptualization

4.2.1 Definition

Symptoms refer to (a) sensations or experiences reflecting changes in a person's biopsychosocial functions; (b) a patient's perception of an abnormal physical, emotional, or cognitive state; or (c) the perceived indicators of change in normal functioning as experienced by patients (Henry et al., 1999; Holzemer et al., 1999; Rhodes et al., 1998; UCSF Symptom Management Faculty Group, 1994). In a recent article, Dodd and colleagues (2001) defined a symptom as a "subjective experience reflecting changes in the biopsychosocial functioning, sensations, or cognition of an individual."

Symptoms are characterized by their subjective nature. They are experienced by the individual and, thus are private. Therefore, they are difficult to measure objectively and cannot be detected by another person, such as a healthcare professional (Rhodes et al., 1998; UCSF Symptom Management Faculty Group, 1994). In contrast, signs refer to objective abnormality, evidence, or manifestation indicative of illness or disease. Signs are "more or less definitive, obvious, and apart from the patient's impressions" (Rhodes et al., 1998). They can be detected by the patients themselves or by the health care providers (UCSF Symptom Management Faculty Group, 1994).

4.2.2 Conceptualization

Symptoms are experienced or felt by the person. The subjective sensations are perceived by the individual. The individual then evaluates the meaning of the symptom and responds to it (UCSF Symptom Management Faculty Group, 1994).

"Perception of a symptom refers to whether an individual notices a change from the way she or he usually feels or behaves" (Dodd et al., 2001). It is the conscious, cognitive interpretation of the sensations. The recognition or interpretation of symptoms is influenced by a host of personal, environmental, and health- or illness-related variables. Personal variables encompass (a) demographic characteristics, such as age and gender; (b) psychological factors, such as personality traits, cognitive capacity, and motivation; (c) sociological variables, such as family, social support/network, and religion; and (d) physiological factors, such as the person's physical capacity, and patterns of rest and activity. Environmental variables include sociocultural orientation, beliefs, values, and characteristics of the physical and social settings in which the person lives (such as stress in the work environment). Health- or illness-related variables involve perceived health status and presence of disease or injury, and risk factors (Dodd et al., 2001; UCSF Symptom Management Faculty Group, 1994).

The influence of some factors on symptom perception has been supported empirically. The results of a research synthesis indicated that women reported more physical symptoms than men (O'Neill & Morrow, 2001). Culture is posited as having a powerful impact on symptom recognition and on the meaning given to symptoms (MacLeod, 1995). Anastasia and Blevins (1997) reported that very young and elderly patients with cancer receiving chemotherapy on an outpatient basis were the least tolerant of symptoms. Sutcliffe-Chidgey and Holmes (1996) found that patients in palliative care settings did not always perceive the presence of a symptom as a cause of concern. Several factors were believed to have influenced the patients' perception of symptoms, including age, culture, past experiences, and mood. This led the authors to emphasize the individual or unique nature of the symptom experience, a point that Haworth and Dluhy (2001) also reinforced.

Once the persons perceive the sensations and recognize the symptoms, they evaluate them and assign them a meaning. They assess the symptoms in terms of severity or intensity, location, temporal nature, frequency, duration or persistence, and impact. Impact relates to the pattern of disability and the distress associated with the symptom experience. Disability involves the perceived threat posed by a symptom, such as its danger and disability effect (Dodd et al., 2001; UCSF Symptom Management Faculty Group, 1994). It also entails the extent to which the symptom interferes with the person's physical, psychological, and social functioning. Distress is defined as the degree of physical or psychological upset, anguish, or suffering experienced from the symptoms (Hogan, 1997; Rhodes et al., 1998). Persons also assign a meaning to the symptom based on the observed symptom pattern (Johnson et al., 1997). Symptoms could represent usual or normal alterations expected as a result of some activities in which the person engaged. For instance, tiredness and breathlessness are anticipated following excessive, high-intensity, physical exercise. Symptoms are indicative of changes in the person's functioning or the presence of health problems. They may be the first warning of an impending illness, whether acute or chronic. Symptom experience, therefore, brings the problem to the person's attention. The meaning assigned to symptoms is, again, determined by the same set of personal, environmental, and health- or illness-related variables mentioned earlier.

Persons respond to the symptoms they experience. Their response is individual and shaped by their usual coping mechanisms (Johnson et al., 1997). The response to symptoms includes physiological, emotional, and/or behavioral components (UCSF Symptom Management Faculty Group, 1994). The physiological component can be manifested by exacerbation of the symptoms experienced or by the development of physical symptoms reflective of stress. It also can include alterations in functioning (Dodd et al., 2001). The emotional component is reflected by cognitive or affective changes, such as the generation of uncertainty and anxiety. The behavioral component consists of engaging in activities for the purpose of managing the symptom. The activities performed can vary: the patient may ignore the symptom, assume a "wait-and-see" attitude, seek advice from lay persons (i.e., family members and friends) use commonly recommended strategies or folk/home remedies, apply self-initiated treatment based on common knowledge (e.g., over-the-counter medications) or previous experience, or seek care from healthcare professionals. Briefly, individuals engage in self-care/self-management, independently or in collaboration with health care providers, in an attempt to relieve the symptoms experienced.

Symptoms experienced with acute conditions may be successfully managed in a rather short period of time, particularly when the cause of the symptom is clearly identified and appropriate, effective treatment is given. The result is the resolution of the symptoms. Symptoms are commonly experienced with chronic illnesses. But with these conditions, symptoms are not only indicative of changes in health and functioning related to the pathophysiological alterations characteristic of the illness, and are not the only reason for seeking care. Rather, patients with chronic illness "live" with symptoms, which are often debilitating and incapacitating. They are a constant reminder of the illness. Symptoms are also triggered or exacerbated by medical treatments, such as chemotherapy, radiation therapy, or biological therapy. They form the criteria for monitoring and evaluating the effectiveness of treatment, for modifying treatment dosage, and, in some instances, for discontinuing treatment. Last, but not least, symptoms tend to occur with high frequency and intensity towards the end stages of illness, resulting in increased distress and demand for palliative care.

The consequences of uncontrolled symptoms are devastating to the patients, their families, and the healthcare system. Outcomes associated with the symptom experience are conceptualized in terms of the following indicators: symptom status, self-care ability, financial status, comorbidity, mortality, quality of life, health services utilization, emotional status, and functional status (UCSF Symptom Management Faculty Group, 1994). That is, inadequate symptom management results in worsening of the symptom severity, frequency, and distress, which could not be managed effectively with available strategies. Symptoms experienced with high levels of severity are incapacitating and adversely affect individuals' ability to function as usual, to perform activities of daily living, and to care for themselves. Limited physical ability is associated with emotional distress and restricts the person's engagement in work-related, recreational, and social activities. Ultimately, quality of life is affected. Uncontrolled symptoms may lead to comorbid conditions (such as sleep disruption, discomfort, and decreased energy level) and increased utilization of health services. Similar consequences of poorly controlled symptoms have been reported by Hogan (1997), Gantz et al. (2000), Henry et al. (1999), and Holzemer et al. (1999). Munkres, Oberst, & Hughes (1992) found that symptom appraisal and distress significantly predicted the negative affective mood in patients with cancer receiving chemotherapy. In contrast, application of symptom management strategies resulted in significant reduction in perceived symptom severity, depression, and emotional distress; and in a significant increase in self-esteem and well-being in women experiencing severe premenstrual symptoms (Taylor, 1999).

The untoward and debilitating consequences of uncontrolled symptoms underscore the importance of adequately managing symptoms. Management involves (a) identifying and recognizing symptoms, (b) appropriately interpreting symptoms, (c) monitoring and evaluating symptoms, (d) selecting strategies to relieve the symptoms experienced and enhance functioning and well-being, and (e) evaluating the effectiveness of these strategies. This description of how to manage symptoms is similar to what self-care entails, as discussed in the previous chapter. Self-care or self-management of symptoms should aim at controlling or relieving symptoms. Effective management of symptoms begins with a comprehensive and accurate assessment. Such an assessment is also needed to evaluate the effectiveness of self-care/symptom management strategies. However, measuring symptoms presents some challenges, due to their subjective nature.

4.3 Issues in Symptom Measurement

The subjective and private nature of symptoms presents some challenges for their comprehensive and accurate measurement. Four issues are discussed here:

- Identifying the subjective sensation characterizing the symptom to be measured, and stating it in terms that accurately describe it. These terms used should be acceptable and applicable to individuals with various characteristics. This requirement prompted some tool developers to provide a few terms to refer to the same symptom; for example, "fatigue" for feeling tired and "nausea" for feeling sick to the stomach. Others selected words patients supplied themselves in qualitative interviews to describe relevant symptoms.

- Inability to find a criterion for determining the validity of the symptom measure, again because of the subjective, unique, and private nature of symptoms. Objective indicators of some symptoms did not correlate or converge with the subjective indicators. For instance, low hemoglobin level did not correlate consistently with the subjective report of fatigue. Forced expiratory volume was not associated with dyspnea. Similarly, patients' reporting and rating of symptoms differed from those their health care providers supplied. The health care providers' ratings were often based on their clinical observations. In most studies, the health care providers' and the patients' ratings of the symptom experience, intensity, and distress were discrepant. Rhodes et al. (1998) found that nurses working in hospice settings overestimated their patients' experiences of symptoms, whereas nurses in other settings underestimated those of their patients, particularly pain and dyspnea. The incongruence or lack of consistency in nurse-patient assessment of symptoms led the authors to conclude that "reliable and valid assessment tools that measure patients' subjective symptoms and their response are essential to assure the acquisition of patient-sensitive information and to formulate a sound nursing practice." Holzemer et al. (1999) also reported that nurses' ratings of symptoms were consistently shown to underestimate the frequency and intensity of symptoms experienced by patients with HIV disease. They recommended that "the patient is the gold standard for understanding the symptom experience," as "the meaning of the symptom experience can only be captured from the patient's perspective." Similarly, Grande, Barclay, & Todd (1997) reported discrepancies among general practitioners, nurses, and patients in symptom ratings. Maguire, Walsh, Jeacock, & Kingston (1999) also found marked discrepancies between patients, their caregivers (i.e., spouses) and their general practitioners in the assessment of breathlessness, pyrexia, nausea and vomiting, and loss of appetite. Justice, Chang, Rabeneck, and Zachin (2001) reported that health care providers consistently underestimated the frequency and severity of symptoms experienced by persons with HIV infection. These findings point to the incongruence between patients' and others' ratings of symptoms, and to the importance of assessing the patient's perspective as the most valid measure of the symptom experience. Self-report is viewed as the "gold standard" for measuring symptoms (Dodd et al., 2001).

- Multidimensionality of the symptom experience: A comprehensive measurement of the symptom experience should encompass multiple dimensions of the symptoms. These include (a) symptom occurrence, frequency, and duration over a pre-specified time frame, which should not be longer than one week to avoid recall bias; (b) symptom severity or intensity; (c) symptom impact, that is, the disability and distress associated with the symptom; (d) the meaning assigned to the symptom; (e) the response to the symptom; (f) the strategies the patients applied to manage the symptoms and the perceived effectiveness of the strategies used; and (g) factors that aggravate or alleviate the symptoms. Covering all these dimensions is essential for an initial, or baseline, assessment of symptoms (Yancey et al., 1998). It gives a comprehensive picture of the symptom experience, which provides an adequate understanding and informs planning of individualized and appropriate care. Assessing symptom occurrence, frequency, duration, severity, and use and effectiveness of symptom management strategies can be done to monitor symptoms and to assess symptom control following nursing care.

- Measures of symptoms have most often contained one global item, capturing one dimension of the symptom experience. Symptom severity was the dimension most commonly assessed. Although a one-item measure is clinically useful, it may not represent all the domains and dimensions of the symptom that are of concern for planning nursing care. The one item assessing a symptom was either presented as a separate, independent measure of the symptom; incorporated in a multi-item scale measuring a constellation of symptoms; or measuring quality of life, such as the Quality of Life Index (Ferrans & Powers, 1992), Functional Living Index-Cancer (Schipper et al., 1984), European Organization of Research on Treatment of Cancer (Aaronson et al., 1988), Rotterdam Symptom Checklist (de Haes et al., 1990), Medical Outcomes Study—Short Form-36 (Ware et al., 1993), and Quality of Life Survey (Ferrell et al., 1989). A discussion of the symptom subscales within an instrument measuring quality of life is beyond the scope of this review. For details, refer to Irvine and Sidani (1997).

4.4 General Symptom Measures

Several instruments assessing symptoms in different client populations were found. The characteristics of these measures are summarized in Table 4.1. The instruments were designed to measure symptoms in patients with cancer or HIV, patients in palliative care, and women with premenstrual syndrome. Most scales targeted patients with cancer who experienced various symptoms associated with the disease and its treatment. The instruments reviewed consist of a list of symptoms commonly reported by patients. In some, the listed symptoms can be grouped into larger categories, reflective of alterations in a particular body function or anatomical system. Examples of symptom categories are confusion, gastrointestinal distress, and urinary symptoms. Each instrument measures only one symptom dimension, with severity or distress being the most frequently assessed.

Table 4.1. Instruments Measuring General Symptoms

Instrument (author)	Target population	Domains; number of items; response format	Method of administration	Reliability	Validity	Sensitivity to change and nursing care
Symptom Distress Scale (Rhodes et al., 1984; Rhodes et al., 1998)	Patients in hospice care or patients with cancer	Several symptoms (e.g., nausea, pain, anorexia, sleep disturbances, fatigue, difficulty in breathing, coughing, impaired concentration, change in body temperature and in appearance, and restlessness); 31 items; 5-point Likert-type.	Self-administered	ICR: No data available. TRR: Not applicable.	Content: No data available. Concurrent/Construct: No data available.	Sensitivity to change: no data available. Sensitivity to nursing: no data available.
Sign and Symptom Checklist for Persons with HIV Disease (SSC-HIV) Holzemer et al. (1999) adapted this checklist from the HIV Assessment Tool (HAT) developed by Nokes et al. (1994)	Persons with HIV disease	Six clusters of symptoms (fever, fatigue, confusion, nausea/vomiting, psychological distress, shortness of breath, GI discomfort, and diarrhea); 41 items for original version and 26 for reduced version; 3-point Likert scale.	Self-administered	ICR: α of .80 for fever, .78 for fatigue, .82 for confusion, .74 for nausea/vomiting, .76 for psychological distress, .75 for shortness of breath, .72 for GI discomfort, and .76 for diarrhea). TRR: Not applicable.	Content: validated for its relevance by six clinicians. Construct: subscales correlated with relevant subscales of the MOS-SF-36 (Henry et al., 1999; Holzemer et al., 1999).	Sensitivity to change: Changes in scores observed over time (i.e., fewer symptoms reported upon discharge than at admission). Sensitivity to nursing: No data available.
Symptom Distress Scale (SDS) (McCorkle & Young, 1978; modified by Munkres et al. (1992) and Sutcliffe-Chidgey & Holmes (1996)	Patients with cancer	Several symptoms (e.g., pain, fatigue, anorexia, nausea, vomiting, constipation, breathing difficulty, weakness, loss of appetite, disturbances, and insomnia); 10 items; 5-point numeric rating scale (McCorckle & Young, 1978; Sutcliffe-Chidgey & Holmes, 1996) or VAS (Munkres et al., 1992).	Self-administered	ICR: α of .82 to .85 in patients with cancer (Munkres et al., 1992; McCorkle & Young, 1978). TRR: Not applicable.	Content: No information provided. Construct: correlated with affective mood in patients receiving chemotherapy (Munkres et al., 1992); scores differed between patients with cancer with and without metastasis (McCorkle & Young, 1978).	Sensitivity to change: No data available. Sensitivity to nursing: No data available.

Table 4.1 (continued)

Instrument (author)	Target population	Domains; number of items; response format	Method of administration	Reliability	Validity	Sensitivity to change and nursing care
Menstrual Symptom Severity List (MSS) (Mitchell et al., 1991; cited by Taylor, 1999)	Women with premenstrual syndrome	Physical, cognitive, behavioral, and mood symptoms; 51 items; 5-point scale.	Self-administered	ICR: α > .70 (Taylor, 1999). TRR: Not applicable.	Content: No data available. Construct: subscales scores consistent with symptoms severity across menstrual cycles (Taylor, 1999).	Sensitivity to change: No data available. Sensitivity to nursing: No data available.
Breast Cancer Prevention Trial Symptom Checklist (Gantz et al., 1995)	Women with breast cancer receiving adjuvant therapy	Symptoms associated with the menopause and tamoxifen use (e.g., vaginal symptoms, hot flashes, urinary symptoms); 43 items; 5-point Likert-type.	Self-administered	ICR: α of .73 for vaginal subscale, .76 for hot flashes subscale, .76 for urinary subscale, and .50 for total scale (Gantz et al., 2000). TRR: Not applicable.	Content: No data available. Construct: No data were available.	Sensitivity to change: No data available. Sensitivity to nursing: No data available.
Support Team Assessment Schedule (STAS) (Higginson & McCarthy, 1989); Edmonton Symptom Assessment System (ESAS) (Bruera et al., 1991); Palliative Care Assessment (PACA), which is a Modified version of the STAS (Ellershaw et al., 1995).	Patients in palliative care	Twelve core symptoms (pain, mouth discomfort, anorexia, nausea, vomiting, constipation, breathlessness, depression, agitation, confusion, patient psychological distress, and family anxiety); 12 items but varies with version; 4-point rating scale.	Self-administered or completed by the health care provider based on their clinical assessment of the patients' condition	ICR: Not applicable. TRR: Not applicable. IRR: No data available.	Content: core symptoms selected based on clinicians' input. Construct: No data available.	Sensitivity to change: No data available. Sensitivity to nursing: No data available.

Table 4.1 (continued)

Instrument (author)	Target population	Domains; number of items; response format	Method of administration	Reliability	Validity	Sensitivity to change and nursing care
Semi-Structured Interview (Maguire et al., 1999)	Terminally ill patients with colo-rectal cancer	Symptoms of pain, pyrexia, breathlessness, abdominal swelling, constipation, diarrhea, sore mouth, nausea, and vomiting; 9 items; response format not described.	Interview by observer	ICR: Not applicable. TRR: Not applicable. IRR: No data available.	Content: No data available. Construct: No data available.	Sensitivity to change: No data available. Sensitivity to nursing: No data available.
Symptom Reporting Tool (Tucci & Bartels, 1998)	Patients with cancer	Symptoms of pain, nausea and vomiting, numbness/tingling, and diarrhea; diary/log completed by patients at home; 10-point rating scale to rate symptoms and SC strategies.	Self-administered	ICR: Not applicable. TRR: Not applicable. IRR: No data available.	Content: No data available. Construct: No data available.	Sensitivity to change: No data available. Sensitivity to nursing: No data available.
Symptom Report Form (White, 1992)	Patients with cancer receiving biotherapy	Cluster of symptoms related to cardiovascular condition, dietary intake, fatigue, oral integrity, skin manifestations, flu-like syndrome; unclear number of items; 4-point number of items; 4-point rating scale.	Administered by interviewer	ICR: Not applicable. TRR: Not applicable. IRR: No data available.	Content: No data available. Construct: No data available.	Sensitivity to change: No data available. Sensitivity to nursing: No data available.

Table 4.1 (continued)

Instrument (author)	Target population	Domains; number of items; response format	Method of administration	Reliability	Validity	Sensitivity to change and nursing care
Symptom Control Assessment (SCA) (Benor et al., 1998)	Patients with cancer	Several symptoms (e.g., those related to respiration, fluid and food intake, ADLs, rest and sleep, mobility, hygiene, sociability, bacteriologic and physical safety, pain, anxiety, and sexuality); 16 items; 7-point numeric scale (assessing intensity, independence, help, and knowledge).	Self-administered or administered by interviewer	ICR: α of .85 for total scale. TRR: r of .97 for intensity, .90 for independence, .89 for perception of familial help, and .88 for knowledge dimensions. IRR: r of .90.	Content: reviewed by experts in the field. Construct: patients' and nurses' ratings were almost identical (r of .93 to .95 across the items).	Sensitivity to change and to nursing: changes in scores found for the different dimensions following an educative-supportive nursing intervention.
Symptom indexes (Clark & Talcott, 2001)	Patients with prostate cancer receiving therapy	Symptoms related to urinary incontinence and obstruction, bowel and sexual dysfunction.	Self-administered	ICR: α of .86 for urinary incontinence, .65 for urinary obstruction, .73 for bowel symptoms, .80 for sexual dysfunction. TRR: Not applicable.	Content: No data available. Construct: correlated with health-related quality of life.	Sensitivity to change: scores changed over time. Sensitivity to nursing: No data available.

r = correlation coefficient
α = Cronbach's alpha coefficient
ICR = Internal Consistency Reliability
TRR = Test Re-test Reliability
IRR = Inter-Rater Reliability
SC = Self-Care
CVI = Content Validity Index
GI = Gastro-Intestinal

The instruments have been used in a very small number of studies. They demonstrated initial reliability and validity. However, the evidence on their sensitivity to change is limited. Additional research is required before the use of these instruments in practice can be recommended.

In addition, researchers have used individual items to assess symptoms of interest in a particular study. Most often, the participants were asked to report on the presence of the symptoms (e.g., Johnson et al., 1997) and to rate the severity or intensity of the symptoms experienced. Different rating scales were used, such as the Visual Analogue Scale (e.g., Fainsinger et al., 1991) or numeric rating scales.

In the next sections, the conceptualization, measurement, and sensitivity to nursing care of the symptoms of fatigue, nausea and vomiting, and dyspnea are discussed.

4.5 Fatigue

Fatigue is experienced by every human being following heavy or sustained physical or mental work. In these instances, fatigue is effectively relieved by adequate rest and sleep. Fatigue is also frequently reported by individuals with health-related problems. Patients view fatigue as a "warning signal of approaching health disaster" (Morris, 1982). Fatigue is "the seventh most common complaint in primary care, accounting for an estimated 10 million office visits a year and more than $300 million in medical care costs" in the United States (Piper, 1993). It is experienced by patients with acute conditions such as respiratory diseases like pneumonia, flu, and cold, and following surgery. Fatigue is associated with psychological stress and with alterations in mood, primarily depression. It is reported by patients with chronic illnesses such as cancer, cardiac disease, chronic obstructive pulmonary disease, end-state renal disease, HIV/AIDS, and chronic fatigue syndrome. Fatigue is also associated with the treatment of some conditions, such as cancer therapy (chemotherapy, radiation therapy, and biological therapy).

Although fatigue is experienced by a variety of patient populations, it is most prominent in those with cancer. Blesch et al. (1991) reported that up to 99% of cancer patients report fatigue at some point during their illness experience. It occurs during all phases of the cancer experience: diagnosis, surgical treatment, and adjuvant therapy (Richardson, 1995). In addition to its high prevalence, fatigue is rated as a highly distressing experience with an adverse impact on patients. It serves as an indicator for stopping or modifying treatment, limits the patients' ability to maintain normal functioning, interferes with their performance of daily activities and with self-care, disrupts their family life and work, and influences their quality of life (Dean & Ferrell, 1995).

Assisting patients in managing fatigue effectively is, therefore, an instrumental goal of nursing care. Successful relief of this distressing symptom is necessary to regain and/or maintain usual functioning and to improve the patients' quality of life. To be effective in managing fatigue, nursing care should be guided by a clear definition of this symptom and a precise identification of its indicators. It should be based on a comprehensive and systematic assessment of fatigue, and on empirical results of studies that evaluate the effectiveness of interventions for managing the symptom.

In the next section, the literature on fatigue is reviewed with the purposes of (a) defining fatigue and identifying its indicators; (b) evaluating the reliability, validity, and sensitivity to change of instruments for assessing fatigue; and (c) determining the extent to which fatigue is a symptom that is affected by nursing care.

4.5.1 *Theoretical Background*

This section presents the results of a concept analysis undertaken to clarify the definition and the indicators of fatigue. Some differences were noted in the several definitions of fatigue that were advanced. These differences related to difficulty in differentiating among the antecedents, manifestations, and consequences or impact of fatigue, as they are highly interrelated and produce a complex, multidimensional system of cause-effect relationships (Winningham, 1995; Winningham et al., 1994). The differences were associated with some variability in how the manifestations of fatigue were described. Some authors characterized the nature of fatigue as a feeling of tiredness, lack of energy, or lassitude. Others emphasized the perception of reduced capacity for physical and/or mental work; and still others described fatigue in terms of a decrement in actual performance, either physical or mental. Despite these differences, there is general agreement that fatigue is a subjective feeling that is self-recognized and self-evaluated; it is related to stress of a physiological/physical and/or psychological nature (Graydon et al., 1997).

In addition to these theoretical definitions, scholars have been interested in examining the patients' accounts of fatigue. These were obtained from clinical observations (Aistars, 1987; Morris, 1982; Piper, 1993; Winningham et al., 1994) and from a qualitative research study exploring how patients with cancer perceive fatigue (Glaus et al., 1996). Patients described fatigue as being unusually tired, ready to drop, worn out, weary, listless, or pooped; as a sense of weakness, lack of energy, exhaustion, malaise, and lethargy; as inability to concentrate and to think clearly; as decreased physical performance or reduction in activities; and as feeling hampered, having no desire and/or motivation for work.

Essential attributes

Based on these definitions and descriptions of fatigue, the following attributes are considered characteristic of the symptom of fatigue:

- Fatigue is a feeling that is experienced and perceived by the individual.

- Fatigue is characterized as a sense of lack of energy, lassitude, and tiredness, and as a decreased capacity for activity and/or for physical and mental work.

- Fatigue is subjective; that is, it is self-recognized, based on self-assessment and evaluation. It varies in intensity, frequency, and duration.

- The subjective feeling of fatigue is expressed in terms of physical, affective, cognitive, attitudinal, and behavioral experiences.

The subjective manifestations of fatigue are expressed as physical, affective or emotional, cognitive, attitudinal, and behavioral experiences. Fatigue's physical indicators include the following: feeling tired in the whole body, weary, listless, or worn out; having no energy; malaise or discomfort; tiredness or heaviness in the arms, legs, or eyes; tremors and/or numbness in the extremities; and eye strain. The affective or emotional indicators of fatigue include unpleasant feelings, increased irritability, and lack of patience. Fatigue's cognitive indicators include the following: difficulty in thinking or inability to think clearly, decreased attention, inability to concentrate, slowed and impaired perception of environmental stimuli/information, poor judgment, and forgetfulness. The symptom's attitudinal manifestations include decreased interest, decreased motivation, apathy, and being indifferent to the surroundings. The behavioral indicators of fatigue include feeling able to do only a little, requiring more effort to do things, wanting to lie down, having a strong desire to sleep, and exhibiting changes in general appearance and communication pattern.

It is important to note that decreased activity or performance of physical or mental work represents the consequence or impact of fatigue, as will be discussed later.

Antecedents

The experience of fatigue is influenced by several factors; however, the exact mechanisms through which these factors affect fatigue are not well understood. The factors (or antecedents) suggested in the literature include the following:

- Physiological factors related to the nature of the illness condition experienced by the individual and/or the treatment received. Illness conditions result in alterations in fluid and electrolyte balance (e.g., dehydration), accumulation of metabolites (e.g., hydrogen ions), hormone imbalance (e.g., thyroid disorder), and oxygenation, all of which promote fatigue. Treatment of some illness conditions, whether surgical or medical, leads to fatigue (Piper, 1993; Piper et al., 1989). In particular, cancer therapy is associated with the accumulation of toxic waste products (Aistars, 1987; Richardson, 1995; Smets et al., 1993).

- Physical factors, related to the occurrence of other symptoms (such as pain, fever, diarrhea) and to changes in the patterns of activity, rest, sleep, and fluid and food intake (Berger & Walker, 2001; Piper, 1993; Piper et al., 1989; Richardson, 1995; Winningham, 1995).

- Psychosocial factors, related to increased demands of illness and the need to adjust to changes in various aspects of life; to the emotional response to illness and/or treatment characterized by anger, anxiety, and depression; to ineffective coping strategies used by patients; and to prolonged stress (Aistars, 1987; Berger & Walker, 2001; Nail & King, 1987; Piper, 1993; Piper et al., 1989; Richardson, 1995; Smets et al., 1993).

- Environmental or situational factors related to increased noise, changes in temperature, social and life event patterns, sensory deprivation, and informational overload (Aistars, 1987; Cimprich, 1993; Piper, 1993; Piper et al., 1989).

- Innate host factors, such as age, sex, and genetic makeup (Piper, 1993; Piper et al., 1989).

Consequences

Fatigue has untoward effects on the patient. The consequences or impact of fatigue that have been identified in the literature and summarized by Graydon et al. (1997) include:

- Physical consequences: decreased performance of physical activity, yielding to limited performance of self-care activities and impaired functioning.

- Psychosocial consequences: decreased engagement in social activities, leading to impaired self-concept and personal relationships.

- Cognitive consequences: alteration in thought processes and decreased performance of mental work.

4.5.2 Instruments Measuring Fatigue

Various instruments have been used to measure fatigue in research studies. These are grouped into three categories: single-item measures, multiple-item scales capturing one dimension of fatigue (i.e., unidimensional), and multi-item instruments measuring more than one dimension of fatigue (i.e., multidimensional; Graydon et al., 1997). Table 4.2 summarizes the characteristics of single- and multiple-item scales.

Table 4.2. Instruments Measuring Fatigue

Single items standing alone

Instrument (author)	Target population	Domains; number of items; response format	Method of administration	Reliability	Validity	Sensitivity to change and nursing care
Analogue Fatigue Scale (AFS) (Christensen et al., 1982)	Surgical patients	Global rating of fatigue (focus on the physical domain); 1 item; VAS.	Self-administered or administered by clinician	ICR: Not applicable. TRR: .81 over a 2–4 hour interval in post-operative patients (Christensen et al., 1982).	Content: No data available. Construct: correlated with subjective measures of fatigue in surgical patients (Christensen et al., 1982; 1990); with objective measures of fatigue (Christensen et al., 1982), and with state anxiety (Christensen et al., 1986).	Sensitivity to change: responsive to change in level of fatigue observed post-operatively in surgical patients (Christensen et al., 1986; Schroeder & Hill, 1991). Sensitivity to nursing: no data available.
Rhoten Fatigue Scale (RFS) (Rhoten, 1982)	Surgical and cancer patients	Global experience of fatigue (focus on feeling of tiredness and lack of energy); 1 item; VAS.	Self-administered and administered by clinician	ICR: Not applicable. TRR: Not applicable.	Content: No data available. Construct: correlated with CA 125 in patients with cancer; did not discriminate among individuals with different levels of fatigue, i.e., healthy versus cancer patients (Blesch et al., 1991; Pickard-Holley, 1991).	Sensitivity to change: did not detect significant change in fatigue during course of chemotherapy in patients with ovarian cancer (Pickard-Holley, 1991). Sensitivity to nursing: No data available.

Table 4.2 (continued)

	Unidimensional subscales embedded in general instruments					
Instrument (author)	**Target population**	**Domains; number of items; response format**	**Method of administration**	**Reliability**	**Validity**	**Sensitivity to change and nursing care**
European Organization for Research and Treatment of Cancer Quality of Life Questionnaire (EORTC-QLQ) fatigue subscale (Aaronson et al., 1991)	Patients with cancer	Physical domain of fatigue; 3 items; 4-point rating scale.	Self-administered	ICR: $\alpha > .70$ in patients from various countries (Aaronson et al., 1996). TRR: Not applicable.	Content: No data available. Construct: correlated with physical functioning, anxiety, depression, and pain in patients with cancer (Aaronson et al., 1996); discriminated different levels of fatigue in cancer patients with different prognoses (Joly et al., 1996).	Sensitivity to change: responsive to change over course of chemotherapy (Osoba et al., 1996). Sensitivity to nursing: No data available.
Profile of Mood States (POMS) fatigue-inertia subscale (McNair et al., 1981)	General, healthy population; also used in patients with chronic illness	Physical domain of fatigue; 7 items; 5-point Likert-type.	Self-administered	ICR: α of .80 to .95 in various patient populations (Bowling, 1995; McNair et al., 1981; Meek et al., 2000). TRR: r of .74 in patients with cancer (Meek et al., 2000).	Content: No data available. Construct: correlated with other measures of fatigue (Greenberg et al., 1992); with mood, pain, and performance status in patients with cancer (Cassileth, 1985; Glover et al., 1995; Jamar, 1989; Meek et al., 2000); discriminated among cancer patients with different levels of fatigue (Gritz et al., 1988).	Sensitivity to change: scores changed over course of adjuvant therapy (Meek et al., 2000; Stanton & Snider, 1993). Sensitivity to nursing: No data available.

Table 4.2 (continued)

Unidimensional scales

Instrument (author)	Target population	Domains; number of items; response format	Method of administration	Reliability	Validity	Sensitivity to change and nursing care
Pearson-Byars Fatigue Feeling Checklist (PBFFCL) (Pearson & Byars, 1956)	Healthy individuals	Positive aspect (freshness) and negative aspect (tiredness) of fatigue; 10 items; respondents indicate if they feel better than, same as, or worse than the feeling of fatigue described in each item.	Self-administered	ICR: α of .82 to .97 in patients with cancer (Graydon et al., 1995; Greenberg et al., 1992; Jamar, 1989). TRR: Not applicable.	Content: based on the work on fatigue in military aircrew (Pearson & Byars, 1956). Construct: correlated with other measures of fatigue (Greenberg et al., 1992).	Sensitivity to change: scores increased over course of cancer treatment (Graydon et al., 1995; Greenberg et al., 1992). Sensitivity to nursing: No data available.
Fatigue Severity Scale (FSS) (Krupp et al., 1989)	Patients with multiple sclerosis (MS) and systemic lupus erythematosus (SLE)	Impact of fatigue on daily functioning; 9 items; 7-point Likert-type.	Self-administered	ICR: α of .88 in healthy persons, .81 in patients with MS, .89 in patients with SLE; .95 in rural patients with cancer (Winstead-Fry, 1998). TRR: No data available.	Content: based on theoretical considerations and results of factor analysis. Construct: correlated with other measures of fatigue in patients with SLE, MS, healthy persons, and rural patients with cancer (Winstead-Fry, 1998); significant differences in scores between healthy individuals and patients with MS and SLE; correlated with depression (Krupp et al., 1989).	Sensitivity to change: Some changes in scores observed before and after drug therapy for fatigue in patients with MS and SLE (Winstead-Fry, 1998). Sensitivity to nursing: No data available.

Table 4.2 (continued)

Instrument (author)	Target population	Domains; number of items; response format	Method of administration	Reliability	Validity	Sensitivity to change and nursing care
Composite Measure of Fatigue (Buxton et al., 1992)	Surgical patients	Severity of fatigue; 5 items; semantic differential scale with 7 points.	Self-administered	ICR: α > .70 in patients who had elective general surgery. TRR: r > .70.	Content: descriptors selected from the literature. Construct: correlated with other self-report measures and with objective indicators of fatigue (Buxton et al., 1992).	Sensitivity to change and nursing: increase in scores observed from pre-surgery to post-surgery, followed by a decrease during the recovery period.
Fatigue Questionnaire (FQ) (David et al., 1990)	Healthy individuals in a primary care setting	Symptoms of tiredness, need for rest, sleepiness, difficulty to start doing things, weak, getting tired when concentrating, not having enough energy, and strength in muscles; 11 items; 4-point Likert-type.	Self-administered	ICR: Not assessed. TRR: Not applicable.	Content: No data available. Factorial structure: one factor. Construct: persons who reported a brief duration of fatigue had lower scores (David et al., 1990).	Sensitivity to change: No data available. Sensitivity to nursing: No data available.
Multiple-item, multidimensional scales						
Fatigue Impact Scale (FIS) (Fisk et al., 1994)	Patients with chronic fatigue syndrome, hypertension, and multiple sclerosis	Impact of fatigue on quality of life (i.e., cognitive, physical, and psychosocial functioning); 40 items; 5-point Likert-type.	Self-administered	ICR: α > .87 in patients with chronic fatigue syndrome, hypertension, and multiple sclerosis. TRR: Not applicable.	Content: generated from existing fatigue questionnaires and from interviews with patients. Construct: differences in scores across patient groups (highest for patients with chronic fatigue syndrome); positive r with Sickness Impact Profile.	Sensitivity to change: No data available. Sensitivity to nursing: No data available.

Table 4.2 (continued)

Instrument (author)	Target population	Domains; number of items; response format	Method of administration	Reliability	Validity	Sensitivity to change and nursing care
Fatigue Rating Scale (FRS) (Kashiwagi, 1971)	FRS is an observational tool that has been used in Japanese industrial settings	Weakened activation and motivation; 20 items; response format not described.	Observation	ICR: No data available. TRR: No data available. IRR: Not tested.	Content: reviewed by healthy individuals. Factorial structure: two factors, as hypothesized. Construct: No data available.	Sensitivity to change: No data available. Sensitivity to nursing: No data available.
Fatigue Assessment Scale (FAS) (Chalder et al., 1993)	General practice client population	Physical and mental fatigue; 14 items; ratings of better than usual, no more than usual, worse than usual, and much worse than usual.	Self-administered	ICR: α of .89 for total scale, .84 for physical subscale, and .82 for mental subscale, in general practice patients. TRR: Not applicable.	Content: generated from an extensive literature review. Factorial structure: two factors, as hypothesized. Construct: No data available.	Sensitivity to change: No data available. Sensitivity to nursing: No data available.
Fatigue Assessment Instrument (FAI) (Schwartz et al., 1993); it is an extension of the Fatigue Severity Scale (FSS) developed by Krupp et al. (1989)	Patients with chronic fatigue syndrome and multiple sclerosis	Severity, consequences, and responsiveness of fatigue to rest/sleep; 29 items; 7-point Likert scale.	Self-administered	ICR: α of .70 to .92 for the subscales, in ill individuals. TRR: r of .29 for the responsiveness, .62 for consequences, .69 for severity of subscales, in patients with multiple sclerosis.	Content: items drawn drom clinical experience and from patients' responses to interviews. Factorial Structure: four factors, as hypothesized. Construct: discriminated between patients with chronic illness and healthy persons.	Sensitivity to change: No data available. Sensitivity to nursing: No data available.

Table 4.2 (continued)

Instrument (author)	Target population	Domains; number of items; response format	Method of administration	Reliability	Validity	Sensitivity to change and nursing care
Lee Fatigue Scale (LFS) (Lee et al., 1991)	Initially developed for use with individuals having sleep disorders. Also used in patients with chronic conditions	General fatigue and energy; 18 items; VAS.	Self-administered	ICR: α of .91 for fatigue, and .94 for energy subscales, in general practice patients (Lee et al., 1991); .94 to .96 in patients with cancer receiving treatment (Meek et al., 2000). TRR: r of .47 for fatigue and .77 for energy subscales in patients with cancer receiving treatment (Meek et al., 2000).	Content: No data available. Factorial Structure: two factors, as hypothesized (Lee et al., 1991; Meek et al., 2000). Construct: correlated with the POMS-fatigue subscale in general practice patients (Lee et al., 1991); with mood states (e.g., depression) in patients with cancer (Meek et al., 2000).	Sensitivity to change: Changes in scores observed in patients with cancer during periods of expected high and low levels of fatigue (i.e., around exposure to treatment) (Meek et al., 2000). Sensitivity to nursing: No data available.
Fatigue Symptom Checklist (Yoshitake, 1971, 1978)	Healthy individuals	Drowsiness and dullness (e.g., feeling heavy in the head), difficulty concentrating (e.g., difficulty thinking clearly), and physical discomfort (e.g., back pain); 30 items; patients indicate whether or not they experienced the symptoms.	Self-administered	ICR: No data available. TRR: No data available.	Content: No data available. Construct: difficulty concentrating; scores higher in workers involved in mental work; physical discomfort; scores higher in workers involved in physical work; correlated with measures of fatigue.	Sensitivity to change: No data available. Sensitivity to nursing: No data available.

Table 4.2 (continued)

Instrument (author)	Target population	Domains; number of items; response format	Method of administration	Reliability	Validity	Sensitivity to change and nursing care
Piper Fatigue Scale (PFS) (Piper et al., 1989)	Any patient population	Temporal, affective, sensory, and severity; 76 items in original version and 41 or 24 in revised, shorter versions; VAS.	Self-administered	ICR: α of .69 and .95 for subscales; .85 for total scale (Berger & Walker, 2001; Piper et al., 1989). TRR: Not tested.	Content: rated as relevant by experts; dimensions supported by results of cluster analysis. Construct: correlated with POMS subscales and Fatigue Symptom Checklist.	Sensitivity to change: No data available. Sensitivity to nursing: No data available.
Multidimensional Fatigue Inventory (MFI) (Smets et al., 1995)	Patients with various chronic conditions	General, physical, and mental fatigue, reduced motivation, and reduced activity; 20 items; five boxes aligned horizontally and anchored with "Yes, that is true" and "No, that is not true."	Self-administered	ICR: α of .53 to .94 for subscales in patients with cancer receiving radiotherapy, patients with chronic fatigue syndrome, psychology and medical students, and army recruits (Meek et al., 2000; Smets et al., 1996). TRR: r of .50 to .72 (Meek et al., 2000).	Content: derived from a literature review and patient interviews. Factorial structure: hypothesized five factors reported in various client populations (Meek et al., 2000; Smets et al., 1996). Construct: correlated with VAS of fatigue; with measures of mood, ADLs, and emotional distress; discriminated between patients with different levels of fatigue, and between medically ill patients and healthy persons with fatigue (Meek et al., 2000; Smets et al., 1996).	Sensitivity to change: significant changes in subscale scores between times of high and low fatigue associated with exposure to cancer treatment (Meek et al., 2000). Sensitivity to nursing: No data available.

Table 4.2 (continued)

Instrument (author)	Target population	Domains; number of items; response format	Method of administration	Reliability	Validity	Sensitivity to change and nursing care
Multidimensional Assessment of Fatigue (MAF) (Belza et al., 1993)	Patients with arthritis, chronic pulmonary disease, and cancer	Severity, frequency, distress, and interference with ADLs; 16 items; 10-point numeric rating scale.	Self-administered	ICR: α of .88 to .93 for total scale in patients with various conditions (Belza, 1995; Belza et al., 1993; Meek et al, 2000); .88 in rural patients with cancer (Winstead-Fry, 1998). TRR: *r* of .74 to .87 for total scale.	Content: No data available. Factorial structure: two factors, as hyppothesized (Meek et al., 2000). Construct: correlated with other measures of fatigue, anxiety and depression (Belza, 1995; Meek et al., 2000; Winstead-Fry, 1998).	Sensitivity to change: Changes in scores observed during times of high and low fatigue experienced with cancer therapy (Meek et al., 2000). Sensitivity to nursing: No data available.

r = correlation coefficient
α = Cronbach's alpha coefficient
ICR = Internal Consistency Reliability
TRR = Test Re-test Reliability
IRR = Inter-Rater Reliability
SC = Self-Care
CVI = Content Validity Index
GI = Gastro-Intestinal
MS = Multiple Sclerosis
SLE = Systemic Lupus Erythematosus
ADLs = Activities of Daily Living

Single-item measures

Fatigue has been recognized as a symptom associated with physical illness and its treatment, and with psychological disturbances. The interest in assessing this symptom prompted researchers and clinicians to develop single items that capture the patients' perception of fatigue. Two types of single items measuring fatigue were found in the literature: (a) those embedded within scales, and (b) those standing alone as distinct measures.

Single items embedded within scales

Single items measuring fatigue were incorporated in multi-item scales designed to measure general health conditions or quality of life, or in checklists developed to assess symptoms experienced by patients. These scales and checklists are numerous. An exhaustive review of such tools is beyond the scope of this review; however, some examples are provided for illustration.

Examples of scales measuring general health conditions and incorporating a single item to assess fatigue are:

- Self-report instruments of depression, such as the Beck Depression Inventory (Beck & Beck, 1972) and the Hamilton Depression Scale (Schutte & Malouf, 1995)

- Instruments that measure quality of life in patients with cancer, such as the Quality of Life–Cancer Survivors Version (Ferrell et al., 1995) and the Functional Assessment of Cancer Therapy–General Version (Cella et al., 1993)

Examples of symptom checklists including a single item to assess fatigue are:

- Symptom Checklist (SCL-90) (Derogatis, 1994)

- Brief Symptom Inventory (Derogatis, 1993)

- Rotterdam Symptom Checklist (de Haes et al., 1990)

- Symptom Distress Scale (McCorkle & Young, 1978)

- Self-Care Diary (Nail et al., 1991), which assesses the incidence and severity of side effects experienced by patients receiving chemotherapy, and the use and effectiveness of self-care strategies.

The single items embedded within scales or checklists often consist of a term reflecting the symptom of fatigue or a descriptor indicative of fatigue. They inquire about (a) the patients' perception of the symptom's occurrence, with a Yes-No response format; or (b) the patients' perception of the symptom's frequency of occurrence over a specified time frame, with a Likert-type response format with options ranging from *never* to *always*; or (c) the patients' perception of the symptom's severity, with a Likert-type response format with options ranging from *none* to *severe*.

The terms used to describe fatigue in these items differed and included fatigue, tiredness, weakness, lack of energy, and muscle aches. None has been validated as the most accurate reflection of fatigue from the patients' perspective. These terms capture the global experience of fatigue. The items used to quantify fatigue represent only one dimension of the experience, that is, incidence, frequency, or severity. A comprehensive measure of all dimensions may be necessary to adequately assess fatigue, and to guide the evaluation of nursing care effectiveness.

The psychometric properties of these single items could not be evaluated. Therefore, the extent to which they reliably and validly measure fatigue is not known, which renders questionable their use in clinical practice.

Single items standing alone

Since fatigue has been defined as a subjective sensation, some researchers attempted to measure it with single-item scales. Such scales have been useful for assessing the perception of other symptoms, such as pain and dyspnea (Waltz et al., 1991). They capture the individual's perception of the whole phenomenological experience of the symptom.

In most instances, the single-item scales were developed for use in particular research studies (Devlen et al., 1987; Greenberg et al., 1993; Greenberg et al., 1992; Joly et al., 1996; Love et al., 1989; Morant, 1996; Richardson & Ream, 1996). Two single-item scales have been used in more than one study: the Analogue Fatigue Scale (AFS) and the Rhoten Fatigue Scale (RFS, see Table 4.2). The available but limited empirical evidence indicates that the AFS has demonstrated acceptable validity and sensitivity to change, more so than the RFS.

The advantages of these single-item scales relate to their simplicity of use: (a) they can be administered in a very short time period (about one minute), which is suitable for fatigued or sick patients; (b) they are easy to administer (that is, they do not require special instructions or training for using them); and (c) they do not need a complex scoring system and their scores are easy to interpret. The weaknesses of these scales relate several points. First, the item provides an overall, global rating of fatigue. Second, the respondents' answers to a single item may be unreliable, introducing error; thus, it is difficult to evaluate the reliability of one-item scales. Last, the visual analogue scale (VAS) response format may be difficult to use in some patient populations, including children and elders; the VAS reproduction may be inaccurate; and their scoring may be cumbersome, especially if respondents did not precisely follow the instructions for indicating their fatigue level.

Multiple-item, unidimensional instruments

Multiple-item instruments were developed in an attempt to overcome the weaknesses of single-item measures of fatigue: incorporating multiple items improves reliability of measurement. Some of these instruments formed subscales embedded within instruments measuring general conditions or quality of life, whereas others formed separate, independent tools.

Unidimensional subscales embedded in general instruments

Two unidimensional subscales embedded within general instruments were found to measure the symptom of fatigue. The subscales were in the European Organization for Research and Treatment of Cancer Quality of Life Questionnaire (EORTC-QLQ) and the Profile of Mood States (POMS, see Table 4.2). Both measure the severity of fatigue. The EORTC-QLQ fatigue subscale has been used to assess fatigue in patients with cancer. It is reliable, valid, and sensitive to change. The POMS fatigue subscale is well established and has shown reliability, validity, and sensitivity to change in various patient populations.

Unidimensional, independent instruments

Four independent, unidimensional instruments measuring fatigue are reviewed in Table 4.2. These include the Pearson-Byars Fatigue Feeling Checklist (PBFFCL), the Fatigue Severity Scale (FSS), the Composite Measure of Fatigue, and the Fatigue Questionnaire (FQ). Most of these measures were developed for and tested with patients with chronic fatigue syndrome and with surgical patients. Their psychometric properties were evaluated in only one study. They require further testing before their utility in measuring fatigue in clinical practice can be determined. The PBFFCL has been used in different patient populations, and has demonstrated acceptable reliability, validity, and sensitivity to change. Its content, however, may not be relevant in today's social and healthcare systems.

Multiple-item, multidimensional scales

An increasing number of recently developed multi-item, multidimensional scales measuring fatigue has been appearing in the literature. A total of 12 tools were reported and reviewed in Table 4.2.

In addition to the 12 scales reviewed in Table 4.2, three multidimensional tools were recently developed to measure fatigue in patients with cancer. Glaus and colleagues (1996) designed the Fatigue Assessment Questionnaire to measure three dimensions of the subjective experience of fatigue: physical, affective, and cognitive. Minimal details describing the scoring method are available. Although its initial reliability was supported, no data on its validity was reported. The Cancer Fatigue Scale, developed by Schwartz (1997), assesses the physical, emotional, cognitive, and temporal dimensions of fatigue. No information on its scaling and scoring methods was published. It demonstrated initial reliability. Meek, Nail, & Jones (1997) designed the General Fatigue Scale to capture the pattern, general intensity, distress, and impact of fatigue. A 10-point rating scale, anchored by *no* and *greatest possible fatigue,* was used. It demonstrated initial reliability and validity. These three measures should be further tested before their clinical utility is evaluated.

The multidimensional measures of fatigue assess the subjective perception of this symptom, which is consistent with it conceptualization. They cover slightly different dimensions of the fatigue experience. The physical dimension is the most frequently included. Some instruments incorporate items reflecting mental fatigue. None of the tools cover all five dimensions of fatigue identified earlier. All instruments assess the severity of fatigue, and a few assess its frequency. The interest in measuring its impact on everyday functioning led scholars to measure this aspect of the fatigue experience as well.

The evidence of the instruments' psychometric properties is based on the results of the initial testing of the tools. Investigators who used the tools in subsequent studies did not report additional testing of their properties. The MFI and PFS are exceptions, since they were validated in large samples of various clinical and healthy populations, which improves the precision of the estimates. The instruments showed acceptable initial reliability, validity, and acceptability by different patient populations. However, some may be long, which may increase the response burden for patients who already experience fatigue.

4.5.3 *Recommendations for Measuring Fatigue*

The decision about which fatigue instrument to use depends on the purpose of the clinical assessment as well as on the instrument's psychometric properties, and on the characteristics of the patient population. Unidimensional and single-item scales could be used to monitor the severity of fatigue and to evaluate how effective the interventions are in relieving this symptom. Unidimensional scales offer respondents different descriptors of fatigue from which they could choose the one that best describes their experience. A single, global measure of fatigue provides information on the patients' overall perception of the symptom severity, with minimal response burden. Such a measure of fatigue is similar to the one used for assessing pain and other symptoms in clinical practice. Nonetheless, it does not indicate which specific dimension of the fatigue experience is affected. Multidimensional scales present an accurate operationalization of fatigue. They are useful for comprehensively assessing the patients' experience of fatigue, which is helpful for planning care and evaluating its effectiveness.

4.5.4 *Sensitivity to Nursing Care*

The distressing and debilitating experience of fatigue prompted researchers to investigate interventions that could be useful in relieving this symptom. Most of the studies were conducted with patients with cancer who were receiving therapy, as fatigue is most frequently reported in this patient population.

A large number of the studies found were descriptive, aimed at identifying self-initiated strategies for managing fatigue. These strategies included the following:

- Alteration of activity and rest pattern, such as resting and napping, taking things easy, modifying usual activities, and walking or exercising.

- Alteration in sleep and wake pattern, such as going to bed early and taking naps during the day.

- Diversional activities, such as listening to relaxation tapes, listening to music, reading, and watching TV.

- Alternative therapies, such as taking homeopathic remedies and acupuncture.

- Social activities, such as engaging in hobbies, going to movies, and having dinner with family and friends.

- Preservation of normality, such as doing housework, going shopping, and cooking (Dodd, 1984; Graydon et al., 1995; Jamar. 1989; Nail et al., 1991; Richardson & Ream, 1997; Ream & Richardson, 1999)

The studies generally found that the self-initiated strategies were moderately effective in relieving fatigue (Graydon et al., 1997).

Four types of interventions were evaluated for their effectiveness in relieving fatigue in patients with cancer: relaxation, education or psychoeducation, exercise, and attention-restoring activities. The studies are reviewed briefly here:

- Relaxation: Decker, Cline-Elsen, & Gallagher (1992) examined the impact of stress reduction, given in the form of progressive muscle relation and imagery, on fatigue. The design was experimental; patients were randomly assigned to the experimental (i.e., received muscle relaxation and imagery) or the control group. Patients ($n = 82$) with cancer undergoing curative or palliative radiation therapy were included. Fatigue was measured with the POMS-Fatigue subscale at pre- and posttest. Patients in the experimental group experienced no significant change in the level of fatigue, whereas those in the control group showed a significant increase from pre- to posttest. The results indicate that relaxation training may prevent patients from experiencing worsening levels of fatigue during the course of radiation therapy.

- Education or psychoeducation: This type of intervention included (a) providing patients with educational materials about fatigue and its management in addition to six hours of individualized teaching and instruction in progressive muscle relaxation (Fawzy, 1995), and (b) a group education intervention that involved 7–10 patients who met for 1.5 hours a week for six consecutive weeks; the discussion focused on general health education, stress management, problem solving, and psychological support (Fawzy et al., 1990). The participants were randomly assigned to the experimental or the control group. They included patients with Stage 1 or 2 malignant melanoma. The sample sizes were adequate for this type of design (n = 66 and 62, respectively). Fatigue was measured with the POMS-Fatigue subscales. Measurements were obtained before and after treatment completion, with one to two follow-ups. Patients who received the intervention reported a decrease in the severity of fatigue experienced immediately after the intervention; the relief was more significant at follow-up.

- Exercise: The benefits of exercise were examined in two studies involving patients with cancer who were receiving adjuvant therapy. The exercise consisted of (a) a program of walking and a support group delivered throughout the course of chemotherapy (Mock et al., 1994), and (b) a 10-week program of walking (Graydon et al., 1999). The design was experimental with repeated measures in the first study; and pre-experimental, involving one group with repeated measures, in the second study. The sample sizes were 14 and 70, respectively. Fatigue was measured with different self-report tools. Mock et al. reported that women with breast cancer who participated in the program experienced less fatigue at program completion than those who received the usual care. Graydon et al. (1999) found no significant change in the level of fatigue severity over time. The inconsistent findings could be explained by the differences in the research design, nature of the walking program, measures of fatigue, or sample size. In both studies, the attrition rate was rather high, implying that exercise may not be well tolerated by patients with cancer.

- Attention-restoring activities: Cimprich (1993) explored the effects of an intervention on attentional fatigue in women who had surgery for breast cancer. Women were randomly assigned to the experimental (n = 16) or the control group (n = 16). Women in the experimental group engaged in restorative activities (e.g., walking in nature, gardening) for 20–30 minutes three times a week. Attentional capacity was measured 3, 18, 60, and 90 days post-surgery. Significant improvement in attentional capacity was observed in the experimental group over time. However, the small sample size and the initial group non-equivalence present threats to the validity of conclusions.

The results of the studies reviewed here provide initial evidence of the effectiveness of some nursing interventions in managing fatigue in patients with cancer. The beneficial effects of educational interventions were consistent, but cannot be generalized to different patient populations. The evidence suggests that fatigue is potentially responsive to nursing care; however, additional research is needed.

4.6 Nausea and Vomiting

Nausea and vomiting are symptoms that tend to co-occur. They are reported by women in their first trimester of pregnancy and are also experienced in a variety of acute and chronic medical conditions, as well as post-surgery. For instance, nausea and vomiting are experienced with food indigestion, food poisoning, acute inflammation/infection or obstruction of the gastro-intestinal system, and some fluid and electrolytes imbalances that are caused by a disease or dialysis. Nausea and vomiting also have been reported in a few psychological conditions, particularly in patients who use somatization as a coping mechanism. Some patients may experience these symptoms following surgery, depending on the anesthetic agent used. Nausea and vomiting are most frequently reported by patients with cancer receiving chemotherapy. These two symptoms, along with fatigue, have been of primary concern and, consequently, have been extensively studied in this patient population. Most studies have aimed at examining the frequency and pattern of their occurrence, as well as at evaluating the effectiveness of pharmacological and non-medical interventions in relieving nausea and vomiting. Therefore, the following discussion draws primarily on the empirical evidence gathered across studies involving patients with cancer receiving chemotherapy. The discussion focuses on (a) defining these symptoms, (b) assessing the psychometric properties and clinical utility of available measures, and (c) determining the extent to which independent nursing interventions that are non-pharmacological in nature are effective in relieving nausea and vomiting.

4.6.1 Theoretical Background

Almost none of the sources reviewed provided a theoretical or conceptual definition of nausea and vomiting, which limited the operationalization of these two symptoms to single, global items in most empirical studies. Worcester et al. (1991) defined these two symptoms as follows:

- Nausea is a "disagreeable feeling experienced in the back of the throat (epigastrium), and generally culminating in vomiting. It may be accompanied by pallor, cold clammy skin, increased salivation, faintness, tachycardia, and diarrhea."

- Vomiting is "an involuntary reflex causing the forceful expulsion of the contents of the stomach or intestines. Vomiting is immediately preceded by widespread autonomic stimulation resulting in tachypnea, copious salivation, dilation of the pupils, sweating, pallor, and rapid heart rate."

Essential attributes

These definitions imply that (a) nausea and vomiting tend to co-occur, where nausea precedes vomiting; (b) nausea is a subjective sensation that is felt by the affected individual; and (c) vomiting has a rather objective nature that can be detected by another person, in addition to the affected individual.

Antecedents

The causes of nausea and vomiting vary with the physiological and/or pathological alterations underlying the condition in which they are experienced. The causative factors could be physical/physiological and/or psychological in nature. For instance, in patients with cancer receiving chemotherapy, several factors have been considered as contributing to nausea and vomiting, including the type, number, and dose of chemotherapeutic agent; metastasis to the brain or liver; and the conditioning effects of the exposure to and receipt of chemotherapy. This latter psychological factor has been described as a "classical" conditioning process; that is, through their association with pharmacologically induced side effects, various stimuli (e.g., smells, thoughts, tastes) become capable of eliciting nausea, vomiting, and intense emotional reactions (Burish et al., 1987). The presence of nausea and vomiting in such situations has been referred to as conditioned or anticipatory nausea and vomiting.

Consequences

The consequences of nausea and vomiting are essentially related to nutritional deficits, such as loss of fluid and electrolytes, loss of appetite, and loss of weight. These changes ultimately lead to reduced energy and fatigue, which constrains the person's ability to engage in activities of daily living and in self-care.

4.6.2 *Instruments Measuring Nausea and Vomiting*

As mentioned earlier, single, global items have been frequently used to measure nausea and vomiting in empirical, descriptive-correlational, and experimental studies. In most instances, the items were part of instruments or checklists designed to assess the experience of multiple symptoms, or part of a symptom subscale incorporated in a scale measuring quality of life, as discussed in the first part of this chapter. In a few cases, the single item was used independently.

The term most commonly used to describe nausea in these single items, whether embedded in a multi-item scale or used independently, was the word "nausea." It is a word commonly found in lay persons' language, as well as in medical encounters. The items often assessed the perceived severity or intensity of nausea, using Likert-type response options. The response options selected varied across scales and included the following:

- *Mild, moderate,* or *severe* in the Sign and Symptom Checklist for Persons with HIV disease (Holzemer et al., 1999)

- *None* to *severe* in the instruments measuring the symptoms experienced by patients in palliative care settings that were presented early in this chapter (Edmonds et al., 1998)

- A 100 mm horizontal visual analogue scale (Fainsinger et al., 1991)

- A seven-point numeric rating scale ranging from *none* to *most of the time* in the Symptom Control Assessment (Benor et al., 1998)

- A seven-point rating scale anchored with *not at all* and *extremely* (Burish et al., 1987; Burish & Jenkins, 1992; Burish et al., 1991; Carey & Burish, 1987; Lyles et al., 1982; Vasterling et al., 1993)

A few scales were designed to assess the distress associated with nausea. The response options used were:

- A five-point Likert scale in the Symptom Distress Scale (Rhodes et al., 1984)

- A five-point numeric rating scale or a 100 mm horizontal visual analogue scale anchored with *not at all* and *very much so* in the original and modified versions of the Symptom Distress Scale (McCorkle & Young, 1978)

- A 10-point linear analogue scale with three descriptors ranging from *no change in lifestyle* to *unable to maintain lifestyle* (Tucci & Bartels, 1998)

- A four-point scale including *none; mild,* activity not interfered with; *moderate,* activity interfered with; and *severe,* bedridden with nausea for more than two hours, in the Duke's Descriptive Scale used by Cotanch (1983) and Cotanch & Strum (1987).

Grande et al. (1997) measured the perceived difficulty in controlling nausea with a five-point scale ranging from *not at all difficult* to *very difficult.*

The term most commonly used to describe vomiting in the single or multi-item scales mentioned earlier was the word "vomiting," which is again in common use. The same response options were used to assess the severity and distress of vomiting. The Duke's Descriptive Scale was the exception. The four grades to assess vomiting used in this scale were (a) no vomiting 24 hours after chemotherapy; (b) mild: vomiting less than five times within 24 hours after chemotherapy; (c) moderate: 5–10 times within 24 hours after chemotherapy; and (d) severe: greater than 10 times within 24 hours, patient bedridden, possible dehydration (Cotanch, 1983; Cotanch & Strum, 1987). In addition to these dimensions, the frequency of vomiting (i.e., the reported number of vomiting episodes) was assessed in a few instances (e.g., Tucci & Bartels, 1998).

Three multi-item instruments measuring nausea and vomiting were reported in the literature reviewed. Two were used in studies evaluating psychological-behavioral interventions for managing anticipatory nausea and vomiting in patients with cancer who were receiving chemotherapy. These two measures were not used in nursing research; therefore, they will be mentioned only briefly.

The first of these two measures, the Morrow Assessment of Nausea and Vomiting, contains items assessing the frequency, severity, and duration of nausea and vomiting before and after receiving chemotherapy (Morrow, 1982; Morrow & Morrell, 1982). The second instrument, referred to as the Patient Postchemotherapy Nausea and Vomiting Rating Form, was developed by Gard, Edwards, Harris, & McCormack (1988) and modeled after Morrow's assessment form. It contains five items assessing the severity, as well as the frequency and duration, of nausea and vomiting with a semantic differential scale anchored with *very mild* and *intolerable*.

The third multi-item instrument, the Rhodes Index of Nausea and Vomiting (INV-Form 2), was reported and published by Worcester et al. (1991). These authors described it as an outcome measure assessing the occurrence of nausea and vomiting and their perceived intensity and distress. Lay terms were used to describe nausea (sick at my stomach) and vomiting (throw up), which represents an advantage over the previously reviewed measures of these symptoms. The instrument consists of eight items. Each item assesses one dimension of a symptom. That is, one item inquires about the frequency, one about the severity, and one about the distress of nausea and vomiting. Two of the items ask about the frequency and distress of retching. Descriptive statements are provided to reflect varying degrees of frequency, severity, and distress, and the respondents are asked to circle the statement that most clearly corresponds to their experience. The scoring method was not described. No additional source describing this measure was found.

The psychometric properties of the single, global items measuring nausea and vomiting were not evaluated or reported in any of the sources included in this review. While it may be difficult to examine these properties for items incorporated in multi-item instruments, it is possible to examine the validity and sensitivity to change of independent single measures of subjective sensations, as has been reported for single-item indicators of fatigue and dyspnea. Youngblut and Casper (1993) reviewed the psychometric properties of single-item indicators, which are being used increasingly in clinical research to evaluate symptom experience. They concluded that (a) the test-retest reliability of these measures could not be established due to the changing nature of the symptoms experienced; (b) these measures provide a global rating of the phenomenon of interest that has been shown to be valid; and (c) the single, global items were able to detect change over time. Despite these possibilities, single global measures of nausea and vomiting have not been validated. However, they demand minimal burden and time on the part of the respondent when completing them, and they have been used in practice. Therefore, they are clinically useful. Providing descriptors of nausea and vomiting in lay terms will further enhance the clinical utility of these measures, ensuring understanding by, and applicability to, various client populations.

The reliability, validity, and sensitivity to change of the multi-item measures of nausea and vomiting have not been reported. These measures address several dimensions of these symptoms; that is, frequency, intensity, and distress, which gives a comprehensive assessment of the symptom experience. Such an assessment may be useful in understanding the symptom experience and in guiding care planning. The Rhodes INV-Form 2 may be of limited clinical relevance because of the length and complexity of the descriptive statements used. It requires the respondents to have an acceptable reading and comprehension ability, to concentrate, and to compare and contrast the statements before selecting the most appropriate response. These abilities may be limited in patients with chronic illness.

4.6.3 *Recommendations for Measuring Nausea and Vomiting*

From this discussion of the measurement of nausea and vomiting, the use of single, global items assessing the frequency, intensity, and/or distress of these symptoms is recommended for clinical practice. The items should contain lay terms to describe the symptoms and simple numeric scales to quantify the experience (similar to those used to quantify pain). Further validation of these single measures is also needed before their widespread use in everyday practice.

4.6.4 *Sensitivity to Nursing Care*

A variety of independent nursing interventions have been suggested to relieve nausea and vomiting. Most are based on clinical experience or trial and error, and few have been systematically investigated. In addition to administering anti-emetics as prescribed, the following categories of interventions were mentioned:

- Changing the types of food and fluid offered to patients, the amounts taken at any one time, and the frequency of eating (e.g., small frequent meals, dry food, clear fluids)

- Maintaining cleanliness, both personal and environmental

- Encouraging rest periods before and after meals

- Creating pleasant settings around meal time (i.e., preventing strong odors, exposure to fresh air, involving family members)

- Introducing psychological measures, which include relaxation, guided imagery, and distraction such as watching TV, talking, reading, and socializing with the affected person during mealtime (Worcester et al., 1991)

Of these interventions, relaxation and guided imagery have been investigated, primarily in patients with cancer receiving chemotherapy (e.g., Carty, as cited in Smith et al., 1994; Cotanch, 1983; Cotanch et al., 1985; Cotanch & Strum, 1987; Lerman et al., 1990; Scott et al., 1986). Systematic reviews of the effectiveness of these interventions were also conducted. Smith et al. (1994) found that five types of interventions were used to relieve nausea and vomiting in patients with cancer: (a) medication, that is, anti-emetic use (examined in two studies); (b) aerobic exercises (one study); (c) self-hypnosis (one study); (d) relaxation (four studies); and (e) use of ginger in the form of capsules (one study). The effect sizes were as follows: (a) for medication/anti-emetic use, .45–.87; (b) for aerobic exercises, .45; (c) for self-hypnosis, .69; (d) for relaxation, .23–.36 (note: in one study, the reported effect size was –7.39, which is considered an outlier and excluded from further discussion); and (e) for use of ginger, .17. Although the observed effects were positive, implying that all types of interventions were effective in relieving nausea and vomiting, relaxation and the use of ginger had weaker effects than aerobic exercise, self-hypnosis, and medication. Sanzero Eller (1999) conducted a qualitative review of the effects of guided imagery without relaxation on diverse physical and psychological symptoms in adult patients. She reported the results of six studies in which guided imagery was used to relieve anticipatory nausea and vomiting in patients receiving chemotherapy. Guided imagery was implemented by trained psychologists. In all six studies, the intervention was effective in reducing the aversive impact of nausea and vomiting. Similar results were reported by Van Fleet (2000), who also observed that guided imagery is more effective than relaxation in relieving nausea and vomiting.

It should be noted that symptom management appeared to be a component of some psychoeducational interventions that nurses delivered to patients with cancer who were receiving adjuvant therapy (e.g., Benor et al., 1998; Dodd, 1983; Johnson et al., 1997). Symptom distress and the number of symptoms/side effects of chemotherapy or radiation therapy experienced were measured as indicators of the interventions' effectiveness. The results of these studies supported the effectiveness of the interventions in alleviating symptom distress. There is no clear indication of the extent to which psychoeducational interventions addressed strategies to manage nausea and vomiting, nor of how successful they were in relieving these symptoms. However, the instruments used to measure symptom distress have incorporated items assessing nausea and vomiting. Instructing patients about such strategies may be effective in assisting them to manage these symptoms.

The empirical evidence provided in this review indicates that various interventions have shown initial effectiveness in relieving nausea and vomiting, primarily in patients receiving chemotherapy. Although valid, the evidence is not adequate for making any final recommendations. But it suggests that moderate relief of nausea and vomiting can be achieved with some interventions, such as guided imagery and patient education. Using anti-emetics seems to have the strongest effect. Further investigations in clinical settings with different patient populations are needed.

4.7   Dyspnea

The terms "dyspnea" and "breathlessness" have been used interchangeably in the literature, despite their description as two symptoms that differ in the nature of the sensation. Dyspnea involves an unpleasant sensation of difficult or labored breathing. It is this uncomfortable feeling that distinguishes dyspnea from breathlessness. Breathlessness is normally experienced as increased breathing by healthy individuals following excessive exercise. It is relieved soon after the activity is stopped and/or with rest (Carrieri & Janson-Bjerklie, 1986). The uncomfortable sensation that characterizes dyspnea has been described as chest tightness, inability to move air, and increased effort in the act of breathing, culminating in a feeling of suffocation (Carrieri & Janson-Bjerklie, 1986; Mahler, 1990). The uncomfortable sensation interferes with the person's ability to carry out any physical activity (Rosser & Guz, 1981) and leads to an emotional response to the symptom that is often characterized by fear and anxiety (Clark et al., 1985; Dudley et al., 1980). Dyspnea requires prompt relief, which makes this symptom one of primary concern to health care providers.

In this section, a review of the conceptualization and the measurement of dyspnea will be followed by a summary of the results of studies that investigated the effectiveness of interventions in managing this symptom, in an attempt to determine the extent to which it is sensitive to nursing care. Dyspnea can be experienced by patients with various acute conditions, such as pneumonia and injury to the chest. It is, however, most frequently reported by patients with (a) chronic respiratory diseases, such as asthma, and chronic obstructive pulmonary diseases; (b) chronic cardiac diseases, such as congestive heart failure; and (c) end-stage lung cancer, lung metastasis, or HIV. Dyspnea has been studied in patients with chronic respiratory diseases, cardiac diseases, and lung cancer. Therefore, the sources included in this review are drawn from this pool of research.

4.7.1   Theoretical Background

Essential attributes

Dyspnea is the subjective experience of difficult or labored breathing (Altose, 1985; Carrieri & Janson-Bjerklie, 1986; Gift et al., 1986; Mahler, 1990; McCord & Cronin-Stubbs, 1992). The sensations that characterize dyspnea have been described in the following terms, obtained through clinical observations and studies of patients' description of dyspnea:

- Uncomfortable sensation arising from the chest or lungs; an inability to get in enough air or chest tightness and congestion (Mahler, 1990)

- Difficult, labored, uncomfortable breathing; unpleasant breathing (McCord & Cronin-Stubbs, 1992)

- Hard to breathe, short of breath, shallow breathing and needing air; hard to move air; feeling of suffocation or smothering; tightness in the chest (Carrieri & Janson-Bjerklie, 1986)

- Tightness in the chest, feeling smothered, being out of breath, and needing more air (Worcester et al., 1991)

- Chest tightness, suffocation, not getting enough air, choking, and smothering (McCarley, 1999)

Carrieri and Janson-Bjerklie (1986) reported that 97% of patients interviewed described dyspnea as "I just feel short of breath—there is no other way to say it." The term "short of breath" has been frequently used to refer to the experience of dyspnea in clinical assessment and in instruments used to measure this concept in research studies.

As a subjective sensation, dyspnea is conceptualized as involving the actual sensation of shortness of breath, the perception of that sensation, and the individual's reaction to the sensation (Gift, 1990; Lush et al., 1988; Mahler, 1990; Nield, Kim, & Patel, 1989). The actual sensation refers to the awareness of the physiological change; that is, shortness of breath, which characterizes the symptom of dyspnea. Perception involves interpreting the sensation experienced, and the reaction to the sensation consists of the physiological, behavioral, and emotional responses exhibited by the person in relation to the symptom. The physiological responses to dyspnea include an increase in respiratory rate, a change in the depth of breathing, and use of accessory muscles (McCord & Cronin-Stubbs, 1992), as well as diaphoresis and fatigue (Carrieri & Janson-Bjerklie, 1986). The behavioral responses entail restlessness and changes in position, as well as movement or activity, in an attempt to provide an immediate relief to this distressing symptom. The emotional response most frequently observed is fear and anxiety (Carrieri & Janson-Bjerklie, 1986; Mahler, 1990).

Some objective indicators have been proposed to accompany dyspnea, including audible labored breathing, dilated nostrils, protrusion of the abdomen, expanded chest, gasping, rapid respiratory rate, irregular respiration, use of accessory muscles, open mouth or pursed-lips breathing, cough, impaired voice or speech, facial flushing or pallor, decreased breath sounds, wheezing, and changes in respiratory volumes/spirometry (Carrieri & Janson-Bjerklie, 1986;

Mahler et al., 1984; Worcester et al., 1991). It should be emphasized that no consistent relationship was found between the physiological changes associated with dyspnea and the subjective perception and/or evaluation of the symptom. That is, the perceived severity of dyspnea did not correlate with the alterations in respiration (e.g., respiratory rate, FEV1, PaO2) that accompany dyspnea (Gift et al., 1986; Mahler, 1990; van der Molen, 1995). This finding implies that the assessment of dyspnea should be subjective.

Antecedents

Although the exact mechanisms causing dyspnea are not clear, several factors have been suggested to have an influence on the perception of, and the response and reaction to, this symptom. These antecedent factors have been organized into the following categories:

- Physiological: an increased demand for oxygen; type, duration, and frequency of dyspneic attacks (i.e., the perception of dyspnea may decline with prolonged and repeated exposure to the stimulus triggering the symptom, or to repeated experience of the symptom) (Altose, 1985; Janson-Bjerklie et al., 1986; McCord & Cronin-Stubbs, 1992).

- Demographic: age (i.e., younger persons perceive dyspnea more intensely than older persons) (Gottfried et al., 1981; Janson-Bjerklie et al., 1986; Mahler, 1990); gender (i.e., women were found to report more dyspnea than men, especially among those with asthma) (Janson-Bjerklie et al., 1986); sociocultural orientation and beliefs, as well as life experiences, which influence the identification and interpretation of sensations and symptoms (Mahler, 1990; McCord & Cronin-Stubbs, 1992).

- Environmental: factors such as smoke, pollutants, temperature changes, and stress (Mahler, 1990; McCord & Cronin-Stubbs, 1992).

- Psychological/emotional: cognitive status and emotional disturbances such as stress, anger, depression, and anxiety. Of these factors, anxiety has been consistently found to relate to dyspnea, creating a vicious circle where anxiety leads to dyspnea and dyspnea leads to anxiety (Altose, 1985; Clark et al., 1985; Gift, 1990; Gift & Cahill, 1990; Gift et al., 1986; McCarley, 1999).

Consequences

The experience of dyspnea is debilitating because it interferes with people's physical and psychological functioning. Difficult breathing causes people to stop the activity in which they were engaged when it was felt. Patients experiencing frequent dyspnea may limit the amount of activity in which they engage in their daily lives, which may affect their ability to perform activities of daily living and self-care (Haas et al., 1993). Difficult breathing results in tension and apprehension or anxiety (Clark et al., 1985). Chronic dyspnea results in fatigue (McCarley, 1999).

In summary, dyspnea is a subjective sensation. Although it may be associated with changes in respiration that could be observed by another person, the relationship between dyspnea's subjective and objective indicators has not been supported empirically. Just like other symptoms (e.g., pain, fatigue, and nausea), dyspnea is best assessed by self-report measures.

4.7.2 Instruments Measuring Dyspnea

Dyspnea is a symptom that is of interest and has been investigated by healthcare professionals from different backgrounds. Differences in professional focus led to differences in the approaches used to measure dyspnea. Three general approaches that were reported in the literature—psychophysics, dyspnea and activity, and experience of dyspnea—will be reviewed briefly next:

- Psychophysics: In this approach, a psychophysical technique is used to measure the perceived intensity of a sensation produced by a range of physical stimuli presented with varying intensity. This technique is based on Stevens' power law stating that the perceived magnitude of the stimulus is a direct function of its actual intensity, implying that changes in stimulus intensity produce proportional changes in perceived magnitude (Killian, 1985; Mahler, 1990; Nield et al., 1989; van der Molen, 1995). Magnitude estimation is one psychophysical technique that has been applied, primarily in laboratory settings, to study the sensation of dyspnea. External resistive loads, with varying intensity, are added. The person is asked to estimate the magnitude of the resistive loads on a rating scale. The scale could range from 0 to 10 (e.g., modified Borg scale) or from 0 to 100 (e.g., visual analogue scale). The relationship between the intensity of the added resistive load and the magnitude of the dyspnea is then examined. The results of psychophysical studies have supported the relationship between perceived dyspnea and airflow obstruction/effort of breathing (e.g., Killian, 1985; Mahler et al., 1987; Nield et al., 1989). Although this approach was useful in clarifying the relationship of perceived dyspnea to changes in pulmonary function parameters, its application in everyday nursing practice is of limited clinical utility. Such assessment requires (a) intensive training in the use of equipment, administering tests, and interpreting results; (b) availability of specialized equipment and time to conduct the tests; and (c) willingness and effort on the part of patients. It increases the burden on nurses and patients, especially if it is to be performed on repeated occasions. This approach to assessing dyspnea was not designed for and cannot be used as a means for evaluating effectiveness of care.

- Dyspnea and activity: In this approach, dyspnea is assessed in relation to physical activity (Brown, 1985). It is often used in rehabilitation to determine the level of activity at which the patient experiences difficulty breathing for diagnostic and evaluative purposes. The assessment is done either retrospectively, by asking the person to indicate the type of activities that induce dyspnea (e.g., Medical Research Council's questionnaire, Oxygen-Cost questionnaire, American Thoracic Society Dyspnea Scale, Baseline Dyspnea Index, Transition Dyspnea Index, Part 2 of the Shortness of Breath Assessment Tool) or prospectively, by asking the person to engage in physical activity and to report about shortness of breath before, during, and/or after its performance. The physical activity often selected is walking at the person's own pace (e.g., six- or 12-minute walk test, which is frequently used with patients with COPD). Various self-report scales could be used in this approach to assessing dyspnea; however, the Borg scale was commonly used. This approach to assessing dyspnea has been used in nursing research. It is also employed in clinical practice, particularly in respiratory care clinics or rehabilitation settings.

- Experience of dyspnea: In this approach, dyspnea as experienced by patients is assessed, regardless of its association with physical activity. The most frequently measured dimensions of dyspnea are its intensity or severity and its impact. Patients are often asked to rate their current experience (today or past few days). This approach has been used in research and in clinical practice to explore the patients' view and status, and to evaluate the effectiveness of care.

The scales that have been used to identify the activities that induce or are associated with dyspnea and the instruments that capture the experience of dyspnea will be reviewed separately.

Scales measuring activities associated with dyspnea

The scales measuring activities associated with dyspnea are: the Modified Medical Research Council's Scale, the Oxygen Cost Diagram Scale, the American Thoracic Society Dyspnea Scale, the Dyspnea Index, and the Shortness of Breath Assessment Tool (see Table 4.3). Of these scales, the Medical Research Council's Scale and the Dyspnea Index seem promising as reliable and valid measures of activities associated with the perception of dyspnea. They, however, do not assess the perceived severity of this symptom. They could be useful in rehabilitation care. Although they demonstrated initial sensitivity to change, they have not been used extensively in treatment effectiveness research. Their ability to detect changes in dyspnea experience in response to treatment needs further investigation.

Scales measuring the experience of dyspnea

Three scales measuring dyspnea that are described in Table 4.3 are the Modified Borg Scale, the Visual Analogue Scale (VAS), and the Descriptors of Breathlessness. In addition to these, two subscales incorporated in multidimensional instruments were found to measure dyspnea: the dyspnea subscale in the Bronchitis-Emphysema Symptom Checklist, or BESC (Kinsman et al., 1983), and a subscale in the Chronic Respiratory Disease Questionnaire, or CRD (Guyatt et al., 1987). Examples of items in the BESC dyspnea subscale include the following: feel like I need air, hard to breathe, shallow breathing, short of breath, and gasping for breath. These are different subjective descriptors of the sensation of dyspnea, as identified through clinical observations and descriptive studies. Limited data were available about the psychometric properties of the subscales; however, the reviewed evidence supports the reliability and validity of the BESC, and provides initial support for those of the CRD (McCord & Cronin-Stubbs, 1992). A measure that contains multiple descriptors of dyspnea is clinically useful if the nature of this symptom varies across patient populations. Further investigation is needed to determine the BESC's and CRD's sensitivity to change.

Several symptom checklists presented earlier in the chapter include items measuring the severity of dyspnea, such as the Signs and Symptoms Checklist–HIV (Holzemer et al., 1999) and the Palliative Care or Support Team Assessment Schedule (Edmonds et al., 1998).

4.7.3 Recommendations for Measuring Dyspnea

Of the scales reviewed, the Borg scale and the vertical VAS have been well validated. They have shown sensitivity to changes in the level of perceived dyspnea, which makes them useful to monitor changes associated with progression of the illness condition or with treatment. They are simple to use with various patient populations, and they are quick and easy to administer in clinical practice. The Borg scale could be used to assess dyspnea in relation to physical activity in rehabilitation programs, where it has been commonly applied. The vertical VAS could be used to assess this subjective sensation under any condition, such as following treatment. The VAS, in general, has demonstrated ability to detect small changes; however, the reproduction of the 100 mm line should be carefully monitored. Printing and photocopying it may alter its length.

4.7.4 Sensitivity to Nursing Care

The uncomfortable and distressing nature of dyspnea requires prompt relief. Furthermore, the multidimensionality of the dyspnea experience necessitates a comprehensive management that addresses its physiological and psychological

Table 4.3. Instruments Measuring Dyspnea

Scales measuring activities associated with dyspnea

Instrument (author)	Target population	Domains; number of items; response format	Method of administration	Reliability	Validity	Sensitivity to change and nursing care
Modified Medical Research Council's Scale (Fletcher et al., 1959)	Patients experiencing dyspnea (e.g., patients with cardiac or pulmonary disorders)	Incremental grades of breathlessness experienced with physical activities (e.g., hurrying and walking); 5 items; grades range from 0 (not troubled with breathlessness) to 4 (too breathless to leave the house).	Self-administered or administered by an interviewer	ICR: Not applicable. TRR: No data available. IRR: acceptable.	Content: derived from previous scales and results of descriptive studies. Construct: correlated with lung function tests, and with other self-reported measures of dyspnea in patients with COPD, asthma, cystic fibrosis, interstitial lung disease, and cardiac diseases (Mahler, 1990; Mahler et al., 1987; Mahler & Wells, 1988; Mahler et al., 1989).	Sensitivity to change: grades are too coarse and may not be sensitive to small changes in the level of dyspnea (McCord & Cronin-Stubbs, 1992; van der Molen, 1995). Sensitivity to nursing: no data available.
Oxygen cost diagram scale (McGavin et al., 1978)	Patients with dyspnea	Activities representing different levels of perceived oxygen demand (e.g., sleeping, walking); unclear number of items; VAS.	Administered by an interviewer	ICR: Not applicable. TRR: No data available. IRR: No data available.	Content: No data available. Construct: No data available.	Sensitivity to change: No data available. Sensitivity to nursing: No data available.
American Thoracic Society Dyspnea scale (American Thoracic Society, 1978)	Patients with dyspnea	Similar in content and format to the Medical Research Council's scale; 5 items; 5-point rating scale.	Self-administered or administered by an interviewer	ICR: Not applicable. TRR: No data available. IRR: No data available.	Content: No data available. Construct: No data available.	Sensitivity to change: No data available. Sensitivity to nursing: No data available.

Table 4.3 (continued)

Instrument (author)	Target population	Domains; number of items; response format	Method of administration	Reliability	Validity	Sensitivity to change and nursing care
Dyspnea Index (Mahler et al., 1984); modified by Stoller et al., 1986)	Patients with dyspnea	Functional impairment, magnitude of task, and magnitude of effort; unclear number of items; Baseline Dyspnea Index measures dyspnea at a single point in time, using a 4-point rating scale, and Transition Dyspnea Index measures changes in dyspnea using a 7-point rating scale.	Administered by an observer	ICR: Not applicable. TRR: No data available. IRR: acceptable (Mahler et al., 1984; 1985; 1987; Mahler & Wells, 1988; Mahler & Harver, 1989).	Content: derived from research and clinical experiences. Construct: acceptable in patients with cardiac and pulmonary diseases (Mahler et al., 1984; 1985; 1987; Mahler & Wells, 1988; Mahler & Harver, 1989).	Sensitivity to change: acceptable (Mahler et al., 1984; 1985; 1987; Mahler & Wells, 1988; Mahler & Harver, 1989). Sensitivity to nursing: No data available.
Shortness of Breath Assessment Tool (Lareau, 1986)	Patients with dyspnea	Dyspnea at the current moment and activities that produce dyspnea (e.g., body/care movement, eating, home and recreational, social activities); 7 items in original, and 91 in revised version; for dyspnea at current moment, 10-point rating scale, and for activities producing dyspnea, 7-point scale.	Self-administered	ICR: No report found. TRR: No report found.	Content: No report found. Concurrent/construct: No report found.	Sensitivity to change: No data available. Sensitivity to nursing: No data available.

Table 4.3 (continued)

Scales measuring the experience of dyspnea

Instrument (author)	Target population	Domains; number of items; response format	Method of administration	Reliability	Validity	Sensitivity to change and nursing care
Modified Borg Scale (Borg, 1982)	Patients with dyspnea	Perceived exertion and effort during exercise and severity of dyspnea; number of items: 1 Response format vertical, 11-point rating scale (0 = not at all, to 10 = maximal)	Self-administered or administered by an interviewer	ICR: Not applicable. TRR: no report found.	Content: derived from Borg's work with exertion (magnitude estimation) Construct: correlated with FEV1 in patients with asthma (Burdon et al., 1982); intensity of physical exercise in patients with COPD (Bernstein et al., 1994), and healthy individuals (Killian, 1985).	Sensitivity to change: change reported following 12-minute walk test and exercise training in patients with COPD (Goldstein et al., 1994; Guyatt et al., 1984). Sensitivity to nursing: change in score following listening to soothing music in patients with COPD (Sidani, 1991).
Visual Analogue Scale (VAS)	Patients with dyspnea	Severity of dyspnea; 1 item; VAS.	Self-administered or administered by an interviewer	ICR: Not applicable. TRR: acceptable in 30 patients with lung cancer (Brown et al., 1986).	Content: maintained by using lay terms to describe the sensation. Construct: horizontal and vertical VAS correlated highly in patients with asthma (Gift, 1989; Gift et al., 1986); VAS correlated with peak expiratory flow rate (Gift et al., 1986); scores differed under different levels of obstruction (Gift, 1989).	Sensitivity to change: not well supported (McCord & Cronin-Stubbs, 1992). Sensitivity to nursing: No data available.

Table 4.3 (continued)

Instrument (author)	Target population	Domains; number of items; response format	Method of administration	Reliability	Validity	Sensitivity to change and nursing care
Descriptors of Breathlessness (Simon et al., as cited in McCord & Cronin-Stubbs, 1992)	Tested on healthy adults	No report on domain and response format found; 19 items.	Self-administered	ICR: acceptable in healthy adults (McCord & Cronin-Stubbs, 1992). TRR: No report found.	Content: No data available. Construct: acceptable (McCord & Cronin-Stubbs, 1992).	Sensitivity: No data available. Sensitivity to nursing: No data available.

r = correlation coefficient
α = Cronbach's alpha coefficient
ICR = Internal Consistency Reliability
TRR = Test Re-test Reliability
IRR = Inter-Rater Reliability
SC = Self-Care
CVI = Content Validity Index
GI = Gastro-Intestinal
MS = Multiple Sclerosis
SLE = Systemic Lupus Erythematosus
ADLs = Activities of Daily Living

aspects. The vicious circle linking dyspnea, anxiety, and decreased physical activity demands innovative strategies to interrupt it effectively (Carrieri-Kohlman et al., 1993). Different interventions have been suggested to relieve dyspnea. Gift (1993) classified the interventions into the following four categories, each of which addresses one aspect of the dyspnea experience:

- Physiological treatments, which are subdivided into pharmacological therapies (e.g., bronchodilator and opioids), positioning (e.g., sitting in an upright position), pursed-lips breathing, and mechanical therapies (e.g., vibration of respiratory muscles).

- Psychological treatments, which are aimed at relieving the anxiety associated with dyspnea. Relaxation, guided imagery, and distraction are examples of this type of intervention.

- Cognitive therapies, such as cognitive reframing with the purpose of altering the cause or interpretation and beliefs about the sensation of dyspnea.

- Rehabilitation, including exercise training to increase tolerance for physical activity, and teaching how to plan activities at a pace that will not precipitate dyspnea. The goal is to maintain engagement in physical, recreational, work, and role-related activities valued by the person, thereby preventing depression and social isolation.

Although nurses may be involved in the implementation of any of these treatments, they especially have taken initiatives in investigating the effectiveness of psychological interventions. However, only a few published studies were found. They were concerned with evaluating different interventions, and they used different subjective and objective indicators of dyspnea. This variability precluded integrating results across the studies, which limited the ability to reach meaningful conclusions and recommendations for practice.

Renfroe (1988) examined the effects of progressive muscle relaxation on dyspnea and anxiety in patients with COPD. Patients ($n = 20$) were randomly assigned to an experimental or a control group. Those in the experimental group were "instructed to tense each muscle group for 5–10 seconds, while inhaling, holding their breath, then relaxing while exhaling completely." (Patients attended four weekly sessions in a laboratory setting, during which they were given the instructions and feedback on their performance. They were asked to practice muscle relaxation once a day, in between sessions. Patients in the control group were instructed to relax in any way they wished. Dyspnea was measured with a VAS. Significant reductions in the level of perceived dyspnea were reported by the experimental group following each session; the reductions were greater in the experimental group than in the control group. Significant decreases in respiratory rate were also observed in the experimental group from the beginning to the end of each session. Similar changes were reported for state anxiety. The experimental control exerted by the investigators was successful in enhancing the internal validity of the study. However, the small sample size and the high rate of refusal to participate (55%) limit the ability to generalize the findings.

Gift, Moore, & Soeken (1992) conducted a randomized clinical trial to determine the effects of progressive muscle relaxation on dyspnea, anxiety, and airway obstruction in patients with COPD. Patients in the experimental group were (a) seated in a comfortable position in the physician's office room; (b) asked, over a total of four sessions, to listen to a pre-recorded tape giving them instructions on how to perform progressive muscle relaxation; and (c) asked to practice muscle relaxation at home while listening to the tape. Twenty-six patients completed all of the sessions, yielding an attrition rate of 24%. Dyspnea was measured with VAS, and airway obstruction with the peak expiratory flow rate (PEFR). Significant group × time interaction effects were reported for dyspnea and anxiety, and for PEFR. Patients in the experimental group showed a decrease in the perceived level of dyspnea and anxiety, and an increase in PEFR over time, more so than the control group. Initial group non-equivalence on anxiety and smoking history, the small sample size, and the observed attrition rate limit the validity of the results.

Moody, Fraser, & Yarandi (1993) evaluated the effectiveness of guided imagery in relieving dyspnea, anxiety, fatigue, and depression, and in enhancing quality of life in patients with chronic bronchitis and emphysema. A one-group design with repeated measures was used. Nineteen patients attended four sessions, one per week. During the sessions, the group of patients was instructed to close their eyes and imagine a scene described with a standard script. The nature of the scene was not depicted. No significant decrease in dyspnea, anxiety, fatigue, and depression was reported, but some improvement in quality of life was observed over the 4-week intervention period. The lack of a control group and of a clear description of the intervention implementation, as well as the small sample size, present threats to the validity of the study conclusions.

Use of distraction, in the form of listening to music, was examined in four studies for its effectiveness in relieving dyspnea and improving respiration. The target population in all of the studies was patients with COPD. The designs were pre-experimental, involving only one group of patients. The samples included a small number of patients (20 to 36). The music was soothing in two studies (McBride et al., 1999; Sidani, 1991) and of moderate tempo in one (Thornby et al., 1995). Dyspnea was measured with the Borg scale or a VAS. Sidani reported a greater reduction in respiratory rate following 20 minutes of resting while listening to music than following 20 minutes of resting only; no significant decrease in perceived dyspnea, measured with the Borg scale, was observed. McBride et al. found that listening to music for 20 minutes while sitting down resulted in decreased levels of perceived dyspnea, measured with the VAS, and perceived anxiety. Thornby et al.'s findings indicated that patients undergoing treadmill exercise testing reported lower levels of perceived dyspnea, walked about 25% longer, and performed 53% more work when listening to moderate-tempo music than when listening to gray noise (i.e., hum) or silence during the exercise test. The results of these studies are consistent and point to the potentially beneficial effects of music in alleviating dyspnea and anxiety, and in enhancing engagement in physical activity in this patient population. However, most studies were considered pilot tests of this intervention. Further investigation of its effectiveness, with a more rigorous research design, is necessary to develop a sound, relevant knowledge base.

Sassi-Dambron, Eakin, Ries, & Kaplan (1995) evaluated the effectiveness of a treatment program in managing dyspnea in patients with COPD. The program consisted of six weekly group sessions in which the following strategies for coping with dyspnea were discussed and practiced: progressive muscle relaxation, diaphragmatic and pursed-lips breathing, pacing and energy-saving techniques, self-talk and panic control, and stress management. The 89 patients who consented to participate were randomly assigned to the treatment program or to a control condition that consisted of six weekly sessions of general health education. Dyspnea was measured with VAS, as well as with the Borg scale, administered before and after a six-minute walk test. No significant difference in dyspnea was found between the two groups at posttest; however, both groups showed a significant decrease in perceived dyspnea from pre- to posttest. Despite the observed favorable outcome, the results of this study cannot be generalized due to the reported difference in the level of dyspnea between those who dropped out (had more severe dyspnea) and those who completed the study.

The findings of these studies indicate the potential benefits of relaxation and listening to music, as well as a comprehensive educational program, in managing dyspnea. Further research is needed to generate a sound knowledge base about the effectiveness of nursing interventions in relieving this symptom. Until such knowledge is acquired, it is difficult to claim with certainty that dyspnea is sensitive to nursing care.

4.8 Conclusions and Recommendations

The literature reviewed in this chapter provides evidence supporting the following points:

- Symptoms are subjective sensations that reflect a change in normal functioning. They are experienced by individuals with various health or illness conditions, and they represent the reason for seeking health care across the healthcare continuum.

- Symptoms are experienced, perceived, and reacted to by patients. The process of perceiving, interpreting, and responding to symptoms is individual and is affected by a host of personal, environmental, and health-related variables. These should be accounted for when evaluating the effects of nursing care on symptom control.

- Symptoms interfere with the person's physical, psychological, and social functioning. If not managed effectively and controlled, symptoms have a devastating impact on the person, the family, and the healthcare system.

- Nurses are in a good position to assist patients in managing symptoms. This statement is consistent with (a) the caring perspective underlying nursing; (b) the focus of some models or middle-range theories of nursing (e.g., theory of self-care, symptom management model); (c) the emphasis on self-management and active patient participation in care; and (d) clinical observations and informal patient reports explaining that they seek medical care for the diagnosis and treatment of medical problems, and nursing care for assistance in managing day-to-day functioning and symptoms.

- Symptom management is considered an important component of nursing care for different patient populations, but specifically for patients with chronic illness, with the ultimate outcome of relieving or controlling symptoms.

- Various interventions have been applied and evaluated for their effectiveness in managing different symptoms experienced by patients with chronic illness.

- Educational or psychoeducational interventions have been designed to assist patients in adjusting to chronic illness and to provide them with the knowledge and skills to recognize and manage symptoms they may experience. The interventions have addressed multiple physical and psychological symptoms commonly experienced by the target population. They were delivered by nurses and consisted of discussing the patients' symptoms or concerns and the strategies patients could use to manage symptoms. The results indicated that patients who received the psychoeducational interventions reported lower levels of symptom severity at posttest. The interventions' effects on symptom severity were more prominent at follow-up.

- The effectiveness of various specific nursing interventions in relieving the symptoms of fatigue, nausea and vomiting, and dyspnea was also examined in the sources included in this review. The studies used different designs, ranging from experimental to pre-experimental. They included rather small sample sizes. The symptoms were measured with reliable and valid instruments. In general, the results supported the favorable effects of these specific interventions in relieving the severity of symptoms. These findings, however, should be considered with caution due to the possible introduction of bias.

- The evidence reviewed provides initial support for the benefit of nursing interventions in managing symptoms experienced by patients. Symptom control can be considered an outcome that is sensitive to nursing care.

- Symptom control is of utmost importance for patients with chronic illness, and it constitutes a primary focus for nurses providing care to these patients on an inpatient or outpatient basis.

- The symptoms experienced differ across patient populations, based on the nature of the pathophysiological mechanisms underlying the illness condition and on the type of treatment given. For instance, dyspnea is reported more commonly by patients with respiratory or pulmonary and cardiac conditions than by patients undergoing minor surgery.

- Effective symptom management begins with a comprehensive assessment of the symptom experience. It encompasses (a) the occurrence of multiple symptoms that are commonly reported by the patient population to which the patient belongs, and (b) the multiple dimensions of each symptom experienced (i.e., severity, frequency, duration, meaning, impact, response, alleviating and aggravating factors, and strategies used). This comprehensive assessment should inquire about the patient's individual perception of the symptom. It can be completed in a structured and systematic manner that involves using symptom checklists developed for specific patient populations, such as the Signs and Symptoms Checklist for Persons with HIV disease, the Symptom Distress Scale for patients with cancer, the Menstrual Symptom Severity List, or the Support Team Assessment Schedule for patients in palliative care. The checklists measure the symptoms' occurrence and severity.

- Measuring symptoms as outcomes of nursing care is necessary for determining the effectiveness of the care provided in everyday practice. The same checklist used in the initial clinical assessment of symptoms could be used for evaluating the outcome of symptom control.

- The checklists reviewed here have demonstrated initial reliability and validity. They need further testing to determine their sensitivity to change and to generate normative values and/or cut-off scores before they can be used in clinical practice.

- Similar checklists will have to be developed for assessing symptoms commonly reported by other patient populations.

- Fatigue, nausea and vomiting, and dyspnea are symptoms reported by many patients. Assessing these symptoms could become an integral part of routine nursing assessment, as is done for pain. Single items with a 10-point numeric rating scale, ranging from 0 = *not at all* to 10 = *very severe*, are reliable, valid, sensitive, and clinically useful measures of these symptoms.

References

Aaronson, K. K., Ahmedzai, S., Bullinger, M., Crabeels, D., Estape, J., Filiberti, A., et al. (1991). The EORTC core quality-of-life questionnaire: Interim results of an international field study. In D. Osoba (Ed.), *Effects of cancer on quality of life.* : CRC Press.

Aaronson, K. K., Bullinger, M., & Ahmedzai, S. (1988). A modular approach to quality of life assessment in cancer clinical trials. *Recent Results in Cancer Research, 111,* 231–249.

Aistars, J. (1987). Fatigue in the cancer patient: A conceptual approach to a clinical problem. *Oncology Nursing Forum, 14,* 25–30.

Altose, M. D. (1985). Assessment and management of breathlessness. *Chest, 88*(Suppl. 2), S77–S82.

Anastasia, P. J., & Blevins, M. C. (1997). Outpatient chemotherapy: Telephone triage for symptom management. *Oncology Nursing Forum, 24*(Suppl. 1), 13–22.

Beck, A. T., & Beck, R. W. (1972). Screening depressed patients in family practice: A rapid technique. *Postgraduate Medicine, 52*(6), 81–85.

Belza, B. L. (1995). Comparison of self-reported fatigue in rheumatoid arthritis and controls. *Journal of Rheumatology, 22,* 639–643.

Belza, B. L., Henke, C. J., Yelin, E. H., Esptein, W. V., & Gillis, C. L. (1993). Correlates of fatigue in older adults with rheumatoid arthritis. *Nursing Research, 42,* 93–99.

Benor, D. E., Delbar, V., & Krulik, T. (1998). Measuring impact of nursing intervention on cancer patients' ability to control symptoms. *Cancer Nursing, 21,* 320–334.

Berger, A. M., & Walker, S. N. (2001). An explanatory model of fatigue in women receiving adjuvant breast cancer chemotherapy. *Nursing Research, 50,* 42–52.

Bernstein, M. L., Despars, J. A., Singh, N. P., Avalos, K., Stansbury, D. W., & Light, R. W. (1994). Reanalysis of the 12-minute walk in patients with chronic obstructive pulmonary disease. *Chest, 105,* 163–167.

Blesch, K. S., Paice, J. A., Wickham, R., Harte, N., Schnoor, D. K., Purl, S., et al. (1991). Correlates of fatigue in people with breast or lung cancer. *Oncology Nursing Forum, 18,* 81–87.

Borg, G. A. V. (1982). Psychophysical basis of perceived exertion. *Medical Science & Supports Exercise, 14,* 377–381.

Bowling, A. (1995). *Measuring disease: A review of disease-specific quality of life measurement scales.* Buckingham, England: Open University Press.

Brown, M. L. (1985). Selecting an instrument to measure dyspnea. *Oncology Nursing Forum, 12*(3), 98–100.

Brown, M., Carrieri, V., Janson-Bjerklie, S., & Dodd, M. (1986). Lung cancer and dyspnea: The patient's perception. *Oncology Nursing Forum, 13*(1), 19–24.

Bruera, E., Kuehn, N., Miller, M. J., Selsmar, P., & Macmillan, K. (1991). The Edmonton Symptom Assessment System (ESAS): A simple method for the assessment of palliative care patients. *Journal of Palliative Care, 7*(1), 6–9.

Burdon, J. G. W., Juniper, E. F., Killian, F. E., Hargreave, F. E., & Campbell, E. J. M. (1982). The perception of breathlessness in asthma. *American Review of Respiratory Disease, 126,* 825–828.

Burish, T. G., Carey, M. P., Krozely, G., & Greco, A. (1987). Conditioned side effects induced by cancer chemotherapy: Prevention through behavioral treatment. *Journal of Consulting and Clinical Psychology, 55,* 42–48.

Burish, T. G., & Jenkins, R. A. (1992). Effectiveness of biofeedback and relaxation training in reducing the side effects of cancer chemotherapy. *Health Psychology, 11*(1), 17–23.

Burish, T. G., Snyder, S. L., & Jenkins, R. A. (1991). Preparing patients for cancer chemotherapy: Effect of coping preparation and relaxation interventions. *Journal of Consulting and Clinical Psychology, 59,* 518–525.

Buxton, L. S., Frizelle, F. A., Parry, B. R., Pettigrew, R. A., & Hopkins, W. G. (1992). Validation of subjective measures of fatigue after elective operations. *European Journal of Surgery, 158,* 393–396.

Carey, M. P., & Burish, T. G. (1987). Providing relaxation training to cancer chemotherapy patients: A comparison of three delivery techniques. *Journal of Consulting and Clinical Psychology, 55,* 732–737.

Carrieri, V., & Janson-Bjerklie, S. (1986). Dyspnea. In V. K. Carrieri, A. M. Lindsey, & C. M. West (Eds.), *Pathophysiological phenomena in nursing: Human responses to illness* (pp. 191–215). Philadelphia: W. B. Saunders.

Carrieri-Kohlman, V., Douglas, M. K., Gormley, J. M., & Stulbarg, M. S. (1993). Desensitization and guided mastery: Treatment approaches for the management of dyspnea. *Heart & Lung, 22,* 226–234.

Cassileth, B. R., Lusk, E. J., Bodenheimer, B. J., Farber, J. M., Jochimsen, P., & Morrin-Taylor, B. (1985). Chemotherapeutic toxicity: The relationship between patients' pretreatment expectations and post-treatment results. *American Journal of Clinical Oncology, 8,* 419–425.

Cella, D. F., Tulsky, D. S., Gary, G., Sarafian, B., Linn, E., Bonomi, A., et al. (1993). The Functional Assessment of Cancer Therapy Scale: Development and validation of the general measure. *Journal of Clinical Oncology, 11,* 570–579.

Chalder, T., Berelowitz, G., Pawlikowska, T., Watss, L., Wessely, S., Wright, D., et al. (1993). Development of a fatigue scale. *Journal of Psychosomatic Research, 37,* 147–153.

Christensen, T., Bendix, T., & Kehlet, H. (1982). Fatigue and cardiorespiratory function following abdominal surgery. *British Journal of Surgery, 69,* 417–419.

Chritensen, T., Hjortso, N. C., Mortensen, E., Riis-Hansen, M., & Kehlet, H. (1986). Fatigue and anxiety in surgical patients. *Acta Psychiatrica Scandinavia, 73,* 76–79.

Christensen, T., Nygaard, E., Stage, J. G., & Kehlet, H. (1990). Skeletal muscle enzyme activities and metabolic substrates during exercise in patients with postoperative fatigue. *British Journal of Surgery, 77,* 312–315.

Cimprich, B. (1993). Development of an intervention to restore attention in cancer patients. *Cancer Nursing, 16,* 83–92.

Clark, D. M., Salkovskis, P. M., & Chalkley, A. J. (1985). Respiratory control as a treatment for panic attacks. *Journal of Behavioral Therapy & Experimental Psychiatry, 16*(1), 23–30.

Clark, J. A., & Talcott, J. A. (2001). Symptom indexes to assess outcomes of treatment for early prostate cancer. *Medical Care, 39,* 1118–1130.

Cotanch, P. H. (1983). Relaxation training for control of nausea and vomiting in patients receiving chemotherapy. *Cancer Nursing, 8,* 277–283.

Cotanch, P., Hockenberry, M., & Herman, S. (1985). Self-hypnosis as antiemetic therapy for cancer patients. *Oncology Nursing Forum, 12*(4), 41–46.

Cotanch, P. H., & Strum, S. (1987). Progressive muscle relaxation as antiemetic therapy for cancer patients. *Oncology Nursing Forum, 14*(1), 33–37.

David, A., Pelosi, A., McDonald, E., Stephens, D., Ledger, D., Rathbone, R., et al. (1990). Tired, weak, or in need of rest: Fatigue among general practice attenders. *British Medical Journal, 301,* 1199–1202.

Dean, G. E., & Ferrell, B. R. (1995). Impact of fatigue on quality of life in cancer survivors. *Quality of Life—A Nursing Challenge, 4*(1), 25–28.

Decker, T., Cline-Elsen, J., & Gallagher, M. (1992). Relaxation therapy as an adjunct in radiation oncology. *Journal of Clinical Psychology, 48,* 388–393.

de Haes, J. C. J. M., van Knippenberg, F. C. E., & Neijt, J. P. (1990). Measuring psychological and physical distress in cancer patients: Structure and application of the Rotterdam Symptom Checklist. *British Journal of Cancer, 62,* 1034–1038.

Derogatis, L. R. (1993). *Brief Symptom Inventory: Administration, scoring, and procedures manual.* National Computer Systems.

Derogatis, L. R. (1994). *Symptom Checklist-90-R: Administration, scoring, and procedures manual.* National Computer Systems.

Devlen, J., Maguire, P., Phillips, P., Crowther, D., & Chambers, H. (1987). Psychological problems associated with diagnosis and treatment of lymphomas: A retrospective study. *British Medical Journal, 295,* 953–954.

Dodd, M. J. (1983). Self-care for side effects in cancer chemotherapy: An assessment of nursing interventions: Part II. *Cancer Nursing, 6,* 63–67.

Dodd, M. (1984). Patterns of self-care in cancer patients receiving radiation therapy. *Oncology Nursing Forum, 11*(3), 23–27.

Dodd, M., Janson, S., Facione, N., Fawcett, J., Froelicher, E. S., Humphreys, J., et al. (2001). Advancing the science of symptom management. *Journal of Advanced Nursing, 33,* 668–676.

Dudley, D. C., Galse, E. M., Jorgenson, B. N., & Logan, D. L. (1980). Psychosocial concomitants to rehabilitation in chronic obstructive pulmonary disease: Part I. *Chest, 77,* 544–551.

Eaton, M., MacDonald, F., Church, T., & Niewoehner, D. (1982). Effects of theophylline on breathlessness and exercise tolerance in patients with chronic airflow obstruction. *Chest, 82,* 538–545.

Edmonds, P. M., Stuttaford, J. M., Penny, J., Lynch, A. M., & Chamberlain, J. (1998). Do hospital palliative care teams improve symptom control?: Use of a modified STAS as an evaluation tool. *Palliative Medicine, 12,* 345–351.

Ellershaw, J. E., Peat, S. J., & Boys, L. C. (1995). Assessing the effectiveness of a hospital palliative care team. *Palliative Medicine, 9,* 145–152.

Fainsinger, R., Miller, M. J., Bruera, E., Hanson, J., & MacEachern, T. (1991). Symptom control during the last week of life on a palliative care unit. *Journal of Palliative Care, 7*(1), 5–11.

Fawzy, F. I., Cousins, N., Fawzy, N. W., Kemeny, M. E., Elashoff, R., & Morton, D. (1990). A structured psychiatric intervention for cancer patients. *Archives of General Psychiatry, 47,* 720–725.

Fawzy, N. W. (1995). A psychoeducational nursing intervention to enhance coping and affective state in newly diagnosed malignant melanoma patients. *Cancer Nursing, 18,* 427–438.

Ferrans, C. E., & Powers, M. J. (1992). Psychometric assessment of the quality of life index. *Research in Nursing & Health, 15,* 29–38.

Ferrell, B. R., Dow, K. H., Leigh, S., Ly, J., & Gulasekaram, P. (1995). Quality of life in long-term cancer survivors. *Oncology Nursing Forum, 22,* 915–922.

Ferrell, B. R., Wisdom, C., & Wenzl, C. (1989). Quality of life as an outcome variable in the management of cancer pain. *Cancer, 63,* 2321–2327.

Fisk, J. D., Ritvo, P. G., Ross, L., Haase, D. A., Marrie, T. J., & Schlech, W. F. (1994). Measuring the functional impact of fatigue: Initial validation of the Fatigue Impact Scale. *Clinical Infectious Diseases, 18*(Suppl. 1), S79–S83.

Fletcher, C. (1952). The clinical diagnosis of pulmonary emphysema: An experimental study. *Royal Society of Medicine Proceedings, 45,* 577–584.

Gantz, P. A., Day, R., Ware, J. E., Redmond, C., & Fisher, B. (1995). Baseline quality of life assessment in the National Surgical Adjuvant Breast and Bowel Project. *Journal of the National Cancer Institute, 87,* 1372–1382.

Gantz, P. A., Greendale, G. A., Peterson, L., Zibecchi, L., Kahn, B., & Belin, T. R. (2000). Managing menopausal symptoms in breast cancer survivors: Results of a randomized controlled trial. *Journal of the National Cancer Institute, 92,* 1054–1064.

Gard, D., Edwards, P. W., Harris, J., & McCormack, G. (1988). Sensitizing effects of pretreatment measures on cancer chemotherapy nausea and vomiting. *Journal of Consulting and Clinical Psychology, 56,* 80–84.

Gift, A. G. (1989). Validation of a vertical visual analogue scale as a measure of clinical dyspnea. *Rehabilitation Nursing, 14,* 323–325.

Gift, A. G. (1990). Dyspnea. *Nursing Clinics of North America, 25,* 955–965.

Gift, A. G. (1993). Therapies for dyspnea relief. *Holistic Nurse Practice, 7*(2), 57–63.

Gift, A. G., & Cahill, C. A. (1990). Psychophysiologic aspects of dyspnea in chronic obstructive disease: A pilot study. *Heart & Lung, 19,* 252–257.

Gift, A. G., Moore, T., & Soeken, K. (1992). Relaxation to reduce dyspnea and anxiety in COPD patients. *Nursing Research, 41,* 242–246.

Gift, A. G., Plaut, S. M., & Jacox, A. (1986). Psychologic and physiologic factors related to dyspnea in subjects with chronic obstructive pulmonary disease. *Heart & Lung, 15,* 595–601.

Glaus, A. (1993). Assessment of fatigue in cancer and non-cancer patients and in healthy individuals. *Journal of Supportive Care Cancer, 1*, 305–315.

Glaus, A., Crow, R., & Hammond, S. (1996). A qualitative study to explore the concept of fatigue/tiredness in cancer patients and in healthy individuals. *European Journal of Cancer Care, 5* (Suppl. 2), 8–23.

Glover, J., Dibble, S. L., Dodd, M. J., & Miaskowski, C. (1995). Mood states of oncology outpatients: Does pain make a difference? *Journal of Pain and Symptom Management, 10*, 120–128.

Goldstein, R., Gort, E., Stubbing, D., Avendano, M., & Guyatt, G. (1994). Randomized controlled trial of respiratory rehabilitation. *Lancet, 344*, 1394–1397.

Gottfried, S. B., Altose, M. D., Kelson, S. G., & Cherniack, N. S. (1981). Perception of changes in airflow resistance in obstructive pulmonary disorders. *American Review of Respiratory Disease, 124*, 566–570.

Grande, G. E., Barclay, S. I. G., & Todd, C. J. (1997). Difficulty of symptom control and general practitioners' knowledge of patients' symptoms. *Palliative Medicine, 11*, 399–406.

Grant, M., & Kravits, K. (2000). Symptoms and their impact on nutrition. *Seminars in Oncology Nursing, 16*, 113–121.

Graydon, J. E., Bubela, N., Irvine, D., & Vincent, L. (1995). Fatigue-reducing strategies used by patients receiving treatment for cancer. *Cancer Nursing, 18*, 23–28.

Graydon, J. E., Sidani, S., Irvine, D., Vincent, L., Harrison, D., & Bubela, N. (1997). *Literature review on cancer-related fatigue.* Unpublished report: Canadian Association of Nurses in Oncology.

Graydon, J., Vincent, L., Bubela, N., Thorsen, E., Harrison, D., & Sidani, S. (1999). *A physical activity program for cancer-related fatigue.* Unpublished report: Canadian Association of Nurses in Oncology.

Greenberg, D. B., Gary, J. L., Mannix, C. M., Eisenthal, S., & Carey, M. (1993). Treatment-related fatigue and serum interleukin-1 levels in patients during external beam irradiation for prostate cancer. *Journal of Pain and Symptom Management, 8*, 196–200.

Greenberg, D. B., Sawicka, J., Eisenthal, S., & Ross, D. (1992). Fatigue syndrome due to localized radiation. *Journal of Pain and Symptom Management, 7*, 38–45.

Gritz, E. R., Weliish, D. K., & Landsverk, J. A. (1988). Psychological sequelae in long-term survivors of testicular cancer. *Journal of Psychosocial Oncology, 6*(3/4), 41–63.

Guyatt, G., Berman, L., Townsend, M., Pugsley, S., & Chambers, L. (1987). A measure of quality of life for clinical trials in chronic lung disease. *Thorax, 42*, 773–778.

Guyatt, G. H., Pugsley, S., Sullivan, M. J., Thompson, P. J., Berman, L. B., Jones, N. L., et al. (1984). Effect of encouragement on walking test performance. *Thorax, 39*, 818–822.

Haas, F., Salazar-Schicchi, J., & Axen, K. (1993). Desensitization to dyspnea in chronic obstructive pulmonary disease. In R. Casaburi & T. Petty (Eds.), *Principles and practice of pulmonary rehabilitation* (pp. 241–251). Philadelphia: W. B. Saunders.

Haworth, S. K., & Dluhy, N. M. (2001). Holistic symptom management: Modelling the interaction phase. *Journal of Advanced Nursing, 36*, 302–310.

Henry, S. B., Holzemer, W. L., Weaver, K., & Stotts, N. (1999). Quality of life and self-care management strategies of PLWAs with chronic diarrhea. *Journal of the Association of Nurses in AIDS Care, 10*(2), 46–54.

Higginson, I. J., & McCarthy, M. (1989). Measuring symptoms in terminal cancer: Are pain and dyspnea controlled? *Journal of the Royal Society of Medicine, 82,* 264–267.

Hogan, C. M. (1997). Cancer nursing: The art of symptom management. *Oncology Nursing Forum, 24,* 1335–1341.

Holzemer, W. L., Henry, S. B., Nokes, K. M., Corless, I. B., Brown, M. A., Powell-Cope, G. M., et al. (1999). Validation of the Sign and Symptom Checklist for persons with HIV disease (SSC-HIV). *Journal of Advanced Nursing, 30,* 1041–1049.

Irvine, D., & Sidani, S. (1997). *A critical appraisal of the psychological, psychosocial, and psychiatric assessment tools: Utility for assessment and treatment planning for women with breast cancer.* Unpublished report: Health Canada.

Irvine, D., Sidani, S., & McGillis Hall, L. (1998). Linking outcomes to nurses' roles in health care. *Nursing Economics, 16,* 58–64.

Jamar, S. C. (1989). Fatigue in women receiving chemotherapy for ovarian cancer. In S. G. Funk, E. M. Tornquist, M. T. Champagne, L. A. Copp, & R. A. Wiese (Eds.), *Key aspects of comfort: Management of pain, fatigue, and nausea* (pp. 224–228). New York: Springer.

Janson-Bjerklie, S., Carrrieri, V., & Hudes, D. (1986). The sensation of pulmonary dyspnea. *Nursing Research, 35,* 154–159.

Johnson, J. E., Fieler, V. K., Wlasowicz, G. S., Mitchell, M. L., & Jones, L. S. (1997). The effects of nursing care guided by self-regulation theory on coping with radiation therapy. *Oncology Nursing Forum, 24,* 1041–1050.

Johnson, R. (1993). Nurse practitioner–patient discourse: Uncovering the voice of nursing in primary care practice. *Scholarly Inquiry for Nursing Practice: An International Journal, 7,* 143–157.

Joly, F., Henry-Amar, M., Arveux, P., Reman, O., Yanguy, A., Peny, A. M., et al. (1996). Late psychosocial sequelae in Hodgkin's disease survivors: A French population-based case-control study. *Journal of Clinical Oncology, 14,* 2444–2453.

Justice, A. C., Chang, C. H., Rabeneck, L., & Zachin, R. (2001). Clinical importance of provider-reported HIV symptoms compared with patient-report. *Medical Care, 39,* 397–408.

Kashiwagi, S. (1971). Psychological rating of human fatigue. *Ergonomics, 14*(1), 17–21.

Killian, K. J. (1985). Objective measurement of breathlessness. *Chest, 88*(Suppl. 2), S84–S90.

Kinsman, R., Yaroush, R., Fernandez, E., Dirks, J., Shocket, M., & Fukuhara, J. (1983). Symptoms and experiences in chronic bronchitis and emphysema. *Chest, 5,* 755–761.

Krupp, L. B., LaRocca, N. G., Muir-Nash, J., & Steinberg, A. D. (1989). The Fatigue Severity Scale: Application to patients with multiple sclerosis and systemic lupus eythematosus. *Archives of Neurology, 46,* 1121–1123.

Lang, N. M., & Marek, K. D. (1991). Outcomes that reflect clinical practice. In *Patient outcomes research: Examining the effectiveness of nursing practice. Proceedings of the State of the Science Conference* (pp. 27–38). Bethesda: National Institutes of Health.

Lee, K., Hicks, G., & Nino-Murcia, G. (1991). Validity and reliability of a scale to assess fatigue. *Psychiatry Research, 36,* 291–298.

Lerman, C. Rimer, B., Blumberg, B., Cristinzio, S., Engstrom, P. F., MacElwee, N., et al. (1990). Effects of coping style and relaxation on cancer chemotherapy side effects and emotional responses. *Cancer Nursing, 13,* 308–315.

Love, R. R., Leventhal, H., Easterling, D. V., & Nerenz, D. R. (1989). Side effects and emotional distress during cancer chemotherapy. *Cancer, 63,* 604–612.

Lush, M., Janson-Bjerklie, S., Carrieri, V., & Lovejoy, N. (1988). Dyspnea in the ventilator-assisted patient. *Heart & Lung, 17,* 528–535.

Lyles, J. N., Burish, T. G., Krozely, M. G., & Oldham, R. K. (1982). Efficacy of relaxation training and guided imagery in reducing the aversiveness of cancer chemotherapy. *Journal of Consulting and Clinical Psychology, 50,* 509–524.

MacLeod, J. (1995). Symptom management in transcultural nursing. *European Journal of Palliative Care, 2*(3), 124–126.

Maguire, P., Walsh, S., Jeacock, J., & Kingston, R. (1999). Physical and psychological needs of patients dying from colo-rectal cancer. *Palliative Medicine, 13,* 45–50.

Mahler, D. A. (Ed.). (1990). *Dyspnea.* Mount Krisco: Futura Publishing.

Mahler, D., & Harver, A. (1989). Factor analysis demonstrates independence of dyspnea ratings and physiologic function in obstructive airway disease. *American Review of Respiratory Disease, 139,* A243.

Mahler, D. A., Matthay, R. A., Snyder, P. E., Wells, C. K., & Loke, J. (1985). Sustained-release theophylline reduces dyspnea in nonreversible obstructive airway disease. *American Review of Respiratory Disease, 131,* 22–25.

Mahler, D. A., Rosiello, R. A., Harver, A., Lentine, T., McGovern, J. F., & Daubenspeck, A. (1987). Comparison of clinical dyspnea ratings and psychophysical measurements of respiratory sensation in obstructive airway disease. *American Review of Respiratory Disease, 135,* 1229–1233.

Mahler, D. A., Weinberg, D. H., Wells, C. K., & Feinstein, A. R. (1984). The measurement of dyspnea. *Chest, 85,* 751–757.

Mahler, D., & Wells, C. (1988). Evaluation of clinical methods for rating dyspnea. *Chest, 93,* 580–586.

McBride, S., Graydon, J., Sidani, S., & Hall, L. (1999). The therapeutic use of music for dyspnea and anxiety in patients with COPD who live at home. *Journal of Holistic Nursing, 17,* 229–250.

McCarley, C. (1999). A model of chronic dyspnea. *Image: Journal of Nursing Scholarship, 31,* 231–236.

McCord, M., & Cronin-Stubbs, D. (1992). Operationalizing dyspnea: Focus on measurement. *Heart & Lung, 21,* 167–179.

McCorkle, R., & Young, K. (1978). Development of a Symptom Distress Scale. *Cancer Nursing, 5,* 373–378.

McGavin, C. R., Gupta, S. P., & McHardy, G. J. R. (1976). Twelve-minute walking test for assessing disability in chronic bronchitis. *British Medical Journal, 1*, 822–823.

McNair, D. M., Lorr, M., & Droppleman, I. F. (1981). *Profile of Mood States.* San Diego, CA: Educational and Industrial Testing Service.

Meek, P. M., Nail, L. M., Barsevick, A., Schwartz, A. L., Stephen, S., Whitmer, K., et al. (2000). Psychometric testing of fatigue instruments for use with cancer patients. *Nursing Research, 49*, 181–190.

Meek, P. M., Nail, L. M., & Jones, L. S. (1997). Internal consistency reliability and construct validity of a new measure of cancer treatment related fatigue: The General Fatigue Scale (GFS). *Oncology Nursing Forum, 24*, 334.

Mitchell, P. H., Ferketich, S., & Jennings, B. M. (1998). Quality health outcomes model. *Image: Journal of Nursing Scholarship, 30*, 43–46.

Mock, V., Burke, M. B., Sheehan, P., Creaton, E. M., Winningham, M. L., McKenny-Tedder, S., et al. (1994). A nursing rehabilitation program for women with breast cancer receiving adjuvant chemotherapy. *Oncology Nursing Forum, 21*, 899–907.

Moody, L. E., Fraser, M., & Yarandi, H. (1993). Effects of guided imagery in patients with chronic bronchitis and emphysema. *Clinical Nursing Research, 2*, 478–486.

Morant, R. (1996). Asthenia: An important symptom in cancer patients. *Cancer Treatment Reviews, 22*(Suppl. A), 117–122.

Morris, M. L. (1982). Tiredness and fatigue. In C. M. Norris (Ed.), *Concept clarification in nursing* (pp. 263–275). Rockville, MD: Aspen.

Morrow, G. R. (1982). Prevalence and correlates of anticipatory nausea and vomiting in chemotherapy patients. *Journal of the National Cancer Institute, 68*, 585–588.

Morrow, G. R., & Morrell, C. (1982). Behavioral treatment for the anticipatory nausea and vomiting induced by cancer chemotherapy. *The New England Journal of Medicine, 307*, 1476–1480.

Munkres, A., Oberst, M. T., & Hughes, S. H. (1992). Appraisal of illness, symptom distress, self-care burden, and mood states in patients receiving chemotherapy for initial and recurrent cancer. *Oncology Nursing Forum, 19*, 1201–1209.

Nail, L. M., Jones, L. S., Greene, D., Schipper, D. L., & Jensen, R. (1991). Use and perceived efficacy of self-care activities in patients receiving chemotherapy. *Oncology Nursing Forum, 18*, 883–887.

Nail, L. M., & King, K. B. (1987). Fatigue. *Seminars in Oncology Nursing, 3*, 257–262.

Nield, M., Kim, M. J., & Patel, M. (1989). Use of magnitude estimation for estimating the parameters of dyspnea. *Nursing Research, 38*, 77–80.

Nokes, K., Wheeler, K., & Kendrew, J. (1994). Development of an HIV assessment tool. *Image: The Journal of Nursing Scholarship, 26*, 133–138.

O'Neill, E. S., & Morrow, L. L. (2001). The symptom experience of women with chronic illness. *Journal of Advanced Nursing, 33*, 257–268.

Osoba, D., Zee, B., Warr, D., Kaizer, L., Latreille, J., & Pater, J. (1996). Quality of life studies in chemotherapy-induced emesis. *Oncology, 53*(Suppl. 1), 92–95.

Pearson, R. G., & Byars, G. E. (1956). *The development and validation of a checklist for measuring subjective fatigue.* Randolph Air Force Base, TX: School of Aviation Medicine.

Pickard-Holley, S. (1991). Fatigue in cancer patients: A descriptive study. *Cancer Nursing, 14*, 13–19.

Piper, B. F. (1993). Fatigue. In V. K. Carrieri-Kolman, A. M. Lindsey, & C. M. West (Eds.), *Pathophysiological phenomena in nursing: Human responses to illness* (2nd ed., pp. 279–302). Philadelphia: Saunders.

Piper, B. F., Dodd, M. L., Paul, S. M., & Weleer, S. (1989). The development of an instrument to measure the subjective dimension of fatigue. In S. G. Funk, E. M. Tornquist, M. T. Champagne, L. A. Copp, & R. A. Wiese (Eds.), *Key aspects of comfort management of pain, fatigue, and nausea* (pp. 199–208). New York: Springer.

Ream, E., & Richardson, A. (1999). From theory to practice: Designing interventions to reduce fatigue in patients with cancer. *Oncology Nursing Forum, 26*, 1295–1305.

Renfroe, K. L. (1988). Effect of progressive relaxation on dyspnea and state anxiety in patients with chronic obstructive pulmonary disease. *Heart & Lung, 17*, 408–413.

Rhodes, V. A., McDaniel, R. W., & Matthews, C. A. (1998). Hospice patients' and nurses' perceptions of self-care deficits based on symptom experience. *Cancer Nursing, 21*, 312–319.

Rhodes, V. A., Watson, P. M., & Johnson, M. H. (1984). Development of reliable and valid measures of nausea and vomiting. *Cancer Nursing, 7*, 33–41.

Rhoten, D. (1982). Fatigue and the post-surgical patient. In C. M. Norris (Ed.), *Concept clarification in nursing* (pp. 277–300). Rockville, MD: Aspen.

Richardson, A. (1995). Fatigue in cancer patients: A review of the literature. *European Journal of Cancer Care, 4*, 20–32.

Richardson, A., & Ream, E. K. (1996). The experience of fatigue and other symptoms in patients receiving chemotherapy. *European Journal of Cancer Care, 5*(Suppl. 2), 24–30.

Richardson, A., & Ream, E. K. (1997). Self-care behaviors initiated by chemotherapy patients in response to fatigue. *International Journal of Nursing Studies, 34*(1), 35–43.

Rosser, R., & Guz, A. (1981). Psychological approaches to breathlessness and its treatment. *Journal of Psychosomatic Research, 25*, 439–447.

Sanzero Eller, L. (1999). Guided imagery interventions for symptom management. *Annual Review of Nursing Research, 17*, 57–84.

Sassi-Dambron, D., Eakin, E., Ries, A. L., & Kaplan, R. M. (1995). Treatment of dyspnea in COPD: A controlled clinical trial of dyspnea management strategies. *Chest, 107*, 724–729.

Schipper, H., Clinch, J., McMurray, A., & Levitt, M. (1984). Measuring the quality of life of cancer patients: The Functional Living Index–Cancer. Development and validation. *Journal of Clinical Oncology, 2*, 472.

Schroeder, D., & Hill, G. L. (1991). Postoperative fatigue: A prospective physiological study of patients undergoing major abdominal surgery. *Australian and New Zealand Journal of Surgery, 61*, 774–779.

Schutte, N. S., & Malouf, J. M. (1995). *Sourcebook of adult assessment strategies.* New York: Plenum Press.

Schwartz, A. L. (1997). Reliability and validity of the Cancer Fatigue Scale. *Oncology Nursing Forum, 24*, 331.

Schwartz, J. E., Jandorf, L., & Krupp, L. B. (1993). The measurement of fatigue: A new instrument. *Journal of Psychosomatic Research, 37*, 753–762.

Scott, D. W., Donahue, D. C., Mastrovito, R. C., & Hakes, T. B. (1986). Comparative trial of clinical relaxation and an antiemetic drug regimen in reducing chemotherapy-related nausea and vomiting. *Cancer Nursing, 9*, 178–187.

Sidani, S. (1991). *Effects of sedative music on the respiratory status of clients with chronic obstructive airway disease.* Unpublished master's thesis: University of Arizona College of Nursing.

Smets, E. M., Garssen, B., Bonke, B., & de Haes, J. C. (1995). The multidimensional fatigue inventory: Psychometric qualities of an instrument to assess fatigue. *Journal of Psychosomatic Research, 39*, 315–325.

Smets, E. M. A., Garssen, B., Cull, A., & de Haes, J. C. J. M. (1996). Application of the multidimensional fatigue inventory (MFI-20) in cancer patients receiving radiotherapy. *British Journal of Cancer, 73, 241–245.*

Smets, E. M. A., Garssen, B., Schuster-Uitterhoeve, A. L. J., & de Haes, J. C. J. M. (1993). Fatigue in cancer patients. *British Journal of Cancer, 68*, 220–224.

Smith, M. C., Holcombe, J. K., & Stullenbarger, E. (1994). A meta-analysis of intervention effectiveness for symptom management in oncology nursing research. *Oncology Nursing Forum, 21*, 1201–1210.

Stanton, A. L., & Snider, P. R. (1993). Coping with a breast cancer diagnosis: A prospective study. *Health Psychology, 12*(1), 16–23.

Stoller, J., Ferranti, R., & Feinstein, A. (1986). Further specification and evaluation of a new index for dyspnea. *American Review of Respiratory Disease, 134*, 129–134.

Sutcliffe-Chidgey, J., & Holmes, S. (1996). Developing a symptom distress scale for terminal malignant disease. *International Journal of Palliative Nursing, 2*, 192–198.

Taylor, D. (1999). Effectiveness of professional-peer group treatment: Symptom management for women with PMS. *Research in Nursing & Health, 22*, 496–511.

Thornby, M. A., Haas, F., & Axen, K. (1995). Effect of distractive auditory stimuli on exercise tolerance in patients with COPD. *Chest, 107*, 1213–1217.

Tucci, R. A., & Bartels, K. L. (1998). Patient use of the symptom reporting tool. *Clinical Journal of Oncology Nursing, 2*(3), 97–99.

Turner, J., Corkey, K., Eckman, D., Gelb, A., Lipavsky, A., & Sheppard, D. (1988). Equivalence of continuous flow nebulizer and metered-dose inhaler with reservoir bag for treatment of acute airflow obstruction. *Chest, 93*, 476–481.

University of California, San Francisco, School of Nursing Symptom Management Faculty Group (1994). A model for symptom management. *Image: Journal of Nursing Scholarship, 26*, 272–275.

van der Molen, B. (1995). Dyspnea: A study of measurement instruments for the assessment of dyspnea and their application for patients with advanced cancer. *Journal of Advanced Nursing, 22*, 948–956.

Van Fleet, S. (2000). Relaxation and imagery for symptom management: Improving patient assessment and individualizing treatment. *Oncology Nursing Forum, 27*(3), 501–510.

Vasterling, J., Jenkins, R. A., Tope, D. M., & Burish, T. G. (1993). Cognitive distraction and relaxation training for the control of side effects due to cancer chemotherapy. *Journal of Behavioral Medicine, 16*(1), 65–80.

Waltz, C. F., Strickland, O. L., & Lenz, E. R. (1991). *Measurement in nursing research* (2nd ed.). Philadelphia: F. A. Davis.

Ware, J., Snow, K. K., Kosinski, M., & Gandek, B. (1993). *SF-36 health survey: Manual and interpretation guide.* Boston, MA: New England Medical Center, The Health Institute.

White, C. L. (1992). Symptom assessment and management of outpatients receiving biotherapy: The application of a symptom report form. *Seminars in Oncology Nursing, 8*(4, Suppl 1.), 23–28.

Winningham, M. L. (1995). Fatigue: The missing link to quality of life. *Quality of Life—A Nursing Challenge, 4*(1), 2–7.

Winningham, M. L., Nail, L. M., Burke, M. B., Brophy, L., Cimprich, B., Jones, L. S., et al. (1994). Fatigue and the cancer experience: The state of the knowledge. *Oncology Nursing Forum, 21*, 23–35.

Winstead-Fry, P. (1998). Psychometric assessment of four fatigue scales with a sample of rural cancer patients. *Journal of Nursing Measurement, 6*, 111–122.

Worcester, M., Pesznecker, B., Albert, M., Grupp, K., Horn, B., & O'Connor, K. (1991). Cancer symptom management in the elderly. *Home Health Care Services Quarterly, 12*(2), 53–69.

Yancey, R., Given, B. A., White, N. J., DeVoss, D., & Coyle, B. (1998). Computerized documentation for a rural nursing intervention project. *Computers in Nursing, 16*, 275–284.

Yoshitake, H. (1971). Relations between the symptoms and the feeling of fatigue. *Ergonomics, 14*, 175–186.

Yoshitake, H. (1978). Three characteristic patterns of subjective fatigue symptoms. *Ergonomics, 21*, 231–233.

Youngblut, J. M., & Casper, G. R. (1993). Single-item indicators in nursing research. *Research in Nursing and Health, 16*, 459–465.

Zimmerman, B. W., Brown, S. T., & Bowman, J. M. (1996). A self-management program for chronic obstructive pulmonary disease: Relationship to dyspnea and self-efficacy. *Rehabilitation Nursing, 21*, 253–257.

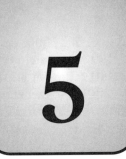

Pain as a Symptom Outcome

Judy Watt-Watson, RN, PhD

5.1 Introduction

Pain is a symptom that has been documented as an indicator of inadequate pain management for almost 30 years, particularly since Marks and Sachar's seminal work in 1973. To establish determinants of this problem, investigators in the 1980s and early 1990s focused primarily on describing health professionals' pain-related knowledge gaps and then later on education programs to solve the problem. However, the intervention's impact on patients' pain was either not measured or findings were equivocal because of methodological problems. In a meta-analysis examining the effectiveness of nonpharmacological interventions for pain management, the strong heterogeneity between studies resulted in a pooled effect size of only 0.06 (Sindhu, 1996). More recently, the question of whether nursing initiatives actually change pain management practices has stimulated an examination of patients' pain as a critical outcome measure. Studies have begun to measure pain as a symptom outcome in order to determine the effect of interventions such as education both for nurses (Dahlman et al., 1999;

Dalton et al., 1999; de Rond et al., 2000; de Rond et al., 1999; de Wit & van Dam, 2001; Francke et al., 1997; Holzheimer et al., 1999; Neitzel et al., 1999) and patients (Ahles et al., 2001; Closs et al., 1999; Clotfelter, 1999; LeFort et al., 1998; McDonald et al., 2001; Neitzel et al., 1999; Ward et al., 2000; Watt-Watson, Stevens et al., 2000). Studies have also begun to measure pain as a symptom outcome in order to determine the effect of interventions such as music, cutaneous stimulation, or therapeutic touch (Broscious, 1999; Good et al., 2001; Keller & Bzdek, 1986; Kubsch et al., 2000; Meehan, 1993; Tanabe et al., 2001).

This chapter reviews pain as a symptom outcome in evaluating nursing care for adults. The review will include a discussion of (a) the theoretical background for the concept of pain, including a definition and factors influencing pain; (b) issues in the assessment of pain; (c) evidence concerning the relationship between nursing and pain as a symptom outcome; (d) evidence concerning approaches to measurement; and (e) recommendations and directions for future research.

The criteria for selecting studies for this review included (a) a pain-related outcome as the major dependent variable being examined, (b) an experimental or quasi-experimental design, (c) a nursing intervention—either analgesic administration or nonpharmacological, (d) an adequate sample size of at least 10 patients per group, and (e) the use of established measures to evaluate nurse-sensitive patient outcomes. After a review of PsychLit (1987–2000), Sociological Abstracts (1963–2000), CINAHL (1982–2000), and MEDLINE (1966–2000), 24 studies were selected. Sources were excluded if (a) pain-related outcomes were not measured as a distinct variable, (b) the intervention was non-nursing or was implemented by non-nurses, or (c) the impact of the intervention on actual practices was not evaluated using patient outcomes.

The key words used in the search were pain, interventions, education, analgesics (non-narcotic/opioid), relaxation (simple/techniques), music (therapy), imagery (simple/guided), and muscle relaxation. These words were combined with the term *nurse* to confine the literature to those sources relevant to nursing. The search yielded a total of 302 relevant sources from which 24, all from journal articles, met the criteria.

5.2 Theoretical Background of the Outcome

Pain continues to be the most common reason people seek help from health professionals. It is also a common cause of disability and diminished quality of life. However, many people with acute and/or chronic pain do not experience the level of adequate pain relief possible through the application of current knowledge about pain and its management. Moreover, unrelieved pain from surgery can precipitate adverse responses, including pulmonary and cardiovascular dysfunction (Benedetti et al., 1984; O'Gara, 1988) and may predispose a patient to long-term pain (Katz, 1997). Also, chronic non-cancer pain is a frequent cause of suffering and disability affecting 3.9 million Canadians (17%) over the age of 15 (Millar, 1996). Therefore, reliable and valid measures to evaluate the effectiveness of pain practices using patient outcomes are critical.

5.2.1 *Definition*

Pain is a subjective phenomenon that varies with each individual and each painful experience (Melzack & Wall, 1965). The International Association for the Study of Pain (IASP) has defined pain as "an unpleasant sensory and emotional experience associated with actual or potential tissue damage, or described in terms of such damage" (Merskey & Bogduk, 1994). This broader definition, which goes beyond solely "pain intensity," was included in only two of the selected studies. The explanatory note with this definition emphasizes the subjectivity of the pain experience, that pain is more than a noxious stimulus, and that patients' self-reports of pain should be accepted even when tissue damage is not clearly evident.

5.2.2 *Pain Theory*

The most prevalent theory from which this definition was developed is Melzack and Wall's (1965) gate control theory. It has been seminal in stimulating new ideas to explain painful phenomena and to explore new therapies for pain relief. They developed their model of pain mechanisms as an alternative to two main theories, the specificity and pattern theories. They challenged von Frey's (1894, as cited in Melzack & Wall, 1965) prevalent specificity theory that pain intensity was proportional to the degree of tissue damage. Gate control theory emphasized that pain was not a simple, sensory experience but a complex integration of sensory, affective, and cognitive dimensions. One of Melzack and Wall's major contributions has been their suggestion that pain perception involves modulation of noxious input at several levels of the central nervous system. The perception of pain and responsiveness to noxious stimuli are variable and unpredictable due to inhibitory mechanisms that include both endogenous neural activity and individuals' unique cognitive factors.

Modulation of pain perception was only minimally described by Melzack and Wall (1965). More recently, researchers have found that changes occur in the peripheral and central nervous systems in response to painful stimuli, particularly if they are prolonged (Basbaum & Jessell, 2000). Peripheral sensitization related to chemicals released from damaged tissues after injury, surgery, or inflammation can decrease the activation threshold of nociceptors. Consequently, nociceptors may discharge spontaneously with a decreased threshold for both noxious and non-noxious stimuli. Prolonged severe and persistent injury, such as with trauma or surgery, stimulates spinal cord neurons in the dorsal horn to respond to all inputs, painful or not, resulting in a phenomenon called central sensitization. This sensitization can result in abnormal interpretation of normal stimuli and chronic pain that lasts long after the original noxious stimulus. Increasing evidence suggests that preventing or minimizing acute pain may reduce the incidence of long-term pain (Dahl et al., 1990; Katz, 1997; Woolf, 1991). Therefore, pain relief after interventions such as opioid analgesia, the cornerstone of acute pain management (AHCPR, 1992), is a very important outcome to measure. Also, additional outcomes that would be helpful in understanding the broader impact of interventions would include improvement in activity and other pain-related quality of life issues.

Melzack and Dennis (1978) developed this conceptualization further by emphasizing that noxious stimuli enter an already active nervous system that is a substrate of past experience, culture, anticipation, and emotions. A person's cognitive processes act selectively on sensory input and motivation to influence pain transmission via the descending tracts to the dorsal horn. As a result, the amount, quality, and impact of pain are determined by individual factors such as previous pain experiences and one's concept of the cause of pain and its consequences. Therefore, pain is a highly personal experience and more than a noxious stimulus. Consequently, researchers have begun to look at outcomes besides pain sensation in order to understand the impact of pain on mood and usual activities, such as sleeping and walking. Their focus, however, has been on pain and its direct impact, and not on the more global experience of suffering. The terms "pain" and "suffering" have tended to be used interchangeably in the literature (Khan & Steeves, 1996). The distinction between the two—that pain is a perception of a sensation related to trauma or disease, whereas suffering takes place at the level of the person's lived experience—has not always been made clear. Spross (1996) defined suffering as being more than a perception or sensation, and as an evaluation of the meaning of pain for the person. Similarly, Kahn and Steeves (1996) emphasized that suffering is determined by the relationship between the self and the event, rather than by the inherent characteristics of the event itself.

In summary, Melzack and Wall (1965) emphasized that pain is a complex subjective phenomenon. Pain perception and responsiveness to a given stimulus are variable and unpredictable because of inhibitory mechanisms that include both endogenous neural activity and cognitive factors that are unique to each person (Fields, 1987). Pain mechanisms have a plasticity in that they can change in response to tissue injury such as surgery; pain perceptions can vary because of factors such as the meaning of pain (Wall, 1996). Although process outcomes such as pain intensity and pain relief are important to measure, they are unidimensional and focus only on pain sensation. Outcomes such as changes in usual activities and abilities reflect broader dimensions beyond the sensory that are important indicators of whether the intervention has been successful. However, almost all studies reviewed focus mainly on pain sensation.

5.2.3 *Conceptual Definition*

Based on the theoretical work in pain, one can conclude that pain is a subjective, multidimensional phenomenon that varies with each individual and each painful experience. The perception of pain and responsiveness to noxious stimuli are variable and unpredictable due to inhibitory mechanisms that include both endogenous neural activity and individuals' unique cognitive factors. Pain sensation and its direct impact are different from the broader concept of suffering.

5.2.4 *Factors that Influence Pain*

Pain perception is influenced by both internal and external factors. The nervous system has a functional plasticity that allows it to react to changing situations by altering its functions (Willis, 1994; Woolf, 1991). As a result, the nervous system does not respond in a fixed way to a given stimulus, but can alter its response properties dynamically. A person's cognitive processes act selectively on sensory input and motivation to influence pain transmission via the descending tracts to the dorsal horn (Melzack & Wall, 1965). Therefore, the amount and quality of pain are determined by individual factors such as previous pain experiences, mood, and one's concept of the cause of pain and its consequences. Also, cultural values can influence how one feels and responds to pain.

With repeated noxious stimuli, receptive fields can expand from the injured peripheral site to surrounding uninjured tissue. Alterations in perceptions of stimuli can occur, for example, so that a normal stimulus such as touch may be felt as painful. Therefore, pain involves not only the periphery, but can result from an altered central nervous system that is interpreting normal signals in an abnormal way. Consequently, a treatment implication is that prevention of pain signals from reaching the central nervous system peri- and postoperatively may reduce immediate pain as well as long-term pain problems (Dahl et al., 1990; Katz, 1997; Woolf, 1991).

5.3 Issues in the Assessment and Measurement of Pain

A broad review of the literature provided considerable evidence that pain assessment and its related management are problematic. Key issues that emerged are the need to (a) use standardized pain measures to guide assessment and related management, (b) control for nurse and patient mediators of effective assessment, and (c) use other outcomes as well as pain intensity to determine the impact of the pain problem and its management.

5.3.1 Using Standardized Pain Measures to Guide Assessment and Related Management

Standardized measures such as the 11-point numerical rating scale for pain intensity or the Brief Pain Inventory (BPI) have not routinely been a component of nursing assessment practices, and patients have not perceived nurses as resources in assessing and managing their pain (Watt-Watson, Garfinkel, et al., 2000). Moreover, nurses have underestimated the pain experienced by their patients, although they believed that mild pain or less was ideal.

Although nurses have identified asking the patient as the most frequently used method of determining pain intensity, fewer than 50% actually regarded it as the most influential factor (Ferrell et al., 1991). Instead, patient behaviors such as movement and verbal expressions like moaning were used to assess pain and determine analgesic interventions. These behaviors were ranked as more important than the patient's self-report. This finding is unfortunate, as patients frequently do not express pain or their need for help with management; instead they realize that their pain will be minimal if they do not move or breathe deeply and cough (Watt-Watson, Garfinkel, et al., 2000). Treating these behaviors as major pain indicators would also mean that patients must have significant return of pain before being given any intervention. Even recently, less than 50% of prescribed analgesia had been given despite patients' reports of moderate to severe pain (Watt-Watson, Garfinkel, et al., 2000; Watt-Watson, Stevens, et al., 2000).

5.3.2 Controlling for Nurse and Patient Mediators of Assessment

Nurses' experience and personal beliefs can influence their pain assessment. Nurses who experienced their own intense pain were more aware of their patients' pain (Holm et al., 1989). In addition, almost three quarters of nurses in Dalton's (1989) study reported that they were more empathic with patients having difficult pain management problems. Also, nurses have inferred greater pain when patients verbalized their discomfort (Baer et al., 1970). Similarly, patients who asked for pain relief were thought to suffer more than other patients (Oberst, 1978).

Patient characteristics such as diagnosis, age, gender, and culture may influence caregivers' perceptions of patients' pain and need for intervention. For example, female patients have received fewer analgesics after surgery than male patients (Calderone, 1990; Faherty & Grier, 1984; McDonald, 1994), older adult patients have received fewer analgesics than younger adult patients (Duggleby & Lander, 1994; Melzack et al., 1987; Winefield et al., 1990), and patients from ethnic minority groups have received less opioid analgesia postoperatively than did Caucasian patients (McDonald, 1994). As well, Bernabei et al. (1998) reported similar data in a study of 13,625 cancer patients aged 65 or more and living in a nursing home; predictors of unrelieved pain and minimal or no analgesic administration included being older, from a minority racial group after language adjustment, cognitively less able, and female. Todd, Samaroo, and Hoffman's (1993) research indicated that Hispanics with long-bone fractures were twice as likely as non-Hispanic Whites to receive no pain medication in emergency departments, although other research has found no racial differences in the amount of analgesia given in emergency departments (Choi et al., 2000). Cleeland et al. (1997) suggested that the inadequate analgesia for Hispanic patients found in their research may relate to patients' concerns about addiction and side effects, but the latter has been consistently documented for all patients (Ward et al., 1993; Watt-Watson et al., 2001).

Patients' own beliefs about pain may influence their seeking and accepting help (Ward et al., 1993); they identified opioid side effects such as constipation and nausea, as well as fears of addiction, as the major reasons for not seeking help with pain or taking analgesics. Several studies have documented that patients do not necessarily tell a caregiver when they are in pain (Carr, 1990; Lavies et al., 1992; Owen et al., 1990; Watt-Watson, Garfinkel et al., 2000); yet nurses have inferred more pain when patients verbalized their discomfort or asked for relief (Baer et al., 1970; Oberst, 1978).

5.3.3 *Using Other Outcomes as Well as Pain Intensity to Determine the Impact of the Pain Problem*

Pain is multidimensional and not directly proportional to tissue damage (Melzack & Wall, 1965). Although sensation is important, other dimensions, such as the quality and impact of pain, also need to be assessed. Only five trials in this review used measures to determine the impact of pain on everyday relationships and activities or health-related quality of life along with pain intensity (Dalton et al., 1999; de Wit & van Dam, 2001; LeFort et al., 1998; Ward et al., 2000; Watt-Watson, Stevens et al., 2000).

The approach to determining a person's pain commonly involves using quantitative measures of pain intensity and its location, and/or temporal features. Documented reports of the pain symptom have included primarily well-established unidimensional ratings to measure pain intensity, such as visual analogue scales (VAS) or numerical rating scales (NRS). The internationally recognized

McGill Pain Questionnaire, or MPQ (Melzack, 1975), developed from gate control theory, expanded pain assessment to include both qualitative and quantitative dimensions of pain sensation. Further development has included multidimensional measures, such as the Brief Pain Inventory (Daut et al., 1983), which are beginning to be documented to examine not only intensity but also pain-related interference in usual activities.

More recently, the paucity of measures to examine patients' expectations and perceptions of their pain management experience has been recognized. However, most of these measures have been utilized in single studies with major design issues and have only rudimentary reliability and validity; therefore, they will not be discussed here. The Barriers Questionnaire, both long and short forms, has established reliability and validity and asks about concerns patients have that would prevent them from taking analgesics or asking for help with pain (Ward et al., 1998; Ward et al., 1993). As concerns are a mediator of pain, but not a direct measure of pain sensation or its impact on everyday activities, this scale will not be included in this review. However, data related to this measure are included in the two studies using concerns as a mediator variable (Ward et al., 2000; Watt-Watson, Stevens, et al., 2000). Well-established health-related quality of life measures such as the MOH-SF36 were used in two studies (de Wit & van Dam, 2001; LeFort et al., 1998) but are discussed in the chapter on functional status in this book.

Therefore, only measures used almost exclusively in the 24 studies selected for this review will be discussed in this chapter. These measures include the visual analogue numerical rating scales, the McGill Pain Questionnaire, and the Brief Pain Inventory.

5.4 Evidence Concerning the Relationship between Nursing and Pain as a Symptom Outcome

The 24 empirical studies that were identified are reviewed in Table 5.1. In all but one of the studies, pain as a primary outcome was operationalized as intensity and measured by VAS or NRS. Fewer researchers used the MPQ or the BPI. In 11 studies, however, additional outcomes along with pain intensity were examined, including pain-related quality of life or activity interference issues ($n = 6$), and/or analgesic prescription and administration ($n = 5$). In one study, analgesic prescription and administration was the primary outcome. The nursing contexts included (a) acute care ($n = 17$ including emergency [2]); (b) home (4) or rural care (1); (c) outpatient or oncology practice (2); or (d) university health service/community (1). Only recently have nurses begun to systematically examine the influence of interventions on patient outcomes related to pain management by using randomized controlled trials. In this review, 16 studies were randomized controlled trials and the remainder had quasi-experimental pre/posttest designs.

The evidence supporting pain as a relevant outcome for measuring nursing interventions is equivocal. The nursing interventions identified in this review include (a) nonpharmacological strategies including music alone or combined with relaxation or ibuprofen (Broscious, 1999; Good et al., 2001; Tanabe et al., 2001), therapeutic touch (Keller & Bzdek, 1986; Meehan, 1993), and cutaneous stimulation (Kubsch et al., 2000); (b) patient education (Ahles et al., 2001; Closs et al., 1999; Clotfelter, 1999; LeFort et al., 1998; McDonald et al., 2001; Neitzel et al., 1999; Ward et al., 2000; Watt-Watson, Stevens et al., 2000); (c) nurses' education (Dahlman et al., 1999; Dalton et al., 1999; de Rond et al., 2000; de Rond et al., 1999; de Wit & van Dam, 2001; Francke et al., 1997; Holzheimer et al., 1999; Neitzel et al., 1999); and (d) nurses' individual feedback related to assessment and pain treatment flowchart (Duncan & Pozehl, 2000). Two studies were also reviewed that reported systematic reviews of the use of relaxation techniques, including imagery, hypnosis, visualization, and cognitive therapy (Seers & Carroll, 1998), and nonpharmacological interventions (Sindhu, 1996).

5.4.1 *Nonpharmacologic Strategies*

Broscious (1999) demonstrated no significant differences in NRS scores for pain intensity with the music intervention group during chest-tube removal for elective open heart surgical patients. Tanabe et al. (2001) also reported no clinically significant pain relief for patients with moderate pain from minor musculoskeletal pain in the emergency department, using standard care (ice, elevation, immobilization) alone or with ibuprofen or music. However, Good et al. (2001) found that music alone or with relaxation, or relaxation alone, did reduce pain at rest and on ambulation for patients following abdominal surgery. Using therapeutic touch, Keller & Bzdek (1986) reported greater pain relief for this group on the MPQ at the first posttest time, which did not last to the four-hour time for university volunteers with tension headaches. In contrast, Meehan (1993) found that therapeutic touch did not make a difference in pain intensity on a VAS for elective abdominal or pelvic surgical patients. However, Kubsch et al. (2000) reported significant reductions in pain intensity and interference scores using a VAS for patients receiving cutaneous stimulation in an emergency setting. In addition, Sindhu (1996) found some evidence that relaxation reduced pain scores, although heterogeneity in design and methods between studies made findings of this meta-analysis difficult to interpret. Similarly, Seers and Carroll (1998) found that three studies with methodological problems did report reduced pain with muscle relaxation with or without imagery; however, four other more rigorously designed studies reported no differences.

Table 5.1. Studies Investigating the Relationship between Nursing Interventions and Pain as a Symptom Outcome

Author/date	Design of study (method of participant assignment, number of measurement occasions)	Characteristics of the sample and response rate (RR) and the setting (acute, community, or long-term care)	Definition of the outcome concept	Nursing interventions being evaluated	Major results	Limitations
Ahles et al., 2001	Pilot RCT, randomized to usual care group or telephone-based pain intervention; baseline screening for pain and mailed outcome assessment at 3- to 6-months post enrollment.	744 patients from four U.S. rural primary care practices with mild to severe pain in last 4 weeks; RR = 32 randomized to usual care (n = 320) or intervention groups (n= 295, RR = 92%), with or without psychosocial problems; mean age = 48; 55% women.	Pain defined as intensity (NRS 0–5), duration, location, and adequacy of treatment; psychosocial functioning (Medical Outcomes Study Short Form, SF-36); Functional Interference Estimate (FIE).	Telephone-based pain assessment and tailored education strategies by phone and mail.	Patients in the intervention group had significantly better scores on SF-36 for Pain, Physical, Emotional, and Social subscales and on the total Functional Interference Scale.	Description of methodology unclear; patient response rate low for study (32%) and final questionnaires (53%); follow-up period post-intervention varied from 3–6 months; despite randomization, significant differences between groups for age, sex, emotional distress, and poor health status.
Broscious, 1999	Experimental, single-blind, pretest/posttest three-group design; random assignment using blinded group chip selection for control, white noise, or music prior to chest tube removal (CTR); pain measured at baseline, 5–7 and 20–22 minutes after CTR.	156/189 patients having elective open heart surgery in U.S. (4 withdrew, 29 became ineligible due to complications or surgery cancellation). Surgeries included 81% coronary bypass graft, 9% valve, and 9% both; chest tubes were mediastinal (100%) plus one (80%) or two (20%) pleural tubes; Mean (SD) age = 66 (9.7) years; 38% women.	Pain intensity measured by a numerical rating scale (NRS 0–10).	Music vs. white noise vs. control; experimental groups listened to tape 10 minutes pre-chest removal, either to the same white noise or to music chosen from 10 options at preadmission testing; controls had standard care not described.	No significant differences at any time period, and mean score for total group 5–7 minutes after procedure was 5.62 ± 2.79.	Further work needed on dosing, timing, and type of music.

Table 5.1 (continued)

Author/date	Design of study (method of participant assignment, number of measurement occasions)	Characteristics of the sample and response rate (RR) and the setting (acute, community, or long-term care)	Definition of the outcome concept	Nursing interventions being evaluated	Major results	Limitations
Closs et al., 1999	Pre/posttrial with a control and intervention ward sample over 9 months; interviewed for 15–30 minutes in A.M. of second day post-surgery.	417 patients from two matched orthopedic wards in four groups in England; convenience sample of elective or trauma patients; excluded if working nights, had terminal disease, confused or cognitively impaired; RR and demographics not stated.	Experience of postop night-time pain defined by pain intensity (verbal rating scale, 0–4), analgesics given, pain documentation, and patient-initiated reports.	Patient information and structured pain assessment to improve pain after surgery at night.	Significant reductions in overnight worst and average pain scores and increase in documented pain assessments; no differences in patients' reporting pain or analgesic administration.	Information intervention did not address toxicity and addiction concerns.
Clotfelter, 1999	Quasi-experimental pretest/posttest design; patients randomly assigned; pain measured at baseline, 2 weeks later twice on same day.	36 elderly people (≥65 years) with cancer from a U.S. private oncology practice; RR = 88% (17 rated pain as zero at 3 time periods and were removed); mean age = 77; 64% women.	Pain intensity measured by visual analogue scale (VAS 0–100).	Education video and booklet; experimental group received booklet and saw video vs. control who received only instructions from office staff.	Significantly less pain for experimental group than for control group (F_{34} = 5.8, $p < 0.02$).	Small sample, although differences significant; use of VAS with elderly may have influenced pain ratings; generalizable to this sample only.

Table 5.1 (continued)

Author/date	Design of study (method of participant assignment, number of measurement occasions)	Characteristics of the sample and response rate (RR) and the setting (acute community, or long-term care)	Definition of the outcome concept	Nursing interventions being evaluated	Major results	Limitations
Dahlman et al., 1999	Pretest/posttest design with two different convenience samples; all patients rated pain daily and were asked for a retrospective review before discharge; one group given open-ended questions pre-study and one group at 3 months post-study.	75 patients (RR = 94%) with thorax surgery via sternotomy in Sweden; no demographic data reported.	Pain intensity using VAS (0–10); satisfaction with pain relief, pain experience, but domains unclear.	A study day for nurses on pain; all nurses in thoracic surgery (N > 75–6 = 69) attended a study day focused on physiology, pharmacology, pain assessment, and treatment strategies.	Patients reported lower pain ratings post-intervention; all pain scores were low but postgroup significantly lower; 95% satisfied with pain relief.	Quasi-experimental with non-equivalent control group; not clear if pain ratings at rest or on movement.
Dalton et al., 1999	RCT, random selection of 6/14 hospitals having interest in an education intervention, and random assignment to experimental or control; data were collected from convenience patient samples and charts at baseline, end of program, and 6 months later on experimental sites.	Cohorts of 50 patients per site at discharge after abdominal, thoracic, or orthopedic surgery in three community hospitals of 100–500 beds in North Carolina; median age = 49; 69% women; 84.5% Caucasian, 14.8% African-American.	Pain defined as an unpleasant sensory and emotional experience arising from actual or potential damage or described in terms of such damage (IASP), pain-related interference, and patient satisfaction using American Pain Society questionnaire.	A pain education program for nurses, physicians, and pharmacists; teams of 10–15 RNs, 1–2 MDs, and 2 pharmacists designated per site for the program; a Delphi-developed program was given in three 4.5-hour sessions over 8 weeks on pain assessment, pharmacology, and patient role in evaluation of relief.	Outcome data to be reported.	No patient outcome data reported.

Table 5.1 (continued)

Author/date	Design of study (method of participant assignment, number of measurement occasions)	Characteristics of the sample and response rate (RR) and the setting (acute, community, or long-term care)	Definition of the outcome concept	Nursing interventions being evaluated	Major results	Limitations
de Rond et al., 2000	Quasi-experimental with non-equivalent control group; interviewed twice: on admission and either before discharge (control) or post-intervention.	480 Dutch patients from two surgical wards and one medical ward from each of three general hospitals; patients stratified for duration of pain (acute/chronic) and type of pain (non-cancer/cancer); $RR = 68\%$; mean (SD) age = 59.5 (16.8); 58.5% female.	Prescribed analgesics by MDs, administered analgesics by RNs, and the discrepancy between the two.	3-hour pain education for nurses and implementation of two daily pain assessments (NRS 0–10).	The Pain Monitoring Program improved nurses' administration of analgesics ($p < 0.05$), particularly with moderate-severe pain; however, the discrepancy between orders and administration did not change; PRN dosing was excluded from this.	Quasi-experimental with non-equivalent control group; excluded PRN analgesia from total administration calculations; some post-intervention interviews completed after discharge at home.
de Rond et al., 1999	Part of larger study using a quasi-experimental, non-equivalent control group design; this study includes the intervention group experiencing daily pain assessments in hospital.	Patients from one medical and two surgical wards in each of three hospitals in the Netherlands; included if in pain or had an analgesic prescription; diagnoses included acute malignant, chronic malignant, acute non-cancer, and chronic non-cancer pain; $N = 315$, $RR = 315/369$: 24 declined as older and female, and 30 older patients left after first interview; mean (SD) age = 58.6 (17.3); 56.2% women.	Feasibility and value of daily pain assessments (NRS, 0–10) as determined by patient opinion; experimental group was asked four open-ended questions about daily pain assessment at second interview.	Nurses' compliance with daily, systematic pain assessment and value for nurses and patients; all nurses working in areas ($n = 227$) were given 3-hour education about pain assessment, NRS, and pharmacological and nonpharmacological management.	75% of patients were positive about using NRS twice daily; instructions confused some patients.	Quasi-experimental with non-equivalent control group; not clear how sites chosen.

Table 5.1 (continued)

Author/date	Design of study (method of participant assignment, number of measurement occasions)	Characteristics of the sample and response rate (RR) and the setting (acute, community, or long-term care)	Definition of the outcome concept	Nursing interventions being evaluated	Major results	Limitations
de Wit & van Dam, 2001	Randomized, longitudinal study with pretest/posttest experimental design; stratified by sex, age, metastatic site; interviewed at baseline and 2, 4, 8 weeks post-discharge.	104 cancer patients with chronic pain at home; at 8 weeks attrition, 20% control vs. 41% intervention group due to deaths; 68.6% women; mean (SD) age = 58.1 (12.4).	Pain intensity (NRS 0–10) and experience (location, time since onset, analgesic use); Quality of Life (EORTC QLQ-C30).	Pain education program tailored for individual patients.	No significant differences between groups for pain.	Despite randomization, groups differed on analgesics administered, physical and cognitive functioning at baseline, and 41% intervention group vs. 20% control group died post-discharge.
Duncan & Pozehl, 2000	Quasi-experimental pretest/posttest design with data collected from two convenience samples of patients over 17 weeks, pre-nurse feedback and post-intervention follow-up over 15 months along with retrospective chart data.	240 patients had a total knee arthroplasty (pre =121, post =119) on a unit where PCA morphine was standard in first 24–28 hours postop in U.S.; 243 patient records were audited postop and 3 excluded due to complications; mean age = 70; 62% women.	Pain intensity (NRS 0–10); analgesic use from chart data: morphine equivalents given during 4-day postop stay, post-analgesic effectiveness (NRS, 0–10).	Intervention involves performance feedback to nurses on patients' postoperative pain outcomes; 30 nurses (23 RNs, 7 LPNs) working on the unit for a minimum of 6 months received individual feedback and a pain treatment flowchart related to their q4h assessment, post-analgesic assessments, follow-up, and documentation of patients' acceptable pain level.	Significant changes from pre- to posttest included a decline in mean pain ratings from 3.59 to 3.16, increase in analgesic use from 12.70 mg to 14.54 mg morphine equivalents, decrease in postanalgesic ratings from 3.07 to 2.68, and decrease in unacceptable levels of pain after analgesia from 1.12 to 0.84.	Quasi-experimental with non-equivalent control group; patient pain outcomes were taken from documented ratings.

Table 5.1 (continued)

Author/date	Design of study (method of participant assignment, number of measurement occasions)	Characteristics of the sample and response rate (RR) and the setting (acute, community, or long-term care)	Definition of the outcome concept	Nursing interventions being evaluated	Major results	Limitations
Francke et al., 1997	Pretest/posttest control group design; in each of five hospitals, one ward randomly allocated to CE Program for nurses or control (no program); data collected for 3 months before and 3–6 months after the program; interviewed the day before about 4:00 A.M., and at 2 and 4 days after surgery.	152 surgical patients with curative resection of colon or breast cancer in five Dutch hospitals in four groups per hospital: pre/post groups on intervention ward and pre/post control groups on control ward; nurse recruiters reported less than 10% refusal rate; mean (SD) age = 68.6 (13.6, colon) and 61.2 (25.5, breast); women = 55.5% for colon and 100% for breast.	Pain intensity NRS (0–10), pain duration during day, and sleep disruption because of pain (two items from McGill Pain Quality of Life Questionnaire).	Continuing pain education program for nurses on surgical cancer units; all qualified nurses on ward team given 8 weekly 3-hour sessions on pain assessment and management and one follow-up session 4 months after the program.	Pain intensity day 2 was less for treatment group, but not day 4 ($p < 0.02$); no differences in pain duration and number of sleepless hours from pain.	Not clear which changes in intervention program were related to decreased patient pain.
Good et al., 2001	Secondary analysis of RCT; random assignment to one of four groups (relaxation, music, combined, and control); baseline and days 1 and 2 post-surgery.	468 abdominal surgery patients in five U.S. hospitals; RR = 76%; mean (SD) age = 45 (11); 84% women.	Pain: used IASP definition, pain intensity (NRS 0–100), distress (NRS 0–100); jaw relaxation as lowering jaw slightly, let tongue rest quietly, allow lips to get soft, breathe slowly, and stop thinking; music types: synthesizer, harp, piano orchestra, or slow modern jazz.	Relaxation and/or music to reduce postoperative pain.	Treatment groups had less pain and distress across days, but interventions were not statistically different in effect.	None noted

Table 5.1 (continued)

Author/date	Design of study (method of participant assignment, number of measurement occasions)	Characteristics of the sample and response rate (RR) and the setting (acute, community, or long-term care)	Definition of the outcome concept	Nursing interventions being evaluated	Major results	Limitations
Holzheimer et al., 1999	Pretest/posttest design using secondary analysis of two studies, one before a nurse intervention and one about 2 years later; measures taken twice for pretest group within 48 hours of admission to hospice care and at week 4, and once for posttest group over a wide range of time periods > 48 hours.	Pretest ($n = 47$) and posttest ($n = 255$) homecare hospice patients with cancer in the U.S.; mean (SD) age for both groups = 71 (10.2–12.1); women = 48–52%.	Pain intensity defined as worst pain in the past week (NRS 0–10); pain relief (NRS 0–10) rated from none to complete relief in past week.	Nurse-focused, hospice-wide, four-part intervention including education, policies and procedures, documentation, and performance evaluation.	Adjusted mean scores improved from 1995 to 1997 for worst pain ($X = 6.7$ to 6.1) and pain relief ($X = 6.0$ to 8.4).	Non-equivalent control group; timing of data collection differed; different pain scales were used for each group.
Keller & Bzdek, 1986	RCT, two-group design with convenience samples; measures taken prior to, 5 minutes after, and 4 hours after intervention.	60 volunteers from a U.S. university with tension headache who were not taking medication 4 hours before the intervention; mean age = 30; women = 75%.	Pain defined as tension headache with no prodrome, neurological deficit, infectious process, or recent head trauma; pain intensity measured using MPQ-Pain Rating Index, number of words chosen, Present Pain Intensity.	Therapeutic touch (TT) vs. placebo; treatment group given a standardized 5-minute therapeutic touch procedure; other group given a mimicked TT (MTT) using counting rather than a meditative state; both groups told to use deep breathing during the post-intervention 5-minute interval.	TT group had greater relief than MTT group at first posttest time (MPQ reduction $X = 70\%$ [TT] vs. 37% [MTT] $p < 0.002$), but no significant differences at 4 hours posttest.	Small sample size; overall results presented as positive, although no significant differences at 4 hours post-intervention; minimized the contribution effect of deep breathing in a 5-minute quiet break.

Table 5.1 (continued)

Author/date	Design of study (method of participant assignment, number of measurement occasions)	Characteristics of the sample and response rate (RR) and the setting (acute, community, or long-term care)	Definition of the outcome concept	Nursing interventions being evaluated	Major results	Limitations
Kubsch et al., 2000	One-group pretest/posttest design with convenience sample having cutaneous stimulation.	50 people entering a U.S. emergency department over a 6-month period, who were experiencing pain due to non-emergent/non-life-threatening conditions and who had not self-medicated for pain in the previous 4 hours. 12 < 18 years; women = 64%.	Pain intensity (NRS 0–10) and VAS, blood pressure, and heart rate.	Cutaneous stimulation; certified emergency nurse was trained and implemented the intervention.	Significant reductions in pain scores ($t = 7.09$, $p<0.0001$), heart rate ($t = 2.79$, $p<0.008$), and BP ($t = 3.42$, $p<0.0013$) after cutaneous stimulation using circular pressure/massage to a localized site (over, contra-lateral, or proximal to pain site).	Small sample size; one-group pretest/posttest design.
LeFort et al., 1998	RCT, consenting adults randomly allocated to one of two conditions; measures at pretreatment and posttreatment 3 months later; 11 programs with 6–10 participants each.	110 people in Newfoundland (treatment = 57, control = 53) with idiopathic chronic non-cancer pain longer than 3 months; 5 from treatment and 3 from control groups did not complete the study; patients self-referred or from pain specialists; women = 75%; mean age = 40; attrition = 7%.	Pain sensation (MPQ-SF, VAS [0–100]); disability: subscale of Survey of Pain Attitudes (SOPA-D) and severity (VAS 0–100); health-related quality of life: Medical Outcomes Study Short Form (SF-36).	A community-based chronic pain self-management psychoeducation program included six 2-hour sessions given by the principal investigator.	Significant improvement in treatment group, who reported reduced severity of pain problem; less disability (SOPA-D) and greater improvement for bodily pain, physical role functioning, and vitality (SF-36).	Examined effect to 3 months only; only one facilitator used.

Table 5.1 (continued)

Author/date	Design of study (method of participant assignment, number of measurement occasions)	Characteristics of the sample and response rate (RR) and the setting (acute, community, or long-term care)	Definition of the outcome concept	Nursing interventions being evaluated	Major results	Limitations
McDonald et al., 2001	Two-group, double-blind RCT; data collected prospectively over three points (pre-surgery, and post-surgery on days 1 and 2).	31 people ≥ 65 years old having elective single total hip or knee replacement; mean (SD) age = 74 (6); 74% women; attrition = 23%.	Pain as measured by MPQ-SF.	A PowerPoint slide show to teach basic pain management, communication skills, and two intensity rating scales.	Patients receiving the intervention reported less postoperative pain over the course of their hospital stay.	Small sample size; asked for first rating the evening of surgery, which may have influenced communication abilities; usual care included pain scales.
Meehan, 1993	A single-blind, three-group design with convenience samples over a 7-month period; measures taken prior to and one hour after intervention during the evening.	N = 108 U.S. patients scheduled for major elective abdominal or pelvic surgery and requesting opioid analgesia during the evening of data collection; age range of 23–79 years; women = 70%.	Pain intensity (VAS 0–100) and verbal descriptor scale of no pain, mild pain, moderate pain, severe pain, and pain as bad as it could be.	Therapeutic touch vs. opioid analgesia vs. placebo; experimental group given a standardized 5-minute TT procedure, the other groups, the standard opioid care or a mimicked TT using counting rather than a meditative state.	Pain intensity reduced only in the group receiving opioid analgesics; 56% of all patients requested opioids.	Control of placebo effect.

Table 5.1 (continued)

Author/date	Design of study (method of participant assignment, number of measurement occasions)	Characteristics of the sample and response rate (RR) and the setting (acute, community, or long-term care)	Definition of the outcome concept	Nursing interventions being evaluated	Major results	Limitations
Neitzel et al., 1999	Pretest/posttest design with convenience samples of patients prior to patient and health professional pain education interventions, and 8 months later with a different sample.	118 patients (57 pre-intervention and 61 post-intervention, having surgery for total knee or hip replacement in the U.S.; 3 pretest patients excluded with incomplete medical record data; age range 30–89.	Patient pain experience defined as pain intensity (VAS 0–10 for current and average), function (VAS 0–10 for walking, sleeping, and relating to others), opioid side effects, and satisfaction.	Education program for health professionals (program, revised orders, & documentation) and patients (information); all nurses on an orthopedic unit ($n = 28$) attended 8 hours of pain education; also, all patients given pain material either before or after surgery.	No decrease in pain and no significant differences in pain, function, side effects, or satisfaction.	Pretest/posttest non-equivalent control group; intervention time variable.
Seers & Carroll, 1998	Systematic review of published studies of relaxation techniques.	Seven RCTs involving 362 patients, of whom 150 received relaxation; 33/40 studies excluded: 11 not RCTs, 22 RCTs for small sample size less than 10/group, combination interventions, and/or no pain outcomes; six settings were after surgery and one during femoral angiography.	Pain (VAS 0–10, MPQ), analgesic data, and length of stay from chart.	Relaxation techniques including imagery, hypnosis, visualization, and cognitive therapy.	Three studies reported less pain and/or distress if muscle relaxation used with or without imagery, but methodology and validity problems; no difference for four remaining rigorously designed studies.	Heterogeneity amongst studies.

Table 5.1 (continued)

Author/date	Design of study (method of participant assignment, number of measurement occasions)	Characteristics of the sample and response rate (RR) and the setting (acute, community, or long-term care)	Definition of the outcome concept	Nursing interventions being evaluated	Major results	Limitations
Sindhu, 1996	Meta-analysis of RCTs assessing the effectiveness of nonpharmacological interventions for pain management.	49 RCTs (14 unpublished) of nonpharmacological therapies in acute pain management with 3,357 patients.	Pain intensity.	Nonpharmacological methods.	Strong heterogeneity between the studies making the pooled effect size of 0.06 (range −2.25 to 1.78) difficult to interpret; subgroup analysis also demonstrated considerable heterogeneity, although some evidence that patient teaching and relaxation reduced pain scores.	Heterogeneity amongst studies; pooled effect size 0.06.
Tanabe et al., 2001	Three-group RCT; prospective data collection at baseline and 30 and 60 minutes post-intervention.	76 patients in an emergency department of a suburban U.S. hospital, with pain rating ≥ 4 (0–10) from minor extremity trauma distal to and including the knee or elbow, mean (SD) age = 41 (18).	Pain intensity (NRS 0–10) and two questions for satisfaction related to total treatment (Likert scale 1–6) and binary yes/no response to immediate attention in triage.	Use of ibuprofen or music along with standard care of ice, elevation, and immobilization.	Standard care alone, or with ibuprofen or music, did not decrease moderate pain with musculoskeletal trauma.	Small sample size and nonrandom assignment.

Table 5.1 (continued)

Author/date	Design of study (method of participant assignment, number of measurement occasions)	Characteristics of the sample and response rate (RR) and the setting (acute, community, or long-term care)	Definition of the outcome concept	Nursing interventions being evaluated	Major results	Limitations
Ward et al., 2000	Randomized two-group pilot over an 18-month period; consenting adults randomly allocated to care-as-usual ($n = 22$) or informational intervention group ($n = 21$); measures at baseline, 1-, and 2-month follow-up after education intervention.	43 women with metastatic gynecological cancers in a U.S. outpatient comprehensive care cancer center; attrition by third interview = 41%; reason given was too ill. No difference in dropout between groups; mean (SD) age = 58 (12); *RR* = 56%.	Pain intensity: now, worst pain, and least pain in last week (BPI-NRS 0–10); congruence between severity of pain and medication used (Pain Management Index); interference in activities (BPI); Concerns by Barriers Questionnaire.	Pain information vs. usual care; individually tailored information about concerns (barriers) and side effect management discussed related to a booklet previously developed; two highest rated concerns then clarified; booster telephone calls given at 1 week post-intervention and post-time two measures.	No differential improvement in outcome evident for any group; both groups reported decrease in barriers and interference because of pain.	Small sample size and attrition = 41%, may be floor effect due to selection bias as refusal related to severe pain; short follow-up; intervention did not explore basis for individual barriers.
Watt-Watson, Stevens et al., 2000	RCT pilot; consenting adults randomly allocated to control (standard care) or two treatment conditions (standard + booklet or standard + booklet and interview) measures at preadmission clinic and days 3 and 5 after surgery.	Of 50 consenting patients, 45 responded at all three periods with 2 from group two too ill at day 3; 3 too ill to complete any measures after surgery; patients were having their first elective coronary artery bypass graft surgery in Toronto; mean (SD) age = 60.46 (9.49), 5 women.	Pain intensity and quality (NRS 0–10 [rest on movement, present, & past 24 hours], MPQ); analgesic data from chart; interference in activities (interference subscale of BPI); concerns measured by short form of Barriers Questionnaire.	Pain education; eight-page, pain-focused booklet given to patients prior to surgery.	No significant differences using ANOVA among three groups for pain including worst 24h NRS day 3: $\overline{X} = 6.63 \pm 2.46$, day 5: $\overline{X} = 6.0 \pm 2.91$; PPI day 3: $\overline{X} = 2.43 \pm 1.07$, day 5: $\overline{X} = 2.29 \pm 1.06$. No differences for interference because of pain or analgesia; intervention groups had significantly fewer concerns ($F_2, 42 = 4.17, p < 0.02$) and were more satisfied with treatment ($F_2, 40 = 2.96, p < 0.06$).	None noted

5.4.2 Patient Education

Ahles et al. (2001) reported that patients from four rural primary care practices who received a telephone-based, nurse-educator pain intervention scored significantly better than controls for pain; physical, emotional, and social SF-36 subscales; and functional interference scores. Also, Closs et al. (1999) demonstrated significant reductions in overnight pain intensity, on a 1 to 5 verbal descriptor scale, for orthopedic patients receiving a pain-education booklet, although analgesic administration did not differ between groups. Clotfelter (1999) also found that older-aged cancer patients who received a booklet and saw a video also reported less pain on a VAS than the control group. LeFort et al. (1998) found that a chronic non-cancer community patient sample participating in a psychoeducation program reported reduced pain severity on the MPQ and a VAS. Similarly, McDonald et al.'s (2001) sample of elderly patients receiving pain education related to communication, management, and intensity scales reported less pain after total hip or knee replacement surgery. Ward et al. (2000) reported that all women with metastatic gynecological cancer in a trial of individually tailored information about concerns and side effect management experienced less pain interference (BPI-interference) at one month, regardless of their randomized group.

In contrast, Neitzel et al. (1999) demonstrated no decrease in pain on a VAS for an orthopedic group receiving a pain booklet. Similarly, Watt-Watson, Stevens et al. (2000) found no significant differences in pain on the MPQ-SF or in analgesic administration for coronary bypass surgical patients receiving a pain education booklet.

5.4.3 Nurses Education

Educational pain-focused programs for nurses have resulted in reduced pain scores for patients having thoracic (Dahlman et al., 1999), colon, or breast surgery (Francke et al., 1977) and for those in a homecare hospice program (Holzheimer et al., 1999). De Rond and colleagues (1999, 2000) concluded from their findings that using a simple numerical rating scale along with pain education for nurses improved the analgesic administration for medical and surgical patients in three Dutch hospitals. De Wit & van Dam (2001) found that district nurses who received additional information about the pain of patients being discharged to them better estimated patients' pain intensity and were more satisfied with patients' pain management, but were no different from the control group on assessing patients' relief. However, Neitzel et al. (1999) demonstrated no statistically significant decrease in pain ratings for an orthopedic patient sample, despite their being given educational material either before admission or postoperatively. Outcome data are yet to be reported for an eight-week program for nurses working with surgical patients (Dalton et al., 1999). Across studies, variability was evident in the length of programs (3–13.5 hours) and duration of teaching (one day to eight weeks).

5.4.4 Individual Nurse Feedback

Duncan and Pozehl (2000) demonstrated a statistically significant decline in mean pain ratings and an increase in analgesic use for orthopedic patients when nurses received performance feedback about their pain management practices (Duncan & Pozehl, 2000). Nurses were evaluated on four practices that included pain assessments every four hours, assessments after analgesic administration, action for unacceptable pain ratings, and documentation of the patient's acceptable pain level. Each nurse received a copy of the feedback and a pain treatment flow chart. Although Holzheimer et al. (1999) included performance improvement monitors as a part of their nurse intervention, this component's effectiveness was not reported.

In summary, a significant improvement in pain following nursing intervention was reported in some of the studies reviewed. However, responses to these pain interventions are equivocal, which may relate more to issues such as the individuality of the pain experience, complexity of the pain management context, and/or methodology issues like uncontrolled designs than to the measures themselves. When the evidence from the most rigorous clinical trials is examined, nursing interventions such as patients' and nurses' education improved patients' pain outcomes. However, the interventions vary considerably in both design and implementation. Nevertheless, based on the evidence from the clinical trials, there is reason to suggest that pain is an outcome that is relevant and sensitive to nursing practice.

5.5 Evidence Concerning Approaches to Measurement

This review included only those measures used to examine the relationship between nursing interventions and patient outcomes related to pain. Three measures of pain sensation and/or pain-related impact on usual activities were identified in this review of the empirical nursing literature. The following characteristics of these measures are summarized in Table 5.2: (a) target population; (b) domains of measurement, number of items, and response format; (c) method of administration; (d) reliability; (e) validity; and (f) sensitivity to nursing intervention.

The approach to assessing pain in all studies was to use the instrument as a self-report measure or interview guide. Therefore, the inclusion criteria for all studies included the ability to speak, read, and understand the primary language

Table 5.2. Instruments Measuring Pain

Instrument (author)	Target population	Domains (number of items and response forms)	Method of administration	Reliability	Validity	Sensitivity to nursing care
Brief Pain Inventory (Cleeland & Syrjala, 1992)	Adults	20 items; pain history, etiology, intensity, location, quality, and interference with activities.	Self-administered	Internal consistency of pain intensity range from 0.80 to 0.86 (McDowell & Newell, 1996); reliability for the interference subscale range from 0.86 to 0.91 (McDowell & Newell, 1996).	Discriminant validity (Cleeland, 1991); Construct validity (McDowell & Newell, 1996).	Sensitivity to change in 5-day postoperative period in a nursing study (Watt-Watson, Stevens, et al., 2000).
McGill Pain Questionnaire (Melzack, 1975, 1987)	Adults	Domains: 1) Body outline for pain location, 2) Present Pain Intensity (6 items), 3) a pain rating index (78 adjectives), 4) pain pattern (9 items)	Self-report or by interview.	Good test-retest reliability (Wilkie et al., 1990).	Construct validity (Lowe et al., 1991) and concurrent validity (Dudgeon et al., 1993).	Sensitivity to change in a nursing evaluation of a pain self-management trial (LeFort et al., 1998).
Visual Analogue Scale (VAS) and numeric rating scales (NRS): numerous author-generated versions (McDowell & Newell, 1996)	Adolescent and cognitively intact adults	One-item measuring, measured with 11-point scale; perceived pain intensity or relief.	Self-administered.	High test-retest reliability (Scott & Huskisson, 1976; Grossman et al., 1991).	Concurrent, construct validity (Grossman et al., 1991; Jansen & McFadden, 1989; Price et al., 1994).	Evidence of sensitivity to change in nursing trials for VAS (Dahlman et al., 1999; Meehan et al., 1993; Seers & Carroll, 1998); and for NRS (Duncan & Pozehl, 2000; Francke et al., 1997; Holzheimer et al., 1999; Kubsch et al., 2000).

of the country (i.e., Dutch, English); patients were excluded if they were cognitively impaired. All patients in this review were adults; since pain is a subjective phenomenon, this approach was appropriate.

The most frequently used approach to examine outcomes has focused on pain intensity, along with its location and/or temporal features. Unidimensional measures to document pain intensity have included visual analogue scales or numerical rating scales that have clinical utility as well as established reliability and validity. In five studies in this review, additional measures were used to examine pain. To assess both the qualitative and quantitative aspects of pain sensation, Melzack (1975) developed the McGill Pain Questionnaire to include not only a VAS for pain intensity but also adjectives that patients could use to describe the sensory, affective, and evaluative components of pain sensation. From the MPQ, Daut et al. (1983) developed the Brief Pain Inventory, a multidimensional measure that examines the impact of pain on mood and usual activities, as well as the person's response to treatment. The use of the longer or shorter versions of the MPQ and BPI depends on the nursing context, that is, shorter forms for more acute care settings.

The three measures that were used almost exclusively in the 24 studies selected for this review include the (a) visual analogue scales and/or the numerical rating scale version, (b) McGill Pain Questionnaire, and (c) Brief Pain Questionnaire.

5.5.1 Visual Analogue Scale/Numerical Rating Scale

The visual analogue scales have been used primarily to measure patients' perceived pain intensity or pain relief. The numerical rating scale is an alternative format that asks patients to verbally choose a number between 0 (no pain) and 10 (worst pain ever), instead of marking their intensity on a line. Scott and Huskisson (1976) established that retest reliability of the VAS was higher (0.94) with literate patients than with nonliterate ones (0.71), whereas the NRS did not differ significantly because of literacy (0.96 and 0.95, respectively). Responses have been defined as mild (1–3), moderate (4–6), or severe (7–10) (Cleeland & Syrjala, 1992).

The sensitivity to change in pain over time was evident in several nursing trials in this review for both VAS (Clotfelter, 1999; Dahlman et al., 1999; Kubsch et al., 2000; Meehan, 1993; Seers & Carroll, 1998; Sindhu, 1996) and NRS (Ahles et al., 2001; Dalton et al., 1999; de Rond et al., 2000; de Rond et al., 1999; Duncan & Pozehl, 2000; Francke et al., 1997; Good et al., 2001; Holzheimer et al., 1999; Kubsch et al., 2000). Although both kinds of measures were used in the studies reviewed, the NRS was used twice as often, perhaps because of its greater clinical utility. NRS are easier to administer and score, require no costs for measures, and have a high rate of correct response regardless of literacy (Ferraz et al., 1990; Guyatt et al., 1987). The majority (75%) of de Rond et al.'s (1999) sample of medical-surgical patients were positive about using the NRS twice daily.

5.5.2 McGill Pain Questionnaire

The long form of the MPQ includes (a) a diagram for pain location; (b) a global pain rating scale (PPI); (c) sensory, affective, and evaluative adjectives (PRI); and (d) adjectives to describe the pattern in relation to duration and frequency of pain. The short form of the MPQ includes a VAS for pain intensity, a global pain rating scale (PPI), and sensory, affective, and evaluative adjectives (PRI). Both forms of the MPQ are easy to score. However, difficulties may arise with interpreting some of the adjectives, particularly where English is not the participant's first language. No manual is available for administration instructions or scoring procedures, which must be gleaned from Melzack's (1975) original paper (Wilkie et al., 1990). The time required to complete the MPQ-LF has been found to be greater than the 10 to 15 minutes reported by Melzack (1975). McGuire (1984) observed that hospitalized cancer patients required an average of 24 minutes to complete the MPQ. Moreover, Cohen & Tate (1989) described the MPQ as too long for their postoperative sample and recommended using a shorter version. The MPQ-SF requires at least five minutes to complete and has been used with acutely ill patients, such as those who have just had surgery (Watt-Watson, Garfinkel et al., 2000). However, the MPQ-SF does not have the clinical utility of an NRS, although the latter has no quality component. Using two numerical rating scales for both pain intensity and unpleasantness of pain would address this issue.

Of the five studies using one or more components of the MPQ, sensitivity to change was evident over time for a continuing education trial of nurses working in acute care (Francke et al., 1997), for a chronic pain self-management trial (LeFort et al., 1998), and for a surgical patient education trial (McDonald et al., 2001). In contrast, Keller and Bzdek's (1986) trial of therapeutic touch and Watt-Watson, Stevens et al.'s (2000) trial of a pain booklet for surgical patients demonstrated no change in MPQ scores over time.

5.5.3 Brief Pain Inventory

The BPI is a multidimensional pain measure that addresses pain history, etiology, intensity, location, quality, and interference with activities. A subscale can be used to measure how much pain interferes with everyday function in the six categories of mood, walking, other physical activities, work, social activity, relations with others, and sleep (BPI-I). The standard measure takes 10 to 15 minutes to complete, and results are comparable for the self- and interviewer-administered versions. The BPI-short form has even more clinical utility because it is short, easy to read, self-administered, and easy to score. The BPI has been recommended as a comprehensive tool in the *Cancer Pain Management Clinical Practice Guidelines* (AHCPR, 1994). The BPI-SF is incorporated in the American Pain Society (APS) Patient Outcome Questionnaire to be used for quality improvement initiatives (APS, 1995). However, only two studies (Ward et al., 2000; Watt-Watson, Stevens et al., 2000) used any form of the BPI in the studies reviewed.

The BPI-I was sensitive to changes over the five-day postoperative period (Watt-Watson, Stevens et al., 2000). However, as Ward et al. (2000) reported, it demonstrated decreased interference for both control and intervention groups of gynecological cancer patients two months after the intervention; the time period may have been too long to detect any immediate change that resulted from the information given. The BPI-SF is incorporated in the American Pain Society Patient Outcome Questionnaire. Dalton et al. (1999) used this measure, but have not yet published the outcome data.

In summary, all measures reviewed have well-established reliability and validity in nursing studies that examined pain and/or its impact with patients in a variety of clinical settings. In addition, these measures have been translated into several languages and are useful for nurses working with multicultural patients. The shorter versions of the MPQ and BPI measures have greater clinical utility than the other forms. However, the NRS, although unidimensional, has demonstrated the most clinical utility of all measures, particularly with people having less education. The BPI is unique in that it examines broader issues of the impact of pain that would be important to assess, particularly for people with persistent pain. Also, the BPI can be used as a long, short, or interference subscale version, all with established reliability and validity. This review affords considerable evidence that visual analogue scales and numerical ratings scales are sensitive to changes in outcomes. In addition, the McGill Pain Questionnaire and the Brief Pain Inventory are both sensitive measures that include important outcomes other than pain intensity. It is noteworthy that the short form of the BPI has been used in acute pain settings as well as with cancer patients in the studies in this review.

5.6 Recommendations and Directions for Future Research

Intervention studies have not always measured patient outcomes, particularly in evaluating the effectiveness of nurses' pain education programs. What nurses say they know and believe about pain may not be reflected in their practices (Watt-Watson, Garfinkel et al., 2000), and changes in knowledge and beliefs in a posttest may not be retained over time (Howell et al., 2000). Therefore, patient outcomes that are responsive to a variety of interventions are critical to changing practices.

In this review, the most frequently chosen pain outcomes were pain intensity and analgesic administration, which reflect nursing pain management practices, particularly with acute pain problems. The measures chosen, mainly VAS/NRS and MPQ, were sensitive to these outcomes, as change was demonstrated in response to nursing interventions. Where change did not occur, outcomes may have been influenced by the complexity of the pain management context or methodological issues; results may not be related to the measure. Several studies used a pretest/posttest design with two different groups, and did not discuss intervening variables that could have confounded the study results.

In the future, multidimensional measures must be used to determine the degree to which interventions affect an outcome, reflecting not only the sensory experience of pain but also its effect on change in usual activities. Pain intensity and function or disability are not necessarily correlated, as tissue damage is not directly proportional to pain (Melzack & Wall, 1965). Therefore, data about other outcomes, such as the degree to which pain-related interference continues despite intervention, would provide a clearer picture of the efficacy and utility of the intervention. Only two studies in this review used interference related to pain as an outcome measure. Pain measures such as the VAS and MPQ are responsive to changes in pain intensity. However, measures such as the BPI allow a multidimensional assessment of pain that would give more direction to nursing interventions and form a better basis for evaluating the effectiveness of nursing care.

Nurse and patient factors can influence pain assessment. Interventions in the future need to be focused to a greater degree on nurses' and patients' beliefs and concerns about pain management, and the impact of any intervention needs to be evaluated by using patient-related outcomes. Further work is needed to examine relationships between outcomes such as pain and analgesic use, and those reflecting pain-related activities and beliefs. While pain outcomes after an intervention did not change in two studies, concerns about taking analgesics were significantly reduced (Ward et al., 2000; Watt-Watson, Stevens et al., 2000). Therefore, we need to include different kinds of outcomes for assessing the effectiveness of nursing interventions within this domain of practice. Pain is one such outcome, but others are relevant, including patients' concerns about following effective treatments.

References

Agency for Health Care Policy and Research (AHCPR). (1992, 1994). *Acute pain management: Operative or medical procedures and trauma (No. 92-0032); Management of Cancer Pain: Clinical Practice Guidelines* (No. 94-0692). Rockville, MD: U.S. Department of Health and Human Services.

Ahles, T., Seville, J., Wasson, J., Johnson, D., Callahan, E., & Stukel, T. (2001). Panel-based pain management in primary care: A pilot study. *Journal of Pain and Symptom Management, 22,* 584–590.

American Pain Society Quality of Care Committee (1995). Quality improvement guidelines for the treatment of acute and cancer pain. *Journal of the American Medical Association, 274,* 1874–1880.

Baer, E., Davitz, L., & Lieb, R. (1970). Inferences of physical pain: In relation to verbal and nonverbal communication. *Nursing Research, 19,* 388–392.

Basbaum, A., & Jessell, T. (2000). The perception of pain. In E. Kandel, J. Schwartz, & T. Jessell (Eds.), *Principles of neural science* (pp. 472–491). New York: McGraw Hill.

Benedetti, C., Bonica, J., & Belluci, G. (1984). Pathophysiology and therapy of postoperative pain: A review. In C. Benedetti, C. R. Chapman, & G. Moricca (Eds.), *Recent advances in the management of pain* (pp. 373–407). New York: Raven Press.

Bernabei, R., Gambassi, G., Lapane, K., Landi, F., Gatsonis, C., Dunlop, R., et al. (1998). Management of pain in elderly patients with cancer. *Journal of the American Medical Association, 279,* 1877–1882.

Broscious, S. K. (1999). Music: An intervention for pain during chest tube removal after open heart surgery. *American Journal of Critical Care, 8,* 410–415.

Calderone, K. (1990). The influence of gender on the frequency of pain and sedative medication administered to postoperative patients. *Sex Roles, 23,* 713–725.

Carr, E. (1990). Postoperative pain: Patients' expectations and experiences. *Journal of Advanced Nursing, 15,* 89–100.

Choi, D. M., Yate, P., Coats, T., Kalinda, P., & Paul, E. (2000). Ethnicity and prescription of analgesia in an accident and emergency department: Cross sectional study. *British Medical Journal, 320,* 980–981.

Cleeland, C. (1991). Pain assessment in cancer: In D. Osoba (Ed.), *Effect of cancer on quality of life* (pp. 293–305). Florida: CRC Press.

Cleeland, C., Baez, L., Loehrer, P., & Pandya, K. (1997). Pain and treatment in minority patients with cancer. *Annals of Internal Medicine, 127*(9), 813–6.

Cleeland, C., & Syrjala, K. (1992). How to assess cancer pain. In D. Turk & R. Melzack (Eds.), *Handbook of pain assessment* (pp. 362–387). New York: Guilford Press.

Closs, S. J., Briggs, M., & Everitt, V. E. (1999). Implementation of research findings to reduce postoperative pain at night. *International Journal of Nursing Studies, 36,* 21–31.

Clotfelter, C. (1999). The effect of an educational intervention on decreasing pain intensity in elderly people with cancer. *Oncology Nursing Forum, 26,* 27–33.

Cohen, M., & Tate, R. (1989). Using the McGill Pain Questionnaire to study common postoperative complications. *Pain, 39,* 275–279.

Dahl, J., Rosenberg, J., Dirkes, W., Mogensen, T., & Kehlet, H. (1990). Prevention of postoperative pain by balanced analgesia. *British Journal of Anaesthesia, 64,* 518–520.

Dahlman, G., Dykes, A., & Elander, G. (1999). Patients' evaluation of pain and nurses' management of analgesics after surgery: The effect of a study day on the subject of pain for nurses working at the thorax surgery department. *Journal of Advanced Nursing, 30,* 866–874.

Dalton, J. (1989). Nurses' perceptions of their pain assessment skills, pain management practices, and attitudes toward pain. *Oncology Nursing Forum, 16*, 225–231.

Dalton, J., Blau, W., Lindley, C., Carlson, J., Youngblood, R., & Greer, S. M. (1999). Changing acute pain management to improve patient outcomes: An educational approach. *Journal of Pain and Symptom Management, 17*, 277–287.

Daut, R., Cleeland, C., & Flanery, R. (1983). Development of the Wisconsin Brief Pain Questionnaire to assess pain in cancer and other diseases. *Pain, 17*, 197–210.

de Rond, M., de Wit, R., van Dam, F., & Muller, M. (2000). A pain monitoring program for nurses: Effect on the administration of analgesics. *Pain, 89*, 25–38.

de Rond, M., de Wit, R., van Dam, F., van Campen, B., den Hartog, Y., Klievink, R., et al. (1999). Daily pain assessment: Value for nurses and patients. *Journal of Advanced Nursing, 29*, 436–444.

de Wit, R., & van Dam, F. (2001). From hospital to home care: A randomized controlled trial of a pain education program for cancer patients with chronic pain. *Journal of Advanced Nursing, 36*(6), 742–754.

Dudgeon, D., Raubertas, R., & Rosenthal, S. (1993). The short-form of the McGill Pain Questionnaire in chronic cancer pain. *Journal of Pain and Symptom Management, 8*, 191–95.

Duggleby, W., & Lander, J. (1994). Cognitive status and postoperative pain: Older adults. *Journal of Pain and Symptom Management, 9*, 19–27.

Duncan, K., & Pozehl, B. (2000). Effects of performance feedback on patient pain outcomes. *Clinical Nursing Research, 9*, 379–401.

Faherty, B., & Grier, M. (1984). Analgesic medication for elderly people post-surgery. *Nursing Research, 33*, 369–372.

Ferraz, M., Quaresma, M., & Aquino, L. (1990). Reliability of pain scales in the assessment of literate and illiterate patients with rheumatoid arthritis. *Journal of Rheumatology, 17*, 1022-1024.

Ferrell, B., McCaffery, M., & Grant, M. (1991). Clinical decision making and pain. *Cancer Nursing, 14*, 289–297.

Fields, H. (1987). *Pain.* New York: McGraw-Hill.

Francke, A. L., Garssen, B., Luiken, J. B., de Schepper, A. M. E., Grypdonck, M., & Abu-Saad, H. H. (1997). Effects of a nursing pain programme on patient outcomes. *Psycho-Oncology, 6*, 302–310.

Good, M., Stanton-Hicks, M., Grass, J., Anderson, G., Lai, H., Roykulcharoen, V., et al. (2001). Relaxation and music to reduce post surgical pain. *Journal of Advanced Nursing, 33*, 208–215.

Grossman, S., Sheidler, V., Swedeen, K., Mucenski, J., & Piantadosi, S. (1991). Correlation of patient and caregiver ratings of cancer pain. *Journal of Pain and Symptom Management, 6*, 53–57.

Guyutt, G., Townsend, M., & Berman, L. (1987). A comparison of Likert and visual analogue scales for measuring change in function. *Journal of Chronic Diseases, 40*, 1129–1133.

Holm, K., Cohen, F., Dudas, S., Medema, P., & Allen, B. (1989). Effect of personal pain experience on pain assessment. *Image, 21,* 72–75.

Holzheimer, A., McMillan, S. C., & Weitzner, M. (1999). Improving pain outcomes of hospice patients with cancer. *Oncology Nursing Forum, 26,* 1499–1504.

Howell, D., Butler, L., Vincent, L., Watt-Watson, J., & Stearns, N. (2000). Influencing nurses' knowledge, attitudes, and practice in cancer pain management. *Cancer Nursing, 23,* 55–63.

Jansen, K., & McFadden, M. (1989). Postoperative nursing management in patients undergoing myocardial revascularization with the internal mammary artery bypass. *Heart & Lung, 15*(1), 48–54.

Jenson, M., Karoly, P., & Braver, S. (1986). The measurement of clinical pain intensity: A comparison of six methods. *Pain, 27,* 117–126.

Jenson, M., Karoly, P., O'Riordan, E., Bland, E., & Burns, R. (1989). The subjective experience of acute pain: An assessment of the utility of 10 indices. *Clinical Journal of Pain, 5,* 153–159.

Katz, J. (1997). Perioperative predictors of long-term pain following surgery. In T. Jensen, J. Turner, & Z. Wiesenfeld-Hallin (Eds.), *Proceedings of the 8th World Congress on Pain: Vol. 8. Progress in pain research and management* (pp. 231–240). Seattle: IASP Press.

Keller, E., & Bzdek, V. M. (1986). Effects of therapeutic touch on tension headache pain. *Nursing Research, 35,* 101–106.

Khan, D., & Steeves, R. (1996). An understanding of suffering grounded in clinical research and practice. In B. Ferrell, *Suffering* (pp. 3–27). Boston: Jones and Bartlett Publishers.

Kubsch, S. M., Neveau, T., & Vandertie, K. (2000). Effect of cutaneous stimulation on pain reduction in emergency department patients. *Complementary Therapies in Nursing and Midwifery, 6,* 25–32.

Lavies, N., Hart, L., Rounsefell, B., & Runciman, W. (1992). Identification of patient, medical and nursing attitudes to postoperative opioid analgesia: Stage 1 of a longitudinal study of postoperative analgesia. *Pain, 48,* 313–319.

LeFort, S. M., Gray-Donald, K., Rowat, K. M., & Jeans, M. (1998). Randomized controlled trial of a community-based psychoeducation program for the self-management of chronic pain. *Pain, 74,* 297–306.

Lowe, N., Walker, S., & McCallum, R. (1991). Confirming the theoretical structure of the McGill Pain Questionnaire in acute clinical pain. *Pain, 46,* 53-60.

Marks, R., & Sachar, E. (1973). Undertreatment of medical inpatients with narcotic analgesics. *Annals of Internal Medicine, 78,* 173–181.

McDonald, D. (1994). Gender and ethnic stereotyping and narcotic analgesic administration. *Research in nursing & health, 17,* 45–49.

McDonald, D., Freeland, M., Thomas, G., & Moore, J. (2001). Testing a preoperative pain management intervention for elders. *Research in nursing & health, 24,* 402–409.

McDowell, I., & Newell, C. (1996). *Measuring health: A guide to rating scales and questionnaires.* New York: Oxford University Press.

McGuire, D. (1984). The measurement of clinical pain. *Nursing Research, 33,* 152–156.

Meehan, T. C. (1993). Therapeutic touch and postoperative pain: A Rogerian research study. *Nursing Science Quarterly, 6,* 69–78.

Melzack, R. (1975). The McGill Pain Questionnaire: Major properties and scoring methods. *Pain, 1,* 277–299.

Melzack, R. (1987). The short-form McGill Pain Questionnaire. *Pain, 30,* 191–197.

Melzack, R., Abbott, F., Zackon, W., Mulder, D., & Davis, M. (1987). Pain on a surgical ward: A survey of the duration and intensity of pain and the effectiveness of medication. *Pain, 29,* 67–72.

Melzack, R., & Dennis, S. (1978). Neurophysiological foundations of pain. In R. Steinbach (Ed.), *The psychology of pain* (pp. 1–26). New York: Raven Press.

Melzack, R., & Wall, P. (1965). Pain mechanisms: A new theory. *Science, 150,* 971–979.

Merskey, H., & Bogduk, N. (1994). *Classification of chronic pain: Descriptions of chronic pain syndromes and definitions of pain terms* (2nd ed.). Seattle: IASP Press.

Millar, W. (1996). Chronic pain. *Health Reports, 7,* 47–53.

Neitzel, J. J., Miller, E. H., Shepherd, M. F., & Belgrade, M. (1999). Improving pain management after total joint replacement surgery. *Orthopaedic Nursing, 18,* 37–64.

Oberst, M. (1978). Nurses' inferences of suffering: The effects of nurse-patient similarity, and verbalizations of distress. In M. J. Nelson (Ed.), *Clinical perspectives in nursing research* (pp. 38–60). New York: Teachers College Press.

O'Gara, P. (1988). The hemodynamic consequences of pain and its management. *Journal of Intensive Care Medicine, 3,* 3–5.

Owen, H., McMillan, V., & Rogowski, D. (1990). Postoperative pain therapy: A survey of patients' expectations and their experiences. *Pain, 41,* 303–307.

Price, D., Bush, F., Long, S., & Harkins, S. (1994). A comparison of pain measurement characteristics of mechanical visual analogue and simple numerical rating scales. *Pain, 56,* 217–226.

Scott, J., & Huskisson, E. (1976). Graphic representation of pain. *Pain, 2,* 175–184.

Seers, K., & Carroll, D. (1998). Relaxation techniques for acute pain management: A systematic review. *Journal of Advanced Nursing, 27,* 466–475.

Sindhu, F. (1996). Are non-pharmacological nursing interventions for the management of pain effective?: A meta-analysis. *Journal of Advanced Nursing, 24,* 1152–1159.

Spross, J. (1996). Coaching and suffering: The role of the nurse in helping people face illness. In B. Ferrell (Ed.), *Suffering* (pp. 173–207). Boston: Jones and Bartlett Publishers.

Tanabe, P., Thomas, R., Paice, J., Spiller, M., & Marcantonio, R. (2001). The effect of standard care, ibuprofen, and music on pain relief and patient satisfaction in adults with musculoskeletal trauma. *Journal of Emergency Nursing, 27*(2), 124–131.

Todd, K. H., Samaroo, N., & Hoffman, J. R. (1993). Ethnicity as a risk factor for inadequate emergency department analgesia. *Journal of the American Medical Association, 269,* 1537–1539.

Wall, P. (1996). Comments after 30 years of the Gate Control Theory. *Pain Forum, 5*(1), 12–22.

Ward, S., Carlson-Dakes, K., Hughes, S., Kwekkeboom, K., & Donovan, H. (1998). The impact of patient-related barriers to pain management on quality of life. *Research in nursing & health, 21*, 405–413.

Ward, S., Donovan, H., Owen, B., Grosen, E., & Serlin, R. (2000). An individualized intervention to overcome patient-related barriers to pain management in women with gynecologic cancers. *Research in nursing & health, 23*, 393–405.

Ward, S., Goldberg, N., Miller-McCauley, B., Mueller, C., Nolan, A., Pawlik-Plank, D., et al. (1993). Patient-related barriers to management of cancer pain. *Pain, 52*, 319–324.

Watt-Watson, J., Garfinkel, P., Gallop, R., Stevens, B., & Streiner, D. (2000). The impact of nurses' empathic responses on patients' pain management in acute care. *Nursing Research, 49*, 1–10.

Watt-Watson, J., Stevens, B., Costello, J., Katz, J., & Reid, G. (2000). Impact of pre-operative education on pain management outcomes after coronary artery bypass graft surgery: A pilot. *Canadian Journal of Nursing Research, 31*, 41–56.

Watt-Watson, J., Stevens, B., Streiner, D., Garfinkel, P., & Gallop, R. (2001). Relationship between pain knowledge and pain management outcomes for their postoperative cardiac patients. *Journal of Advanced Nursing, 36*, 535–545.

Wilkie, D., Savedra, M., Holzemer, W., Tesler, M., & Paul, S. (1990). Use of the McGill Pain Questionnaire to measure pain: A meta-analysis. *Nursing Research, 39*, 36–41.

Willis, W. (1994). Central plastic responses to pain. In G. Gebhart, D. Hammond, & T. Jenson (Eds.), *Proceedings of the 7th World Congress on Pain: Progress in pain research and management*, Vol. 2 (pp. 301–324). Seattle: IASP Press.

Winefield, H., Katsikitis, M., Hart, L., & Rounsefell, B. (1990). Postoperative pain experiences: Relevant patient and staff attitudes. *Journal of Psychosomatic Research, 34*, 543–552.

Woolf, C. (1991). Central mechanisms of acute pain. In M. Bond, E. Charlton, & C. Woolf (Eds.), *Proceedings of the 6th World Congress on Pain* (pp. 25–34). Amsterdam: Elsevier Science Publishing.

6

Patient Safety Outcomes

Peggy White, RN, MN

Project Manager, Nursing and Health Outcomes Project
Ministry of Health and Long-Term Care

Linda McGillis Hall, RN, PhD

Assistant Professor
Faculty of Nursing, University of Toronto &
New Investigator, Canadian Institutes of Health Research

6.1 Introduction

Patient safety is a rising concern in health care today. People enter the healthcare system trusting that the system will not harm them. However, increasing evidence suggests that this may not always be true. While serious problems in the quality of health care are infrequent compared to the amount of care provided, when they do occur they can have devastating consequences for patients and their families (Kohn et al., 2000). Recently released reports on errors and adverse events in the U.S. and the U.K. depict a system that is fragmented and prone to errors. These documents have heightened awareness of patient safety (Kohn et al., 2000; National Health Services, 2000), and led to an increased focus on the prevention of adverse events in health care.

6.2 Definition of the Concept of Patient Safety

Patient safety has been defined as freedom from accidental injury (Kohn et al., 2000). Much of the literature has operationalized patient safety in relation to adverse occurrences, which can include falls, pressure ulcers, medication errors, nosocomial infections, treatment errors, and mortality (American Nurses Association, 1995; Pierce, 1997). Measures of adverse occurrences are usually obtained from secondary data sources.

In the United States, the Institute of Medicine (IOM) (Kohn et al., 2000) examined two studies of adverse events among large samples of hospitalized patients and estimated that health care error may have accounted for close to 100,000 patient deaths (Kohn et al., 2000). In U.K. hospitals, adverse events were found to occur in around 10% of admissions, or at a rate in excess of 850,000 a year (National Health Services, 2000). In a study examining the health records of over 30,100 patients admitted to 51 acute care hospitals in New York state, adverse events occurred in 3.7% of admissions (Brennan et al., 1991). Wilson et al. (1995) reported adverse events in 16.6% of admissions to Australian hospitals, of which 13.7% resulted in permanent disability and 4.9% in death. A New Zealand study reported adverse events in 12.9% of admissions to public hospitals (Davis et al., 2001). All of these reports emphasized that the majority of health services are of a very high standard and that serious failures are uncommon.

Canada has no consistent approach to identifying and tracking health care errors within the system, although individual organizations monitor adverse occurrences. A recent study has been funded by the Canadian Institute for Health Information (CIHI) and the Canadian Institutes of Health Research (CIHR) to examine adverse events in Canadian hospitals. In addition, Affonso and Doran have developed a theoretical framework that is being used to foster a transdisciplinary approach to patient safety research among a recently funded team of scholars at the University of Toronto. These initiatives should help address the lack of understanding of the depth of the problem and the absence of a coordinated approach to addressing the issue.

While the reports on adverse events examined errors and the system issues that contribute to them, they did not explore nursing's role in patient safety. As a profession, nursing is accountable for enhancing health and promoting quality outcomes. Patient safety outcomes are an essential component of quality. Buerhaus and Norman (2001) maintain that efforts to improve quality will continue to shape health care delivery and that nurses need to be knowledgeable in the "theories, methods and practices of quality improvement." To achieve this goal, nurses will require good data on the measures of quality. Research on the relationship between nursing and patient safety outcomes can provide nurses with the evidence to advocate for safe patient care.

This chapter includes a discussion of adverse occurrences as patient safety outcomes that are sensitive to nursing. An analysis of the current nursing research on patient falls, pressure ulcers, nosocomial infections, medication errors, and mortality will be conducted to explore the association between these outcomes and nursing. Factors that influence patient safety outcomes, including perceptions about error and system issues, and a review of the empirical research on the relationship between nursing structural variables and patient safety outcomes are presented. This chapter also addresses issues with the state of the science in relationship to nursing and patient safety outcomes research, and makes recommendations for future research in this area. The literature review examines literature relating to the current state of thinking in the area of patient safety outcomes—specifically, patient safety outcomes in relationship to nurse staffing from 1985 to the present.

6.3 Linking Patient Safety Outcomes to Nursing

Medication errors, nosocomial infections, patient falls, and pressure ulcers are patient safety outcomes that consistently appear in the nursing literature as being theoretically linked to aspects of nursing practice (American Nurses Association, 1995, 1996, 1997, 2000; Blegen et al., 1998; Kovner & Gergen, 1998; Lichtig et al., 1999; McGillis Hall et al., 2001; Needleman et al., 2002a, 2002b; Sovie & Jawad, 2001; Taunton et al., 1994). There is also some evidence that mortality can be linked to nursing (Aiken et al., 1994; Hartz et al., 1989; Tourangeau et al., 2002).

6.3.1 Medication Errors

A medication error can occur at any of three stages: when the drug is prescribed, when it is dispensed, and when it is administered. A prescribing error is the result of a physician ordering the incorrect drug or dosage, a dispensing error is a mistake made by pharmacy staff when distributing medication to nursing units, and an administration error occurs when a nurse administers the drug incorrectly (American Nurses Association, 1995). Leape et al. (2000) found that 39% of medication errors occurred in the prescribing stage, 12% during pharmacy dispensing, and 38% in the nurse administration stage.

In acute-care hospitals and long-term care facilities the administration of medications is primarily a nursing role; therefore, the administration error rate may be associated with the availability and quality of nursing staff (American Nurses Association, 1995). Given that approximately one-third of these errors were attributed to nursing, it is important for nurse researchers to understand the factors that contribute to these, and to develop strategies to manage them.

Medication administration errors can occur in many forms, including omitting doses; giving extra doses; administering a wrong dose; administering a drug not ordered; or administering a drug at the wrong time, through the wrong route, or at an incorrect rate (Mark & Burleson, 1995). Nurses are responsible for administering the correct dosage of the prescribed drug through the appropriate route to the right patient at the right time. In an American Nurses Association survey (1995), nurses reported that short staffing, particularly to the extent that it leads to increased workload and frequent interruptions, can result in medication administration errors. Other factors, such as inexperienced staff and limited knowledge or skills, may also increase the risk of a nurse making a medication administration error (American Nurses Association, 1995).

When exploring linkages between nursing and medication errors, it is important to consider the source and definition of the medication error. The research on medication errors is hampered by a lack of reliable data on the number and type of errors. Investigations have shown that the vast majority of medication errors are not recorded on the patients' charts. Wakefield et al. (1999a, 1999b) surveyed nurses in two Iowa hospitals to determine their perceptions of why medication errors occur, why they are not reported, and what percentage of medication errors are reported. According to the results, nurses perceived that approximately 60% of medication errors are reported. The rationale for underreporting included fear, administrative response, disagreement over error, and reporting effort (Wakefield et al., 1999b). Needleman and Buerhaus (2000) suggested that, in some organizations, medication errors are only documented if something happens to the patient that requires medical attention. Iezzoni et al. (1994) found that even medication errors that are recorded internally on the patient's chart are often not recorded on the discharge abstract of the patient's chart. The lack of reliable data has been noted in nursing, although studies have demonstrated that data on medication error could be collected consistently (Mark & Burleson, 1995).

The literature on the relationship between medication errors and the quality of nursing care reveals varied results. According to Fuqua and Stevens (1988), stress, nursing shortages, and distractions while administering medication contribute to error. The authors also reported on a study in Pennsylvania that found that medication errors decrease as nursing experience increases. Prescott, Dennis, Creasia, & Bowen (1985) found that when fewer nurses were available for patient care, monitoring of patients decreased, treatment omissions and delays occurred, and medication errors increased. McGillis Hall et al. (2001) found that units with a higher proportion of regulated professional nursing staff had fewer medication errors. Other studies did not find a direct correlation between the adequacy of nurse staffing or nurse workload and the incidence of medication errors (Taunton et al., 1994). The literature on medication administration errors suggests that medication errors may be linked to some aspects of nursing, although a direct causal link has not been established (American Nurses Association, 1995, Blegen et al., 1998). The American Nurses Association (1995) suggests that each error may be influenced by a unique set of factors and that more research is needed to understand these factors and how they influence medication administration errors.

6.3.2 *Nosocomial Infections*

Nosocomial infections are infections originating in a healthcare organization (Centers for Disease Control, 2000). The most common types of hospital-acquired infections are: urinary tract infections, surgical wound infections, bloodstream infections, and pneumonia (Weinstein, 1998).

Nosocomial infections are considered a quality indicator, yet methodological issues such as the need for complex risk adjustment and differences in the intensity of surveillance in different settings have limited the use of nosocomial infection rates as a quality indicator in the past (Flood & Diers, 1988; Larson et al., 1988). Mark and Burleson (1995), in a study to determine consistency in the collection of patient outcome data, reported challenges with consistently collecting data on nosocomial infections.

According to Weinstein (1998), one third of nosocomial infections are preventable. Certain patient care practices, such as proper aseptic and antiseptic techniques in hand washing, skin preparation, wound dressing, and prudent monitoring of invasive medical devices, are under the scope of nursing practice. Nurses minimize the risk of spreading infection in their daily practice by using aseptic techniques when changing dressings to prevent wound infections, and in the care and maintenance of tubing such as catheters and chest tubes. Hand washing is considered the most effective preventative practice with respect to nosocomial infections (Larson et al., 1988). Registered nurses also perform a role in the assessment and monitoring of risk factors for infection, such as age, nutritional status, and medical treatment (American Nurses Association, 1995). Given nursing's pivotal role in infection control practices, the incidence of nosocomial infections can be expected to reflect the availability and quality of nursing care (American Nurses Association, 1995).

Flood and Diers (1988) found that units with inadequate staffing had higher levels of complications such as general infections and urinary tract infections. While Taunton et al. (1994) found no relationship between urinary tract infections and nursing workload, they did find evidence that nosocomial infection rates were related to registered nursing staff absenteeism. The authors surmised that staff absenteeism may interrupt continuity of care.

A study conducted by Fridkin, Pear, Williamson, Galgiani, & Jarvis (1996) found that a higher nurse-to-patient ratio was an indicator of a bloodstream infection in patients with a central venous line. The authors hypothesized that an increase in the nurse-to-patient ratio, as well as an increase in the number of central lines, may have placed time constraints on the nursing staff, preventing them from taking proper care of the catheters. American Nurses Association-funded studies piloting quality indicators eliminated the nosocomial infection indicator (central/peripheral line infection) because it occurred so infrequently (Grobe et al., 1998; Langemo et al., 2002). Recent studies have examined nosocomial infections (urinary tract infections, pneumonia) and found a relationship between nurse staffing and these nosocomial infections (American Nurses Association, 2000; Kovner & Gergen, 1998; Lichtig et al., 1999; McGillis Hall et al., 2001; Needleman et al., 2002a, 2002b; Sovie & Jawad, 2001). Further research is needed to understand how these nursing-related variables influence the incidence of nosocomial infections.

6.3.3 *Patient Falls*

A fall is defined as unintentionally coming to rest on the floor or other lower level, but not as a result of syncope or overwhelming external force (Agostini et al., 2001). In Canada, falls are the sixth leading cause of death among older adults and cost the Canadian healthcare system approximately $2.8 billion annually (SMARTRISK, 1998). A previous fall is one of the strongest predictors of falls (Agostini et al., 2001). Rawsky (1998) contends that the effect of patient falls extends beyond physical injury and cost, because older people who fall fear a subsequent fall and may reduce their activities to prevent further falls, which leads to a reduction of independence and further functional decline.

Morse (1993) suggests most falls in institutions are not random events, but the result of a pattern and that, therefore, the opportunity exists to reduce their incidence. In the acute-care, long-term care, and home care setting, nurses are responsible for identifying patients who are at risk for falls, and developing and implementing a plan of care to minimize risk and reduce the number of falls.

The American Nurses Association feasibility studies addressed whether patients were assessed for risk of fall on admission, patients who had previous falls were identified as 'at risk', and fall protocols were in place prior to falls (Grobe et al., 1998; Langemo et al., 2002). Grobe et al. (1998) argue for the use of standardized fall-risk scales and severity scales to add validity to the data. This study also highlights the variation in data on the number and types of injuries associated with falls, the lack of data on the level of patient activity prior to the fall, and whether restraints were in use at the time of the fall. The authors suggest that this information is required to ensure reliable reporting and to allow comparison of rates of falls within units and across organizations.

In an effort to reduce the number of falls, many hospitals, long-term care facilities, and communities have implemented fall-prevention programs as part of quality improvement efforts. However, there are limited studies exploring the effect of fall-prevention programs and the assessment of risk for falls on the number of falls within organizations (Rawsky, 1998). According to Hernandez and Millar (1986), many older patients fall in institutions when getting up to use the bathroom. A study by Bakarich, McMillan, and Prosser (1997) found that significantly fewer falls occurred in an 'at risk' group who were assessed for confusion and mobility status, and toileted on a regular basis, than in the 'at risk' group who were assessed but not toileted. Whedon and Shedd (1989) found that patient acuity, the use of supplemental staffing or inexperienced nursing staff, and a discrepancy between recommended and actual hours of staffing contributed to an increased number of falls. Some studies found no relationship between nursing staffing variables and patient falls (Morse et al., 1987; Taunton et al., 1994; Tutuarima et al., 1993), while others found that units with a higher proportion of registered nurses (RNs) had lower fall rates (Blegen & Vaughan, 1998; Sovie & Jawad, 2001).

Many factors, such as patient characteristics, the onset of acute illness, medical treatments, new medications, or an alteration of medication regimen, increase the risk for falls (Agostini et al., 2001). Current methods for collecting data on falls are inadequate. Further research is required to better understand the relationship among nurse staffing, nursing interventions, and patient falls. This research needs to be grounded with consistent definitions that capture the level of activity, whether the patient was assessed about 'risk for falls', and whether restraints were in place.

6.3.4 *Pressure Ulcers*

Pressure ulcers are localized areas of tissue damage or necrosis that develop due to pressure over a bony prominence (Agostini et al., 2001). Pressure ulcers have been linked to a 50% increase in nursing care time, increased length of stay, higher hospital costs, increased co-morbidity, sepsis, and a fourfold increase in mortality in cases developing bacteremia (American Nurses Association, 1995). Current clinical practice guidelines for the management of pressure ulcers include systematic skin inspection at least once per day, routine skin cleansing, reduction of pressure by positioning, and minimizing skin exposure to moisture. Even with these practices in place, patients may still develop skin breakdown because of underlying pathologic conditions (National Pressure Ulcer Advisory Panel, 1992). Nursing plays a significant role in assessing the skin condition, implementing treatment plans aimed at reducing pressure, and minimizing exposure to moisture.

The National Pressure Ulcer Advisory Panel has developed clear definitions for staging pressure ulcers that are reflected in current clinical practice guidelines. There is corroboration for capturing the incidence and prevalence of Stage 2–4 pressure ulcers (National Pressure Ulcer Advisory Panel, 1992; Registered Nurses Association of Ontario, 2002). Frantz, Gardner, Specht, and McIntire (2001) cite a National Pressure Ulcer Advisory Panel recommendation to exclude Stage 1 pressure ulcers, as the reliability of the identification of Stage 1 ulcers has not been substantiated. However, the feasibility study conducted by the Texas Nurses' Association (Grobe et al., 1998) contends that valuable data was lost by excluding Stage 1 pressure ulcers. Although identifying Stage 1 ulcers presents a challenge, it may be beneficial to include them in future studies.

Most studies of pressure ulcers have examined the impact of different interventions, rather than the influence of nurse staffing in relation to assessment (Bostrum et al., 1996; Frantz et al., 1995; Lyder, 2002; Hopkins et al., 2000). However, some studies (American Nurses Association, 2000; Blegen et al., 1998; Lichtig et al., 1999) found that nursing staff mix was related to lower pressure ulcer rates.

Many organizations have implemented quality improvement initiatives, such as practice guidelines, aimed at preventing the incidence of skin breakdown. The translation of these clinical practice guidelines into routine practice has been problematic, as studies have limited the scope of evaluation to short-term effects of the quality improvement initiatives rather than evaluating whether these strategies are sustained within organizations (Frantz et al., 2001). Researchers who evaluated the integration of a research-based pressure ulcer treatment protocol five years after its implementation at a Veterans Hospital found consistency in the way the protocol had been maintained. Unique factors in this organization included: higher staff salaries and benefits, higher total hours of nursing care, above-average levels of nursing personnel, and less staff turnover compared to national averages (Frantz et al., 2001). The organization was also known for promoting autonomy and accountability in individual nurses, and involving nurses in decision-making about patient care.

While the current evidence on the impact of nurse staffing on pressure ulcers is limited, nursing is responsible for assessing patients and implementing protocols to prevent and treat pressure ulcers (Mark & Burleson, 1995). Changes in the staff mix and/or the number and type of nurses may affect the nurses' capacity to assess patients and implement treatment plans (American Nurses Association, 1995).

To understand the relationship between nursing and the incidence of pressure ulcers, accurate data are required. Grobe et al. (1998) argue for standardization of data collection and risk assessment using a recognized scale. This information would facilitate future research to inform decisions about the nursing inputs required to prevent and/or reduce pressure ulcers.

6.3.5 Mortality

Several studies have examined mortality in relation to nursing over the past two decades, and the results have been varied. Knaus, Draper, Wagner, and Zimmerman (1986) investigated the relationship between mortality and nursing-related hospital characteristics in intensive care units. Hospitals with the lowest mortality ratios had a comprehensive nursing educational support system, such as a master's degree-prepared clinical nurse specialist who focused on staff nurses' education and development, and excellent communication between physicians and nursing staff (Knaus et al., 1986).

Shortell and Hughes (1988) examined data from over 214,839 patients within 981 U.S. hospitals, and found that the percentage of registered nurses in hospitals was associated with lower mortality rates, but the relationship was not statistically significant.

Hartz et al. (1989) examined 30-day mortality rates from 3,100 hospitals and found that lower mortality rates were associated with a higher percentage of registered nurses. Aiken et al. (1994) found that "magnet" hospitals (i.e., hospitals that have a significantly higher ratio of registered nurses to other nursing personnel, as well as a slightly higher nurse-to-patient ratio, and are known as good places to practice nursing) had lower mortality rates than matched hospitals (i.e., similar to "magnet" hospitals in other organizational dimensions, but not known as settings that place a high institutional priority on nursing). The mortality rate was significantly lower in hospitals with the highest ratio of RNs to licensed practical nurses (LPNs) and unlicensed personnel (Aiken et al., 1994).

Blegen et al. (1998) assessed the relationship between nurse staffing and adverse patient outcomes. While the study findings support a relationship between a higher skill mix and mortality, the results were not statistically significant. The researchers controlled for patient acuity but did not control for patient characteristics such as age, sex, and co-morbidities. Needleman et al., (2002a, 2002b) found no association between increased levels of staffing by registered nurses and the rate of in-hospital deaths. In contrast, Tourangeau et al. (2002) examined the effects of nursing-related variables on 30-day mortality rates in 75 acute-care hospitals. The authors found that a richer skill mix of RNs was associated with lower 30-day mortality rates, and that units that had more experienced nurses had lower 30-day mortality rates. They concluded that nurses who had experience with a specific patient population were better able to detect problems and intervene to prevent complications.

In the recent nursing literature, the use of mortality as a measure of patient outcomes with nursing care has been challenged because of inconsistent research reports and questions about the appropriateness of this variable. Brooten and Naylor (1995) suggest that mortality data is not informative for understanding the effects of nursing interventions, and argue that mortality is influenced most by medical care. Blegen et al. (1998) also argue that mortality may not be the best indicator of the quality of nursing care. Mitchell and Shortell (1997) conducted a review of 81 research studies that linked organizational structures or processes to mortality and determined that the studies were inconclusive. The authors suggest that adverse events are more closely related to organizational features of care delivery, thereby making them the most appropriate outcomes to refine and test further. Despite these challenges, Tourangeau et al. (2002) reason that nurse staffing is one component that affects mortality, and that there may be other determinants of 30-day mortality. To be able to link mortality to nursing care interventions, more research involving multiple sites and large data sets is required.

In summary, substantial empirical research supports relationships between nursing and patient safety outcomes in the areas of medication errors, nosocomial infections, patient falls, and pressure ulcers. Some authors have already described these indicators as nurse-sensitive (Needleman et al., 2002b). Consistent evidence for the use of mortality as an outcome of nursing care practice is less apparent.

6.4 Factors that Influence Patient Safety Outcomes

According to the literature, a number of factors influence patient safety outcomes, including perceptions about error and systems issues in the healthcare environment.

6.4.1 Perceptions about Error

Recent reports provide evidence that some errors can be prevented (Kohn et al., 2000; National Health Services, 2000). Leape et al. (1991) maintain that more than two-thirds of adverse events are preventable, which means they are caused by an error. These adverse occurrences do not happen intentionally. In their daily practice, healthcare workers do not plan to commit errors. These errors are the result of the complicated interface between providers and technology, providers and the system; and the complex interaction among the many different healthcare providers (Leape et al., 2000). Furthermore, adverse events do not necessarily signal poor-quality care. For example, Brennan et al. (1991) point out that, while a drug reaction in a patient who has been appropriately prescribed a specific drug for the first time is, by definition, an adverse event, this type of error is not preventable.

Organizational culture significantly affects the number and type of errors reported. Researchers acknowledge that, because of under-detection and under-reporting by healthcare professionals, only a fraction of the true incidence of errors is known (Fuqua & Stevens, 1988). While the current focus is on creating cultures of safety, healthcare organizations have typically handled errors by taking disciplinary action against the individual involved (Keepnews, 2000). This 'culture of blame' has discouraged individuals from reporting errors, which leads to underreporting and, ultimately, a failure to identify or correct systems problems that cause or contribute to errors. Meurier (2000) examined the clinical errors for 20 registered nurses and found that nurses are reluctant to report and discuss errors because of fear of disciplinary action.

Organizations that promote a 'culture of safety' acknowledge the high-risk and error-prone nature of health care, and encourage individuals to report errors. Within these organizations, executives and clinicians work together to change practice, develop systems to monitor quality, and commit resources to support these changes (Wakefield & Maddox, 2000). Organizations that encourage open reporting and balanced analysis, both in principle and in practice, are able to have a positive and quantifiable impact on quality outcomes (National Health Services, 2000).

6.4.2 System Issues

In a systems approach to errors, humans are viewed as fallible and errors can occur even in good organizations (Reason, 2000). Researchers have learned that the reason people make errors is often largely due to the way that work is designed (Nolan, 2000). From this perspective, if a person makes a mistake, the question should not be "who committed the error?" but rather "why did it happen and is there a way to redesign the work so that it will not happen again?" (Reason, 2000). Moreover, there is evidence that, even when processes are well designed, there will be situations where mistakes occur (Nolan, 2000). Cognitive psychologists and human factor engineers confirm that people make mistakes when they are rushed, under pressure, overworked, emotionally distraught, or working in a difficult environment (Buerhaus, 1999). The current environment, in which nurses are caring for patients with complex needs and are being pressured to work overtime and extra shifts while being short-staffed, has the potential to impact patient safety outcomes (Foley, 1999).

A major role of registered nurses involves coping with the complexity of patient care and, in particular, the gaps that complexity generates. Cook, Render, and Woods (2000) define these gaps as "discontinuities in care" that appear in diverse ways, such as losses of information or interruptions in delivery of care. In daily practice, these gaps rarely lead to an adverse event because expert clinicians are able to anticipate, recognize, and bridge these gaps. The authors characterize some bridges to manage these gaps as robust and reliable, while others are frail and brittle. It is easier to manage these gaps in a stable milieu than in a complex environment, characterized by numerous admissions and discharges, complex patients, increased nurse-to-patient ratios, frequent interruptions, and staffing patterns that may involve inexperienced staff or relief staff (Cook et al., 2000). Expert nurses are able to manage gaps better than are novice nurses (Cook et al., 2000). Nurses report that as they gain more experience they develop better ways of managing errors and learning from their mistakes (Meurier et al., 1997). With the introduction of unregulated workers, nurses have had to change how they structure their work. In addition to having more patients to manage, they also have to supervise the work of these unregulated workers (Sovie & Jawad, 2001). This further increases the potential for gaps in patient care.

Decision-making by senior management may create conditions that contribute to adverse occurrences. For example, inadequate systems to support communication, lack of orientation and/or ongoing training, and the failure to supply and maintain equipment required to deliver care can provide conditions that could jeopardize patient safety (Meurier, 2000). In the past, healthcare organizations have failed to address systems problems such as written orders that are illegible, medications that have a similar name or are packaged in a similar way, and potentially dangerous medications that are part of floor stock (Keepnews, 2000). Decreased operating budgets have led to a reduction in nurse managers, educators, and clinical nurse specialists—roles which ensure the structure and expertise to support patient safety and quality (Foley, 1999).

The quality of working environments and quality of interactions with other professionals distinguishes hospitals with lower mortality and complications from those with higher adverse events (Sovie & Jawad, 2001; Mitchell & Shortell, 1997; Aiken et al., 1994; Knaus et al., 1986). In terms of working environments, registered nurses are dissatisfied with their working conditions. They report that they are spending less time taking care of patients with more complex needs (Aiken et al., 2001), and they believe that the safety and quality of care is deteriorating. In terms of the quality of interactions with other professionals, communication among the diverse disciplines managing patient care has been shown to affect patient outcomes (Sovie & Jawad, 2002; Shortell et al., 1994).

6.5 Relationships between Nursing Structural Variables and Patient Safety Outcomes

Nightingale was one of the first nurse researchers to recognize the importance of data collection and the impact that measurement has on patient outcomes. Nightingale logged infection rates and implemented interventions based on her findings (Reed, Blegen, & Goode, 1998).

As rapid changes have occurred within health care, many organizations have re-engineered or redesigned work in order to maximize the expertise and productivity of registered nurses as a means of controlling costs. Many studies have examined different models of care delivery and their affect on staff and organizational outcomes. While these studies have demonstrated that care delivery changes affect organizational outcomes, such as cost, their impact on patient outcomes are inconclusive (Lengacher & Mabe, 1993; Grillo-Peck & Risner, 1995; Kraphol & Larson, 1996; Blegen et al., 1998; McGillis Hall, 1998; Barter et al., 1999; Tourangeau et al., 1999). Recent nursing research is beginning to fill the gap in our understanding of how structural indicators influence quality indicators.

A 1996 report by the Institute of Medicine concluded that there was a lack of empirical evidence to draw conclusions about nurse staffing in hospitals and that, while the "literature on the effect of registered nurses on mortality and on factors affecting the retention of nursing staff is available, there is a serious paucity of recent research on the definitive effects of structural measures, such as specific staffing ratios, on the quality of patient care in terms of patient outcomes when controlling for all other likely explanatory or confounding variables" (Wunderlich, Sloan, & Davis, 1996). This report argued that rigorous research on the relationship between nursing variables and quality of care would have significant payoffs for administrators, decision-makers, and policy-makers. Since that report, a number of studies have provided evidence that links nurse staffing variables to quality of care and patient outcomes (American Nurses Association, 2000; Blegen et al., 1998; Blegen & Vaughan, 1998; Flood & Diers, 1988; Kovner & Gergen, 1998; Lichtig et al., 1999; McGillis Hall et al., 2001; Needleman et al., 2002a, 2002b; Sovie & Jawad, 2001). See Table 6.1.

One of the early studies to examine the effect of nurse staffing levels on patient outcomes compared two medical units with similar capacities, patient mix, and staff mix to assess the effect of nurse staffing levels on patient complications, acuity level, length of stay, and cost (Flood & Diers, 1988). The authors found that the unit with adequate staffing had fewer complications, including infections, length of stay, and decreased patient requests for pain medication, than the unit with less-than-adequate staffing. This study controlled for the case mix of patients and was conducted in a single setting using organizational-specific definitions for understaffing.

Taunton et al. (1994) examined whether adverse occurrences, such as bloodstream and urinary tract infections, patient falls, or medication errors, were correlated with staff nurse absenteeism, staff nurse separation from the work unit by resignation or transfer, and nursing workload. This study, which was conducted in four large acute care urban hospitals, found an association between patient infections and staff nurse absenteeism. The authors hypothesized that absenteeism and the replacement of staff by nurses who are less skilled may disrupt continuity of care and affect patient safety. Although data for this study were collected from hospital documents, and each hospital participated in defining the study outcomes, the authors maintain that there may have been under-reporting, measurement errors, errors related to the operational definitions, and inconsistent adherence to reporting schematics (Taunton et al., 1994).

Kovner and Gergen (1998) examined the relationship between nurse staffing and the adverse events of patient mortality, medication-error rate, and nosocomial infections for 589 acute care hospitals. Controlling for case mix, the researchers collected information on hospital-level variables such as teaching status, ownership, bed size, hospital resources, and region. The researchers examined outcomes that could theoretically be linked to nursing, as well as outcomes that did not have a theoretical link to nursing. They found a strong relationship between full-time-equivalent RNs per adjusted day and urinary tract

Table 6.1. Studies Investigating the Relationship Between Nursing Structural Variables and Patient Safety Outcomes

Author/date	Design	Sample characteristics/ setting	Independent variables	Outcomes being investigated and approach to measurement	Results	Limitations
American Nurses Association (2000)	Correlational	All-payor sample of more than 9.1 million pts in almost 1,000 hospitals; Medicare sample of more than 3.8 million pts in over 1,500 hospitals across 9 U.S. states.	RN Hrs/NIW adjusted day; licensed Hrs/NIW adjusted day; % RN licensed hrs.	Mix of RNs, LPNs, and UAPs = % of RN care hours as a total of all nursing care hours (acute care units); total nursing care hours provided per patient day = total number of productive hrs worked by nursing staff with direct pt. care responsibilities per patient day; pressure ulcers = # of pts with NPUAP-AHCPR Stage I, II, III or IV ulcers/# of pts in a prevalence study. Patient falls = the rate per 1,000 pt days at which pts experience an unplanned descent to the floor during the course of the day (total # of pt falls x 1,000/total # of pt days). Patient satisfaction with pain management: Nosocomial infections = # of laboratory confirmed bacteremia associated with sites of central lines/1,000 pt days per unit.	Secondary bacterial pneumonia, post-operative infection, pressure ulcers and UTI infection rates were lower in hospitals with higher RN skill mixes and in some instances with greater staffing levels.	Poor quality of nurse staffing data: 1) FTEs rather than paid & worked hours; 2) does not report where nurses work in site; 3) may include psychiatry and rehab units in some sites.
Blegen et al. (1998)	Correlational	42 inpatient units (21,783 discharges); one large 880-bed university hospital (U.S.).	Hours of care per pt day from all nursing personnel = RN/LPN/NA hrs direct/unit PD for month; hours of care provided by RNs = RN hrs direct pt care/ unit PD for month; RN proportions = RN hours PD/ all hours PD.	Decubiti = incidences of skin breakdown secondary to pressure or exposure to urine/feces. Infections = nosocomial infections not present or incubating at the time of admission (only UTIs and respiratory infections were included). Patient falls = suddenly and involuntarily leaving a position and coming to rest on the floor or some object. Medication errors = wrong dose, duplication, omission, transcription, wrong route/pt/solution/ time (per 10,000 doses).	RN proportion was inversely related to rates of medication errors, decubiti, and pt complaints. As RN proportions increased, rates of adverse outcomes decreased up to a staff mix of 87.5%.	Concern re: the rigor of incident reports for the reporting of medication errors and pt falls on pt care units; acuity measure may not have been sensitive to higher levels of acuity for pts in critical care and intensive care units. Results are less generalizable as single-site study.

Table 6.1 (continued)

Author/date	Design	Sample characteristics/ setting	Independent variables	Outcomes being investigated and approach to measurement	Results	Limitations
[Blegen et al. (1998) continued]				Patient complaints = both pt and family complaints about aspects of the pt's care such as nursing care, medical care, food, and housekeeping (standardized as rate per 1,000 pt days). Mortality rates per 1,000 pt days.		
Blegen & Vaughn (1998)	Correlational	39 hospital units in 11 hospitals (U.S.).	Hours of care = all hours of care (RN/LPN/NA) per pt day; RN Proportion = proportion of those hours of care delivered by RNs.	Data from comparative occurrence reporting system (CORS): medication administration errors (MAE), pt falls, and cardiac arrest. MAEs = both oral and intravenous medications and includes: omissions, wrong method, wrong pt, wrong dose, inappropriate continuation, wrong drug, administrations to pts with allergies, and adverse drug reactions. (MAE = # of errors on the unit in the quarter per 1,000 pt days, and # of errors on the unit in the quarter per 10,000 doses.) Patient falls = # of pt falls on the unit during the quarter per 1,000 pt days. Cardiac arrests = # of cardiac arrests on the unit during the quarter per 1,000 pt days of care (did not include pts with DNR orders).	Units with higher proportion of RNs had lower rates of pt falls; nurse staffing was not related to cardiac arrest.	Data abstracted retrospectively from hospital records may lead to under-reporting, measurement errors at initial data point, measurement error in relation to operational definitions of variables. Patient outcomes data collected from chart reviews. Dose-based denominators for medication errors were not available for capturing ratios.

Table 6.1 (continued)

Author/date	Design	Sample characteristics/ setting	Independent variables	Outcomes being investigated and approach to measurement	Results	Limitations
Flood & Diers (1988)	Descriptive	482-bed university teaching hospital (northeast U.S.); 2 medical units; Unit B with adequate staffing and Unit A with less-than-adequate staffing as defined by the hospital; $N = 497$ pts (199 male, 298 female).	Staffing Workload Index = Number of required nursing personnel and number of available nursing personnel per shift/per unit, as defined by the hospital.	Patient complications listed on the Uniform Hospital Discharge Data Summary (infections, heart conditions, and GI disorders). Acuity levels range from 1, requiring minimal care, to 4, requiring intensive nursing care (San Joaquin PCS). LOS; cost (room and board charges plus nursing) for pts > or < geographic mean LOS.	Unit A: the frequency and mean number of complications per pt were higher; generalized infections ($N = 88$) & UTI ($N = 62$) were the most common complications. Unit A had a slightly greater LOS than Unit B when controlled for DRG. Unit A had a higher % PD at acuity level=3 (Unit A = 75%; Unit B=57%). Unit A projected to have a greater loss in net revenues.	Study did not measure the amount of care received by pts on both units. It only examined pt complications. It may be that the pts on Unit A had DRGs that were more complex/required more nursing care.
Kovner & Gergen (1998)	Correlational	589 acute-care community hospitals in 10 U.S. states.	# of FTE RNs working in the hospital and outpatient departments per adjusted pt day.	Nine post-surgical outcomes based on ICD-9-CM codes. Nurse-sensitive indicators: Venous thrombosis or pulmonary embolism after major surgery and after invasive vascular procedure, excluding from the at-risk population discharged pts with venous thrombosis as principle diagnosis; UTIs after major surgery, excluding from the at-risk population discharged pts in MDC 11 (Renal), MDC 12 (Male genital), or MDC 13 (Female genital); Pneumonia after major surgery excluding from the at-risk population discharged pts in MDC 4 (Respiratory), with cancer, or with AIDS;	Significant inverse relationships between FTE RNs per adjusted inpt day (RNAPD) & UTIs after major surgery ($p < 0.0001$); pneumonia after major surgery ($p < 0.001$); thrombosis after major surgery ($p < 0.01$); pulmonary compromise after major surgery ($p < 0.05$).	Coding inconsistencies may have occurred in the nine indicators and/or discharge abstracts. Selection process eliminated pts with multiple diagnoses who may have responded differently to nurse staffing.

Table 6.1 (continued)

Author/date	Design	Sample characteristics/ setting	Independent variables	Outcomes being investigated and approach to measurement	Results	Limitations
[Kovner & Gergen (1998) continued]				Pneumonia after invasive vascular procedure, excluding from the at-risk population discharged pts in MDC 4 (Respiratory), with cancer, or with AIDS. Non-nurse sensitive indicators: Pulmonary compromise after surgery (pulmonary congestion, lung edema, or respiratory insufficiency or failure), excluding from the at-risk population discharged pts in MDC 4 (Respiratory), or MDC 5 (Cardiovascular); Acute MI after major surgery, excluding from the at-risk population discharged pts in MDC 5 (Cardiovascular); GI hemorrhage or ulceration after major surgery, excluding from the at-risk population discharged pts in MDC 6 (Gastrointestinal), or MDC 7 (Hepatobiliary), mechanical complications because of device, implant, or graft.	Increased nurse staffing related to decreased UTIs, pneumonia, thrombosis, & pulmonary compromise after surgery.	
Kovner et al. (2002)	Descriptive, cross-sectional	13 U.S. states; HCUP data.	# RN FTEs/PD adjustment; # LPN FTEs/PD adjustment.	Venous thrombosis or pulmonary embolism after major surgery: discharges with venous thrombosis or pulmonary embolism in any secondary diagnosis/all non-maternal/non-neonatal discharges age 18 or older with major surgery procedure on day 1 or 2 of admission; Pulmonary compromise after major surgery; discharges with pulmonary congestion, lung edema, or respiratory insufficiency or failure in any secondary diagnosis/all non-maternal/non-neonatal discharges age 18 or older with major surgery procedure on day 1 or 2 of admission; UTIs after major surgery = discharges with UTIs in any secondary diagnosis/all non-maternal/non-neonatal discharges age 18 or older with major surgery procedure on day 1 or 2 of admission; Pneumonia after major surgery = discharges with pneumonia in any secondary diagnosis/all non-maternal/non-neonatal discharges age 18 or older with major surgery procedure on day 1 or 2 of admission.	# RN hrs/PD adjusted significantly inversely related to pneumonia.	Data do not distinguish between RN direct care providers & indirect or management roles. Data reflect paid hours and may overestimate productive hours. Data excludes UAPs.

Table 6.1 (continued)

Author/date	Design	Sample characteristics/ setting	Independent variables	Outcomes being investigated and approach to measurement	Results	Limitations
Lichtig et al. (1999)	Correlational	Hospitals: California (*N* = 462) and New York (*N* = 229); patients: California = 3.5 million discharges, New York = 2.5 million discharges.	RN hours as a percentage of total nursing hours; total nursing hours per NIW-adjusted pt day.	Collected from Discharge Data Abstract using ICD-9-CM codes that appeared as a secondary diagnosis: pressure ulcers; pneumonia; UTIs; postoperative infections; LOS; rates calculated by DRG for each hospital & for each state > or < statewide average outcome rates.	Nursing skill mix related to lower pressure ulcer rates; higher mix of RNs associated with lower levels of pneumonia. In California only, higher % RNs associated with lower postoperative infections. Nursing skill mix related to UTI rates.	Quality of data was inconsistent, especially reported nursing hours; in some instances there was non-reporting of nurse staffing data. Possible underreporting and inaccurate coding of secondary diagnoses.
McGillis Hall et al. (2001)	Descriptive repeated measure	19 Canadian teaching hospitals, 77 units; 2,046 pts.	Proportion of regulated staff (RNs & RPNs) = # RNs & RPNs on unit x 100/# total nursing personnel on unit; Proportion of RNs on unit x 100/# total nursing personnel on unit.	Data on medication errors, wound infections, urinary tract infections, and pt falls collected from chart review. Other outcomes collected by survey: functional status; perceptions of pain; patient satisfaction with nursing care; medication errors; wound infections; UTIs; patient falls.	Higher proportion of RNs/RPNs in the staff mix associated with better functional health and pt satisfaction outcomes at discharge and with lower unit rates of medication errors and wound infections.	Missing data within the health records for secondary data.
Needleman et al. (2002a, 2002b)	Correlational	799 hospitals from 11 states; 5,075,969 medical pts & 1,1104,659 surgical pts.	# of hours per pt for RNs, LPNs, aides, individually & totalled; proportion (%) of total RN hours & LPN hours; # hours/day by licensed nurses; RN hrs as a proportion of licensed nurse hours.	All pts administrative data: UTIs; pressure ulcers; hospital-acquired pneumonia; deep vein thrombosis/pulmonary embolism; upper GI bleed; central nervous system complications; sepsis; shock/cardiac arrest; mortality; failure to rescue. Additional outcomes for surgical pts only: surgical wound infection; pulmonary failure; metabolic derangement.	Medical patients: consistent relationships between nurse staffing variables and five pt outcomes (UTIs, pneumonia, LOS, upper GI bleed, and shock). Surgical patients: relationship between failure to rescue.	Concerns about the quality of discharge abstract data, i.e., missing data or data recorded incorrectly, staffing data collected from diverse data sets, and data not consistently available.

Table 6.1 (continued)

Author/date	Design	Sample characteristics/ setting	Independent variables	Outcomes being investigated and approach to measurement	Results	Limitations
[Needleman et al. (2002a, 2002b) continued]					and nurse staffing was strong and consistent (weaker evidence was found for UTIs and pneumonia). Stronger evidence of an association between pt outcomes and levels of RN staffing compared to the evidence linking pt outcomes to mix of LPNs.	
Sovie & Jawad (2001)	Correlational	29 U.S. teaching hospitals with more than 300 beds; 1 medical unit & 1 surgical unit per site.	FTEs for each type of nursing staff; skill mix; hours worked per pt day for all staff and for selected categories of staff (i.e., RNs, UAPs, and a category that included other roles such as licensed practical nurses, clerks, and managers; LPNs were included in the other category due to the small number of LPNs in these organizations); labor costs per discharge.	Patient falls = any fall or slip in which a pt came to rest unintentionally on the floor, whether it resulted in injury or was witnessed. Multiple falls by the same pt were considered separate events. (# of falls in a unit x 1,000/# of pt days). NPUs = lesions caused by unrelieved pressure, thus resulting in damage to underlying tissue; had to involve broken skin, thus excluding Stage I ulcers in which skin is intact defined as # of pts with NPUs in the unit or hospital/Total # of pts evaluated in the area—unit or hospital—and expressed as an annual rate). UTIs = nosocomial if there was no evidence that the infections were present or incubating at the time of admission to the hospital or within 72 hours after admission, and if the infection met the criteria for symptomatic bacteriuria or asymptomatic bacteriuria, established by the Centers for Disease Control National Nosocomial Infection Surveillance System (UTIs data operationally defined as number of infections × 100/number of patients discharged).	Fall rate declined as # RNs/PD increased. NPU rates declined on surgical unit, remained constant on medical units; not related to nurse staffing. UTI rates increased on both units; not related to nurse staffing.	CMI used for adjustment at hospital level; no risk adjustment at unit level.

Table 6.1 (continued)

Author/date	Design	Sample characteristics/setting	Independent variables	Outcomes being investigated and approach to measurement	Results	Limitations
Taunton et al. (1994)	Correlational	4 large acute care hospitals (Midwest U.S.), one teaching hospital; 65 pt care units.	Absenteeism (Individual staff RN variable averaged for work unit) = total days absent per quarter/total days scheduled per quarter x 100; unit separation (resignation or transfer) = # staff RNs leaving work unit per quarter/# staff RNs on unit at beginning of quarter x 100; workload = required pt care hours/actual pt care hours.	UTI = monthly average for UTIs per quarter/monthly average for pt days per quarter x 1000. Bloodstream infections = monthly average for BSIs per quarter/monthly average for pt days per quarter x 1000. Falls = total pt falls per quarter/total pt days per quarter x 1000. Medication errors = total medication errors per quarter/total nursing care hours per quarter x 10000.	An association between UTIs and staff RN absenteeism, and between BSIs and RN absenteeism; no meaningful relationships between falls and medication errors and any of the organizational variables that were examined.	Data abstracted retrospectively from hospital records may lead to under-reporting; measurement errors at initial data point; measurement error in relation to operational definitions of variables; patient outcomes data collected from chart reviews; dose-based denominators for medication errors were not available for capturing ratios.

Notes:
Hrs = hours
NIW = nursing intensity weight
pt = patient
FTE = full time equivalent
NAP or UAP = unlicensed assistive personnel
BSIs = blood stream infection
UTI = urinary tract infection
LOS = length of stay
NPU = nosocomial pressure ulcer
DRG = diagnosis related group
CMI = case mix index
PD = patient day
HCUP = Health Care Utilization Project

infections and pneumonia after surgery, and a less robust relationship between full-time-equivalent RNs per adjusted day and thrombosis after surgery. The researchers found no relationship between nurse staffing and pneumonia or venous thrombosis. The authors caution that coding inconsistencies and inaccuracies in discharge abstracts may have influenced the results of the study. Also, the selection process eliminated patients with multiple diagnoses, who may have responded differently to nurse staffing.

Blegen et al. (1998) examined the role of nurse staffing on patient outcomes. Data were collected from hospital records on 42 inpatient units on the following outcomes: patient falls, medication errors, pressure ulcers, patient complaints, respiratory and urinary tract infections, and mortality. The researchers controlled for patient severity by using nursing acuity system data. They found that units with higher-than-average patient acuity had lower rates of medication errors and patient falls. They also found that these same units had higher rates of other adverse occurrences such as skin breakdown, patient and family complaints, infections, and deaths. When they controlled for average patient acuity, the proportion of hours of care delivered by RNs was inversely related to the unit rates of medication errors, decubiti, and patient complaints. Total hours of care from all nursing personnel were associated directly with the rates of decubiti, complaints, and mortality. This study also reported an unexpected finding: the relationship between registered nursing staff proportion of care was curvilinear. As the registered nurse proportion increased, rates of adverse outcomes decreased up to 87.5%. At that level, as registered nurse proportion increased, adverse occurrences also increased. The authors theorized that their indicator for acuity might not have been sensitive enough to control for the sharply higher acuity levels in critical care units and intermediate care units.

Blegen and Vaughan (1998) conducted a multisite study to describe the relationship between nurse staffing and the following outcomes: medication errors, patient falls, and cardiopulmonary arrests. They collected unit-level data and controlled for patient acuity. They found that units with a higher proportion of RNs had lower rates of patient falls. An interesting finding in this study was the "non-linear" relationship between the proportion of RNs in the staff mix and medication administration errors. Medication errors declined as the proportion of RNs increased up to 85%; however, any further increase in the proportion of RNs resulted in increased medication administration errors. The authors suggest that further research is required to explain these findings.

Lichtig et al. (1999) examined the impact of nurse staffing on adverse events for hospitals in California and New York. Using state-wide data collected in the Uniform Hospital Discharge Data Set, they collected information on the following outcomes: pressure ulcers, pneumonia, urinary tract infections, postoperative infections, and length of stay. They found that the higher the percentage of registered nursing staff and, to a lesser degree, the more nursing hours per acuity-adjusted day, the better the patient outcomes.

In 1994, the American Nurses Association initiated the Patient Safety and Quality Initiative, a multi-faceted approach to examining the impact of staffing changes on the quality of patient care. It included a focus on research of large databases to identify indicators that have a strong relationship to patient outcomes, as well as an education component to teach nurses about quality. The indicators selected for the Patient Safety and Quality Initiative were specific to nursing, could be tracked over time, and had a strong link to nursing quality. After an extensive literature review, expert consultations, and focus groups, the initiative identified 21 nursing quality care indicators for potential use in a report card for nursing. The American Nurses Association experienced difficulties in measuring and tracking these indicators and, in a pilot study conducted in 48 hospitals in California and New York, collected information on only seven indicators: total nursing care hours per nursing intensity weight, registered nurse hours as a percentage of all nursing hours, length of stay, pressure ulcers, pneumonia, urinary tract infections, and postoperative infections. According to the findings, a higher proportion of RNs was significantly associated with lower length of stay and lower rates of pressure ulcers, pneumonia, postoperative infection, and urinary tract infections (American Nurses Association, 1997).

One component of the American Nurses Association initiative is the development, testing, storage, and evaluation of nursing-sensitive indicators by the University of Kansas School of Nursing and Medical Center Research Institute (Midwest Research Institute, 1999). To support a National Database of Nursing Quality Indicators, which is housed at the University of Kansas, the American Nurses Association conducted six pilot projects with State Nursing Associations in Arizona, California, Virginia, Minnesota, North Dakota, and Texas, and collected data on the following indicators: nursing hours per patient day, nursing skill mix, pressure ulcers, falls, nosocomial infections, patient satisfaction with pain management, patient satisfaction with educational information, patient satisfaction with nursing care, patient satisfaction with overall care, and nurse job satisfaction. More than 256 hospitals across 37 states are currently participating in this initiative (Rowell, 2001).

A second American Nurses Association study examined the relationship between nurse staffing and five outcome measures: length of stay, pneumonia, postoperative infections, pressure sores, and urinary tract infections (American Nurses Association, 2000). Nursing Intensity Weights (NIWs) were used to identify the differences in patients' acuity of need for nursing care. This study found that secondary bacterial pneumonia, postoperative infections, pressure ulcers, and urinary tract infections were lower in hospitals with higher registered nurse skill mixes and, in some instances, greater staffing levels. In examining adverse occurrences, the American Nurses Association also considered two other factors that influence healthcare practice: hospital teaching status (primary medical school affiliate, other teaching, or non-teaching) and setting (defined as large urban, urban, or rural) health care. The American Nurses Association report highlights the difficulty of obtaining data measuring the amounts and type of nursing care provided. Researchers found that nurse staffing data are not collected universally on a comprehensive basis.

McGillis Hall et al. (2001) assessed the composition and mix of nursing care staff in 19 teaching hospitals on patient, nurse, and system outcomes. Over 2,046 patients, 1,116 nurses, 63 unit managers, and 50 senior executives participated in the study. The authors controlled for other possible determinants of health outcomes, such as case mix, baseline health status, patient age, gender, and complexity of illness. Unit-level data were collected from the discharge abstract database of patient health records on patient falls, medication errors, urinary tract infections, and wound infections, using consistent definitions. Nursing staff mix was found to be a significant predictor of four patient health outcomes (functional independence, pain, social functioning, and satisfaction with obstetrical care) and two quality outcomes (medication errors and wound infections). This study is significant, as it measured outcomes at the individual patient level, rather than at the inpatient unit or hospital level. The authors of this study also expressed concern about the availability and quality of nurse staffing data. Given that the secondary data for patient falls, pressure ulcers, and nosocomial infections was collected from the health records, it is impossible to know if data were missing or recorded incorrectly.

Needleman et al. (2002a, 2002b) conducted an analysis of the discharge records of more than six million patients, of which five million were admitted to hospital because of a medical diagnosis and one million for a surgical problem. This study examined whether there was a correlation between the levels of registered nurses and patient outcomes. In hospitals with higher registered nurse staffing, patients' stays were 3% to 5% shorter, and patient complication rates 2% to 9% lower, than in hospitals with lower staffing. Researchers found that a higher proportion of hours of care by registered nurses was associated with lower rates of pneumonia, shock and cardiac arrest, upper gastrointestinal bleeding, sepsis, and deep venous thrombosis. For surgical patients, the higher the proportion of care provided by registered nurses, the lower the rate of urinary tract infections; and the greater the number of hours of care per day provided by a registered nurse, the lower the rate of "failure to rescue." No association was found between increased levels of staffing by registered nurses and the rate of in-hospital death, or between increased staffing by licensed practical nurses or nurses' aides and the rate of adverse events. The study underscored the weaknesses of currently available data. Nurse staffing data is inconsistent in data sets. When using secondary diagnosis, it is not always possible to ascertain whether the conditions were present on admission. Discharge abstract data are vulnerable to missing data or data that are recorded incorrectly.

Sovie and Jawad (2001) collected data from 29 teaching hospitals to evaluate the impact of hospital restructuring initiatives on outcomes. Data were collected on: rate of patient falls, nosocomial pressure ulcers, urinary tract infections, and patient satisfaction. The data were collected from incident reports (patient falls), prevalence studies (nosocomial pressure ulcers), and hospital infectious disease reports or quarterly retrospective chart audits (urinary tract infections). Researchers found that increased RN hours worked per patient day were associated with lower fall rates. They also reported a strong relationship between RN staffing and urinary tract infections. In this study, the prevalence of pressure ulcers decreased and the authors surmised that this was the result of monthly prevalence surveys which resulted in increased assessment and planning by nurses. While case mix index was available at the hospital level, the authors argue that, for risk adjustment purposes, this information is required at the unit level.

Kovner, Jones, Zhan, Gergen & Basu (2002) examined the impact of nurse staffing on four post-surgical events: venous thrombosis/pulmonary embolism, pulmonary compromise after surgery, urinary tract infection, and pneumonia. To limit variation in severity in this study, the authors eliminated data for patients admitted from nursing homes, other hospitals, and elsewhere. They report a significant inverse relationship between RN hours per adjusted patient day and pneumonia. The authors point to the limitations of available staffing data. Databases do not differentiate between direct care providers and indirect care providers. Also, only paid hours are captured. This may diminish the relationship between nurse staffing and adverse events.

6.6   Issues with Nursing Research on Patient Safety Outcomes

This critical review of the current literature exploring the relationship between nursing and patient safety has highlighted a number of important concerns. Most of the challenges relate to methodological concerns with the collection of data and the quality of patient safety data. The studies on adverse occurrences are based on chart reviews of the antecedents of these occurrences and whether an error occurred that led to the event (Hayward & Hofer, 2001). Much of the literature on medical errors is hampered by the lack of workable operational definitions, imprecision in measurement, and conceptual overlap of the terms used to discuss adverse events (Hofer et al., 2000).

One of the limitations with the work to date had been the limited use of conceptual frameworks to guide the field of patient safety research. A number of conceptual models exist that could serve as a framework. For example, Irvine, Sidani, & McGillis Hall (1998) developed the Nursing Role Effectiveness model that conceptualizes nurses' contribution to health care in terms of the roles they assume in health care, and relates those roles to patient outcome achievement. Patient safety can be a result of the quality of nurses' independent roles (e.g., precision in patient assessment), medical care related roles (e.g., nurses' clinical judgment and implementation of a medical order), or interdependent roles (e.g., accurate and timely communication among members of the healthcare team). Affonso and Doran (2002) developed a theoretical framework that conceptualizes patient safety in terms of four cornerstones: (a) building technological tools to create safer ways for dealing with drugs and devices (Kohn et al., 2000); (b) applying human-factors designs to create healthy work environments; (c) reforming the organizational culture to foster critical thinking for decision-making and teamwork; and (d) delivering processes to optimize safe care via precision in assessments, monitoring and tracking patient responses, and ongoing evaluations of processes to prevent errors from occurring.

Comparisons of adverse occurrences are limited by variations in patient characteristics. Of particular concern are characteristics, such as comorbidities, that can affect the probability of an adverse outcome. Mitchell, Heindrich, Moritz, and Hinshaw (1997) argue for the inclusion of risk adjustment when examining adverse occurrences. Without adjusting for variations in these characteristics, it is impossible to determine whether a seemingly bad outcome (e.g., a high number of pressure ulcers) reflects a substandard quality of care or whether it results from the treatment of a disproportionate number of patients with high-risk characteristics. Blegen et al. (1998) report that many studies examining nurse-sensitive outcomes use adjustments for severity at the hospital level (i.e., case-mix adjustments), but these cannot reflect severity of patients on separate units (i.e., an obstetrical unit versus an acute medical unit). As the impact of nurse staffing is at the unit level, future research on adverse occurrences should adjust for acuity at this level.

Nursing research continues to be limited by the variables captured in existing databases. There is a lack of reliability in how the data are reported within and among sites. In the early work on testing the American Nurses Association indicators, challenges were encountered with diverse definitions within organizations, lack of agreed-upon instrumentation for measuring outcomes, and difficulty capturing data at the unit level (Mowinski Jennings et al., 2001). Many early empirical studies on outcomes were conducted in single settings, which affects the ability to compare the role of nursing on various patient outcomes across settings. Researchers are beginning to conduct large-scale examinations of patient outcomes. Multi-site research needs to be grounded in consistent and comparable definitions of outcomes that are of interest to nursing and incorporate standardized, sensitive acuity measures (Blegen et al., 1998; Mark & Burleson, 1995). Rowell (2001) asserts the need for cost-effective databases and data retrieval systems to capture nursing indicator data.

To provide variables that will assist researchers in understanding how different numbers and types of nurses affect patient safety outcomes, the quality of the nursing structural variables in databases needs to be improved. Currently, the nursing variables in administrative databases are inconsistent. The variables include all nurses in the organization, rather than only the nurses who provide direct care (Blegen el al., 1998). This limits the ability to understand the relationships between nurse staffing and patient safety outcomes. To understand the relationship between nurse staffing and adverse patient occurrences, researchers need to know the direct nurse staffing hours by skill level and cost center.

Pierce (1997) warns that studying outcomes alone will be insufficient if they are analyzed in isolation. Donabedian's (1982) framework for measuring the quality of care through structure, process, and outcomes indicators continues to underlie how we view nursing's role in adverse occurrences. Within healthcare organizations, the relationship between the structure of nursing and outcomes of care is not clearly understood. In addition, nursing practice is situated within an increasingly complex environment. A working group on the relationship between nurse staffing and health-care-associated infections suggested that the inconsistencies in nursing research may be reflective of a systems layer that has not yet been identified (Jackson et al., 2002). This should not preclude us from moving forward with the collection of data on patient safety outcomes. Further research requires consistent reliable data to explore the links between nursing inputs, processes of care, and outcomes of care. Also, future research must collect data on organizational variables that shape nursing environments.

To date, much of the nursing research on patient safety outcomes has occurred in acute-care settings. This reflects the availability of staffing data in this sector. However, health care occurs across a continuum of community care, acute care and long-term care. As the population ages, its need for health care changes, and many people move through these different sectors. As nursing plays a role in health care across the continuum of care, future research should examine the relationship between nursing and safety outcomes in all healthcare sectors. This will require administrators, policy-makers, researchers, and funders to identify the staffing and nursing-sensitive outcome variables required to support research.

6.7 Conclusion

Recent reports have raised awareness about patient safety within the healthcare system (Davis et al., 2001; Kohn et al., 2000; National Health Services, 2000; Wilson et al., 1995). These initiatives will direct consumer demands for information about safety in the healthcare system. As the one healthcare provider who is with the patient twenty-four hours a day, seven days a week, nurses play an important role in patient safety. Further research is required to understand the relationship between nursing and patient safety outcomes. Structuring nursing to create an optimum practice environment to promote patient safety is and will continue to be of concern to administrators, decision-makers, policy-makers, and the public.

References

Affonso, D., & Doran, D. (2002). Cultivating discoveries in patient safety research: A framework. *Journal of International Nursing Perspectives*.

Agostini, J. V., Baker, D. I., & Bogardus, S. T. (2001). In *Making Health Care Safer: A Critical Analysis of Patient Safety Practices*. Agency for Healthcare Research and Quality. Evidence Report/Technology Assessment, Number 43. AHRQ Publication No. 01-E058, July 2001. Retrieved [June 6, 2002] from http://www.ahrq.gov/clinic/ptsafety/index.html.

Aiken, L. H., Smith, H. L., & Lake, E. T. (1994). Lower medicare mortality among a set of hospitals known for good nursing care. *Medical Care, 32*(8), 171–187.

Aiken, L. H., Clarke, S. P., & Sloane, D. M. (2001). Hospital restructuring: does it adversely affect care and outcomes? *Journal of Health and Human Services Administration, Spring, 23*(4), 416–442.

American Nurses Association. (1995). *Nursing report card for acute care*. American Nurses Publishing: Washington, DC.

American Nurses Association. (1996a). *Nursing quality indicators*. American Nurses Publishing: Washington, DC.

American Nurses Association. (1996b). *Nursing quality indicators: Guide for Implementation*. American Nurses Publishing: Washington, DC.

American Nurses Association. (1997). *Implementing nursing's report card*. American Nurses Publishing: Washington, DC.

American Nurses Association. (2000). *Nurse staffing and patient outcomes in the inpatient hospital setting*. American Nurses Publishing: Washington, DC.

Bakarich, A., McMillan, V., & Prosser, R. (1997). The effect of a nursing intervention on the incidence of older patient falls. *Australian Journal of Advanced Nursing, 15*(1), 26–31.

Barter, M., McLaughlin, F. E., & Thomas, S. A. (1997). Registered nurse role changes and satisfaction with unlicensed assistive personnel. *Journal of Nursing Administration, 27*(1), 29–38.

Blegen, M. A., & Vaughan, T. (1998). A multisite study of nurse staffing and patient occurrences. *Nursing Economic$, 16*(4), 196–203.

Blegen, M. A., Goode, C. J., & Reed, L. (1998). Nurse staffing and patient outcomes. *Nursing Research, 47*(1), 43–50.

Bostrum, J., Mechanic, J., Lazar, N., Michelson, S., Grant, L., & Nomura, L. (1996). Preventing skin breakdown: nursing practice, costs, and outcomes. *Applied Nursing Research, Nov, 9*(4), 184–188.

Brennan, T. A., Leape, L. L., Laird, N. M., Herbert, L., Localio, R., Lawthers, A. G., et al. (1991). Incidence of adverse events and negligence in hospitalized patients. *New England Journal of Medicine, 324*(6), 370–376.

Brooten, D., & Naylor, M. D. (1995). Nurses' effect on changing patient outcomes. *Image: Journal of Nursing Scholarship, 27*(2), 95–99.

Buerhaus, P. I. (1999). Lucian Leape on the causes and prevention of errors and adverse events in health care. *Image: Journal of Nursing Scholarship, 31*(3), 281–286.

Buerhaus, P. I., & Norman, L. (2001). It's time to require theory and methods of quality improvement in basic and graduate nursing education. *Nursing Outlook, 49*(2), 67–69.

Centers for Disease Control (2000, *March 3) Monitoring Hospital-Acquired Infections to Promote Patient Safety—United States, 1990–1999.* Retrieved [July 25, 2002] from www.cdc.gov/epo/mmwr/preview/mmwrhtml/mm4908al.htm.

Cook, R. I., Render, M., & Woods, D. D. (2000). Gaps in the continuity of care and progress on patient safety. *British Journal of Medicine, March 18, 320,* 791–794.

Davis, P., Lay-Yee, R., Briant, R., Schug, S., Johnson, S., & Bingley, W. (2001). *Adverse Events in New Zealand Public Hospitals: Principal Findings from a National Survey.* Ministry of Health, Wellington, New Zealand: ISBN 0-478-26268. (Internet) http://www.moh.govt.nz/moh.nsf/49ba80c00757b8804c256673001d47d0/d255c2525480c8a1cc256b120006cf25.

Donabedian, A. (1982). Quality, cost and health: an integrative model. *Medical Care, 20 October* (10), 975–992.

Flood, S. D., & Diers, D. (1988). Nurse staffing, patient outcome and cost. *Nursing Management, 19*(5), 35–43.

Foley, M. (1999). Written testimony of the American Nurses Association before the Senate Committee on health education, labor, and pensions on medical errors. Retrieved [April 30, 2000] from www.nursingworld.org/gova/federal/legis/testimon/2000/mf0126.htm.

Frantz, R. A., Berquist, S., & Specht, J. (1995). The cost of treating pressure ulcers following implementation of a research-based skin care protocol in a long term care facility. *Advanced Wound Care, Jan–Feb, 8*(1), 36–45.

Frantz, R. A., Gardner, S., Specht, J. K., McIntire, G. (2001). Integration of pressure ulcer treatment protocol into practice: Clinical outcomes and care environment attributes. *Outcomes Management for Nursing Practice, 5*(3), 112–120.

Fridkin, S. K., Pear, S. M., Williamson, T. H., Gallgiani, J. N., & Jarvis, W. R. (1996). The role of understaffing in central venous catheter-associated bloodstream infections. *Infection Control and Hospital Epidemiology, 17,* 150–158.

Fuqua, R. A., & Stevens, K. R. (1988). What we know about medication errors. A literature review. *Journal of Nursing Quality Assurance, 3*(1), 1–17.

Grillo-Peck, A. M., & Risner, P. B. (1995). The effect of a partnership model on quality and length of stay. *Nursing Economic$, 13*(6), 367–372, 374.

Grobe, S. J., Becker, H., Calvin, A., Biering, P., Jordan, C., & Tabone, S. (1998). Clinical data for use in assessing quality: lessons learned from the Texas nurses' association report card. *Seminars for Nurse Managers, 6*(3), 126–138.

Hartz, A. J., Krakauer, H., Kuhn, E. M., Young, M., Jacobsen, S. J., Gay, G., et al. (1989). Hospital characteristics and mortality rates. *New England Journal of Medicine, 321*(25), 1720–1725.

Hayward, R. A., & Hofer, T. P. (2001). Estimating hospital deaths due to medical errors. Journal of the AMA, *286*(4). Retrieved [July 25, 2001] from: http://jama.ama-assn.org/issues/v286n4/abs/joc02235.html.

Hernandez, M., & Millar, J. (1986). How to reduce patient falls. *Geriatric Nursing, 7*(2), 97–102.

Hofer, T. P., Kerr, E. A., & Hayward, R. A. (2000). What is an error? *American College of Physicians Online.* Retrieved [June 19, 2002] from: www.acponline.org/journals/ecp/novdec00/hofer.htm.

Hopkins, B., Hanlon, M., Yauk, S., Sykes, S., Rose, T., & Cleary, A. (2000). Reducing nosocomial pressure ulcers in an acute care facility. *Journal of Nursing Care Quality, 14*(3), 28–36.

Iezzoni, L. I., Daley, J., Heeren, T., Foley, S. M., Hughes, J. S., Fisher, E. S., et al. (1994). Using administrative data to screen hospitals for high complication rates. *Inquiry, 31,* 40–55.

Irvine, D. M., Sidani, S., & McGillis Hall, L. (1998). Linking outcomes to nurses' roles in health care. *Nursing Economic$, 16*(2), 58–64, 87.

Jackson, M., Chiarello, L., Gaynes, R. P., & Gerberding, J. L. (2002). Nurse staffing and healthcare-associated infections: proceedings from a working group meeting. *Journal of Nursing Administration, 32*(6), 314–322.

Keepnews, D. (2000). A systems approach to health care errors: experts say we'll need a 'culture of safety' to reduce errors. *American Journal of Nursing, 100*(6), 77–78.

Knaus, W. A., Draper, E. A., Wagner, D. P., & Zimmerman, J. E. (1986). An evaluation of outcomes from intensive care in major medical centers. *Annals of Internal Medicine, 104,* 410–418.

Kohn, L. T., Corrigan, J. M., & Donaldson, M. S. (2000). *To Err is Human: Building a Safer Health System.* National Academy Press, Washington, DC.

Kovner, C., & Gergen, P. (1998). Nurse staffing levels and adverse events following surgery in U.S. hospitals. *Image: Journal of Nursing Scholarship, 30*(4), 315–321.

Kovner, C., Jones, J., Zhan, C., Gergen, P. J., & Basu, J. (2002). Nurse staffing and postsurgical adverse events: An analysis of administrative data from a sample of U.S. hospitals, 1990–1996. *HSR: Health Services Research, 37*(3), 611–629.

Kraphol, G. L., & Larson, E. (1996). The impact of unlicensed assistive personnel on nursing care delivery. *Nursing Economic$, 14*(2), 99–109.

Langemo, D. K., Anderson, J., & Volden, C. M. (2002). Nursing quality outcome indicators. The North Dakota study. *Journal of Nursing Administration, 32*(2), 98–105.

Larson, E., Oram, L. F., & Hedrick, E. (1988). Nosocomial infection rates as an indicator of quality. *Medical Care, 26*(7), 676–684.

Leape, L. L., Brennan, T. A., Laaird, N., Lawthers, A. G., Logalio, A. R., Barnes, B. A., et al. (1991). The nature of adverse events in hospitalized patients. *The New England Journal of Medicine, 324*(6), 377–384.

Leape, L. L., Kabcenell, A. I., Gandhi, T. K., Carver, P., Nolan, T. W., & Berwick, D. M. (2000). Reducing adverse drug events: lessons from a breakthrough series collaborative. *Joint Commission Journal on Quality Improvement, June 26* (6), 321–331.

Lengacher, C. A., & Mabe, P. R. (1993). Nurse extenders. *Journal of Nursing Administration, 23*(3), 16–19.

Lichtig, L. K., Knauf, R. A., & Milholland, D. K. (1999). Some impacts of nursing on acute care hospital outcomes. *Journal of Nursing Administration, 29*(2), 25–33.

Lyder, C. H. (2002). Pressure ulcer prevention and management. *Annual Review of Nursing Research, 20*, 35–61.

Mark, B. A., & Burleson, D. L. (1995). Measurement of patient outcomes. Data availability and consistency across hospitals. *Journal of Nursing Administration, 25*(4), 52–59.

McGillis Hall, L. (1998). The use of unregulated workers in Toronto hospitals. *Canadian Journal of Nursing Administration, 11*(1), 9–31.

McGillis Hall, L., Irvine, D., Baker, G. R., Pink, G., Sidani, S., O'Brien Pallas, L., Donner, G. (2001). *A Study of the Impact of Nursing Staff Mix Models & Organizational Change Strategies on Patient, System & Nurse Outcomes.* Toronto, ON: Faculty of Nursing, University of Toronto and Canadian Health Services Research Foundation/Ontario Council of Teaching Hospitals.

Meurier, C.E. (2000). Understanding the nature of errors in nursing: using a model to analyse critical incident reports of errors which had resulted in an adverse or potentially adverse event. *Journal of Advanced Nursing, 32*(1), 202–207.

Meurier, C. E., Vincent, C. A., & Parmar, D. G. (1997). Learning from errors in nursing practice. *Journal of Advanced Nursing, 26*, 111–119.

Midwest Research Institute. (1999). *National Database for Nursing Quality Indicators.* Kansas City, MO. Retrieved [July 1, 2002] from www2.mriresearch.org/health/ndnqi.html

Mitchell, P. H., & Shortell, S. M. (1997). Adverse outcomes and variations in organization and delivery of care. *Medical Care, 35*(11), NS19–NS32 (Supplement).

Mitchell, P. H., Heindrich, J., Moritz, P., & Hinshaw, A. S. (1997). Outcome measures and care delivery systems. *Medical Care Supplement, 35*(11), NS19–NS32 (Supplement).

Morse, J. M. (1993). Nursing research on patient falls in health care institutions. *Annual Review of Nursing Research, 11*, 299–316.

Morse, J. M., Tylko, S. J., & Dixon, H. A. (1987). Characteristics of the fall prone patient. *The Gerontologist, 27*(4), 516–522.

Mowinski Jennings, B., Loan, L. A., DePaul, D., Brosch, L. R., Hildreth, P. (2001). Lessons learned while collecting ANA indicator data. *Journal of Nursing Administration, 31*(3), 121–131.

National Health Services. (2000). *An organisation with memory: Report of an expert group on learning from adverse events in the NHS.* Retrieved [October 16, 2002] from www.doh.gov.uk/orgmemreport/index.htm.

National Pressure Ulcer Advisory Panel (1992). *Statement on Pressure Ulcer Prevention.* Retrieved [June 5, 2000] from www.npuap.org.

Needleman, J., & Buerhaus, P. I. (2000). Nurse staffing and quantity of care in inpatient units in acute care hospitals: Phase one report. Health Resources Services Administration: Contract No. 230-99-0021.

Needleman, J., Buerhaus, P., Mattke, S., Stewart, M., & Zelevinsky, K. (2002a). Nurse-staffing levels and the quality of care in hospitals. *New England Journal of Medicine, 346*(22), 1715–1722.

Needleman, J., Buerhaus, P., Mattke, S., Stewart, M., & Zelevinsky, K. (2002b). Nurse staffing and patient outcomes in hospitals. Final report. Boston: Harvard School of Public Health.

Nolan, T. W. (2000). System changes to improve patient safety. *British Medical Journal, 320*, 771–773.

Pierce, S. F. (1997). Nurse-sensitive health care outcomes in acute care settings: An integrative analysis of the literature. *Journal of Nursing Quality, 11*(4), 60–72.

Prescott, P., Dennis, K. E., Creasia, J., & Bowen, S. (1985). Nursing shortage in transition. *Image: Journal of Nursing Scholarship, 18*, 127–133.

Rawsky, E. (1998). Review of the literature on falls among the elderly. *Image: Journal of Nursing Scholarship, 38*(1), 47–52.

Reason, J. (2000). Human error: models and management. *British Medical Journal, 320*, 768–770.

Reed, L., Blegen, M., & Goode, C. S. (1998). Adverse patient occurrences as a measure of nursing quality. *Journal of Nursing Administration, 28*(5), 62–69.

Registered Nurses Association of Ontario (2002). *Risk Assessment and Prevention of Pressure Ulcers*. Toronto, Canada: Registered Nurses Association of Ontario.

Rowell, P. (2001). Lessons learned while collecting ANA indicator data: The American Nurses Association responds. *Journal of Nursing Administration, 31*(3), 130–131.

Shortell, S. M., & Hughes, E. F. X. (1988). The effects of regulation, competition, and ownership on mortality rates among hospital inpatients. *New England Journal of Medicine, 318*, 1100–1107.

Shortell, S. M., Zimmerman, J. E., Rousseau, D. M., Gillies, R. R., Wagner, D. P., Draper, E. A., et al. (1994). The performance of intensive care units: Does good management make a difference? *Medical Care, 32*(5), 508–525.

SMARTRISK. (1998). *The economic burden of unintentional injury in Canada.* Retrieved [July 15, 2002] from www.smartrisk.ca/PDF/main_study_canada.pdf.

Sovie, M. D., & Jawad, A. F. (2001). Hospital restructuring and its impact on outcomes. *Journal of Nursing Administration, 31*(12), 588–600.

Taunton, R. L., Kleinbeck, S. V., Stafford, R., Woods, C. Q., & Bott, M. J. (1994). Patient outcomes: Are they linked to registered nurse absenteeism, separation, or workload? *Journal of Nursing Administration, 24*(4S), 48–55.

Tourangeau, A. E., White, P., Scott, J., McAllister, M., & Giles, L. (1999). Evaluation of a partnership model of care delivery involving registered nurses and unlicensed assistive personnel. *Canadian Journal of Nursing Leadership, 12*(2), 4–20.

Tourangeau, A. E., Giovannetti, P., Tu, J. V., & Wood, M. (2002). Nursing-related determinants of 30-day mortality for hospitalized patients. *Canadian Journal of Nursing Research, 33*(4), 71–88.

Tutuarima, J. A., de Haan, R. J., & Limburg, M. (1993). Number of nursing staff and falls: a case-control study on falls by stroke patients in acute-care settings. *Journal of Advanced Nursing, 18*, 1101–1105.

Wakefield, D. S., Wakefield, B. J., Borders, T., Uden-Holman, T., Blegen, M., & Vaughn, T. (1999a). Understanding and comparing differences in reported medication administration error rates. *American Journal of Medical Quality, 14*(2), 73–80.

Wakefield, D. S., Wakefield, B. J., Uden-Holman, T., Borders, T., Blegen, M., & Vaughn, T. (1999b). Understanding why medication administration errors may not be reported. *American Journal of Medical Quality, 14*(2), 81–88.

Wakefield, M. K., & Maddox, P. J. (2000). Patient quality and safety problems in the U.S. heath care system: challenges for nursing. *Nursing Economics, Mar–Apr 18*(2), 58–62.

Weinstein, R. A. (1998). Nosocomial infection update. Emerging Infections Diseases. Retrieved [February 28, 2000] from www.cdc.gov/ncidod/eid/vol4no3/weinstein.htm.

Whedon, M., & Shedd, P. (1989). Prediction and prevention of patient falls. *Image: Journal of Nursing Scholarship, 21*, 108–114.

Wilson, R. M., Runciman, W. B., Gibberd, R. W., Harrison, B.T., Newby, L., & Hamilton, J. D. (1995). The quality of Australia health care study. *The Medical Journal of Australia, 163*(6), 458–476.

Wunderlich, G. S., Sloan, F. S., & Davis, C. K. (Eds.) (1996). *Nursing staff in hospitals and nursing homes: Is it adequate?* National Academy Press: Washington, DC.

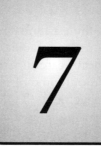

Patient Satisfaction as a Nurse-Sensitive Outcome

Heather K. Spence Laschinger, RN, PhD

Joan Almost, RN, MScN

School of Nursing
The University of Western Ontario

7.1 Introduction

Arguably, patient satisfaction has always been the goal of professional health care because health professionals are guided by, and required to maintain, standards of care thought to be necessary for optimal, high-quality, safe patient care. According to Donabedian (1988), patient satisfaction can be considered an element of health status and, thus, a fundamental component of any measure of quality. In response to calls for accountability for escalating healthcare costs over the past two decades, both healthcare funders and researchers have scrutinized patient satisfaction as a valued outcome of patient care quality.

The Total Quality Management (TQM) movement in the 1980s was a major initiative aimed at improving patient care processes to maximize effectiveness and efficiency in healthcare settings. The expected outcomes of the TQM approach were lower costs and more satisfied clients. At the same time, managed care approaches to healthcare delivery were becoming more prevalent. The competitive nature of these systems made patient satisfaction an important outcome to consider as healthcare businesses struggled for survival in the healthcare market. In the 1980s and 1990s, as the public gained greater access to previously difficult-to-obtain information regarding health and disease, a cadre of more knowledgeable and demanding healthcare consumers required healthcare providers to pay more attention to their needs and opinions. Consequently, the notion of patient as healthcare consumer became prominent.

There are few well-developed conceptual descriptions of patient satisfaction in the literature (Sitzia & Wood, 1997; Thomas & Bond, 1996). Existing instruments have varying degrees of comprehensiveness and, in many cases, no known reliability and validity. Institutions wishing to evaluate patient satisfaction as part of their quality improvement programs often have developed measures locally. Consequently, studies replicating their use have not been conducted. As a result, research in this field has been disadvantaged by inconsistent conceptualization of the phenomenon and a lack of comparable results across settings.

Patient satisfaction has been conceptualized broadly as a patient's overall response to the total healthcare experience, as well as more specifically in relationship to particular aspects of care, such as nursing and medical care or admission and discharge processes. A key component in these definitions has been the notion of a match between patients' expectations of care and what they actually received during the episode of care. When care fails to meet expectations, patients are dissatisfied with what they perceive to be poor-quality care (Ludwig-Beymer et al., 1993). Thus, patient satisfaction is one of several indicators of service quality, an important determinant of accreditation for healthcare institutions.

There are many conceptual and methodological problems in measuring patient satisfaction. Chang (1997) argues that current measures of patient satisfaction fail to capture key nursing actions, and thus are poor indicators of nursing care quality. This makes it difficult to meaningfully link nursing actions to patients' perceptions of the quality of nursing care. Pascoe (1983) pointed out that patients often have difficulty differentiating nursing personnel from other healthcare workers in hospital environments, which confounds their ratings of satisfaction with nursing care. As a result, the measures have questionable reliability and validity. Patient satisfaction ratings are usually positively skewed with a constricted range of values. These data characteristics affect statistical analyses and make it difficult to determine true effects that may exist. As a result, policy changes cannot be justified based on high-quality evidence. Finally, there is no standardization of measures of satisfaction with nursing care, making it impossible to compare results across settings.

Several authors (Bond & Thomas, 1992; Lynn & Moore, 1997) have pointed out that the majority of patient satisfaction measures reflect issues important to providers and do not include the patient's perspective. This is problematic because numerous studies have demonstrated provider/patient differences in importance ratings of various elements of satisfaction. More recently, researchers have begun to determine patient expectations of care and incorporate these perspectives into measures of patient satisfaction (Lynn & McMillen, 1999). Instruments that include both nurse and patient perspectives of good nursing care quality are more likely to yield meaningful results that can be used as a basis for quality improvement initiatives.

To summarize, there are several reasons for the intensified interest in measuring patient satisfaction with nursing and health care: (a) the demand for public accountability for healthcare outcomes and the need to provide evidence of quality, (b) incentives to tie government funding to standards of quality in health care delivery, (c) the Total Quality Management movement to monitor efforts to reduce costs and maintain quality, (d) a shift from the notion of patients as passive recipients of care to one of informed healthcare consumers who are willing and able to choose healthcare services based on their perceptions of quality provided, (e) the managed competition approach to healthcare delivery in the United States with its associated market share implications, and (f) the changing mix of healthcare workers in acute-care settings. As a result of these changes, patient satisfaction has emerged as an important indicator of healthcare quality that has implications for the survival of healthcare organizations and the well-being of patients under their care.

This chapter reviews the available literature on patient satisfaction viewed as a concept reflecting an outcome of nursing care. The purposes of the review were to:

- Clarify the concept of patient satisfaction at the theoretical and empirical levels

- Identify instruments measuring patient satisfaction that demonstrated acceptable reliability, validity, and sensitivity to change

- Determine structural and process factors that influence patient satisfaction

- Determine the extent to which patient satisfaction is an outcome-sensitive/responsive to nursing care

The methodology used to identify the relevant literature, as well as the criteria to select and systematically review it, was discussed in Chapter 1. A systematic search of the nursing and healthcare databases yielded a total of 400 sources that were either empirical or conceptual papers addressing patient satisfaction. One hundred and sixty of these met the pre-set inclusion and exclusion criteria, and are reviewed in this chapter.

7.2 Theoretical Background: Definition of the Concept

This section summarizes the results of a concept analysis that we conducted to clarify the concept of patient satisfaction at the theoretical and operational levels. The strategies we adopted involved the following:

- Carefully reading each article selected on the basis of the inclusion and exclusion criteria

- Abstracting the theoretical definitions of patient satisfaction that were provided in theoretical/conceptual sources, and in the framework or literature review section of empirical sources

- Comparing and contrasting the essential attributes that define the concept of patient satisfaction, as comprised in the theoretical definitions

- Summarizing the essential attributes that are common and consistent across the definitions and the conceptualizations of patient satisfaction

- Identifying the antecedents and consequences of patient satisfaction

7.2.1 Definitions of Patient Satisfaction

Patient satisfaction is frequently defined as the extent to which patients' expectations of care matched the actual care received (Abramowitz, Cote, & Berry, 1987; Hill, 1997; Linder-Pelz, 1982; Ludwig-Beymer et al., 1993; Petersen, 1988; Risser, 1975; Swan, 1985). In a thorough concept analysis of patient satisfaction, Eriksen (1995) defined patient satisfaction with nursing care as "the patients' subjective evaluation of the cognitive-emotional response that results from the interaction of the patients' expectations of nursing care and their perception of actual nurse behaviors/characteristics." Cleary and McNeil (1988) proposed a similar definition in the health services literature. However, Williams (1994) noted that few studies have actually found empirical support for this conception of satisfaction. Many argue that patient satisfaction is a general affective response to the overall healthcare experience, rather than a focused assessment of distinct aspects of the care episode (Chang et al., 1984; Taylor, 1994; Williams, 1994).

In the health services marketing literature, there is considerable debate about the importance of distinguishing between the concepts of patient satisfaction and patient perceptions of quality of care (Cronin & Taylor, 1992; Taylor, 1994). The argument is based on the notion that, although related, they are really distinct concepts and should be measured separately. Patient satisfaction is viewed as a mediator between patient perception of quality and future intentions to reuse the service or recommend the service to others (Woodside et al., 1989). Taylor defined perceived quality as a long-term attitude developed over time. On the other hand, patient satisfaction is defined as a short-term response to a specific experience. According to Taylor, it is important to be able to measure the two concepts separately in order to enable healthcare marketers to determine which of their marketing strategies are most effective. This debate was not evident in the nursing literature reviewed, most likely because of a differing perspective on the goal of collecting patient satisfaction data. Nursing is more concerned with using the data to improve the patients' health status and less concerned about patients' future intentions to choose a particular healthcare setting or recommend the organization to others (a logical interest of healthcare marketers).

Several researchers have found consistent differences in the importance ratings of aspects of care reported by nurses and patients, which suggests that nurses' and patients' definitions of satisfaction with patient care quality differ. In several studies, nurses consistently overestimated the importance of emotional care for patients (Farrell, 1991; von Essen & Sjoden, 1991, 1995; Young, Minnick, & Marcantonio, 1996). However, patients gave higher ratings to the importance of technical care, such as monitoring and following through, and providing explanations regarding their condition and care. These findings are consistent with those of Kovner (1989) and Larson (1987). Kovner's results are important since she found that the less patients and nurses disagreed on desirability of outcomes, the more satisfied patients were with their care. These results, which led to a concern that what was being measured in these surveys reflected provider perspectives, provided the impetus for a variety of qualitative studies to ascertain patients' perspectives of high-quality care (Bond & Thomas, 1992; Lynn & Moore, 1997; Webb & Hope, 1995).

7.2.2 Determinants of Patient Satisfaction

Researchers have identified many factors that have an impact on patient satisfaction. Personal characteristics of patients, such as cultural background and availability of a supportive network, as well as patient age, sex, and education have been shown to be related to patient satisfaction ratings in several studies (Conbere et al., 1992). However, others have found no relationship between patient satisfaction and demographic variables (Rubin et al., 1990). Patients' perceptions of the quality of their interactions with nurses are also important determinants of patient satisfaction. Among the many interpersonal factors identified are (a) involving patients in decisions about their care and supporting their right to convey their thoughts or opinions about care options (Andaleeb, 1998; Chang et al., 1984; Cleary & McNeil, 1988; Forbes, 1996; Kovner, 1989; Krouse & Roberts, 1989); (b) providing information about patients' conditions and explanations of symptoms they may experience (Bowling, 1992; Cleary & McNeil, 1988; Cottle, 1989; Fosbinder, 1994, Mahon, 1996); (c) using a compassionate caring approach (Cleary & McNeil, 1988; Cottle, 1989; Forbes, 1996; Fosbinder, 1994; Lewis & Woodside, 1992); and (d) creating an equitable relationship that ensures fairness (Swan, 1985). Other important determinants of patients' satisfaction with care include prompt attention to patient concerns and efficient execution of therapeutic interventions (Cottle, 1989; Denton, 1989; Thompson et al., 1996).

Several structural factors, including patients' perceptions of nurses' competency (Andaleeb, 1998; Cottle, 1989; Hanan & Karp, 1989) and the methods used to deliver nursing care, such as primary nursing, critical pathways, case management, and professional practice models, have been shown to affect patient satisfaction with nursing care (Goode, 1995; Hayes, 1992; Heinemann et al., 1996; Mahon, 1996; Twardon & Gartner, 1991). Advanced practice nurses, such as nurse practitioners in nurse-led clinics and clinical nurse specialists in inpatient settings, have also been associated with positive patient satisfaction ratings (Baradell, 1995; Graveley & Littlefield, 1992; Hill, 1997; Knaus et al., 1997).

The impact of nurses' job satisfaction on patient satisfaction with nursing care has been demonstrated (Atkins et al., 1996; Kaldenberg & Regrut, 1999; Leiter et al., 1998; Weisman & Nathanson, 1985). However, methodological problems limit the generalizability of these studies. Numerous studies have failed to establish this relationship (Niedz, 1998; Goodell & Van Ess Coelling, 1994). Thus, strong empirical evidence for the link between nurse job satisfaction and patient satisfaction does not exist (Kangas et al., 1999). Methodological difficulties and the complex nature of patient care quality may account for this situation.

7.2.3 Consequences of Patient Satisfaction with Nursing Care

Several health service researchers have studied the consequences of patient satisfaction with nursing care. Patient satisfaction with nursing care has been shown to be strongly related to overall satisfaction with the healthcare encounter in many studies (Abramowitz et al., 1987; Batalden & Nelson, 1990; Carey & Posavac, 1982; Hays et al., 1990). Some researchers have identified adherence to medically prescribed regimens as an outcome of patient satisfaction with nursing care (Swan & Carroll, 1980; Weisman & Nathanson, 1985). Davidow and Uttal (1989) argued that more satisfied patients are more cooperative with their caregivers, although this claim was not supported by empirical evidence. Finally, there is evidence to support the relationship between patient satisfaction with nursing care, patients' intentions to use a service in the future, and their likelihood of recommending the service to others (Abramowitz et al., 1987; Rubin et al., 1988). This outcome is particularly important in U.S. managed care settings, but is less salient in the Canadian healthcare context.

7.2.4 *Conceptual/Theoretical Models of Patient Satisfaction*

Few systematic attempts have been made to develop explanatory models of patient satisfaction (Abramowitz et al., 1987). Particularly in early studies, the concept seems to have been seen as self-explanatory; consequently, numerous idiosyncratic tools were developed locally to measure it. The models that have been proposed have not been widely tested. By far the most common model found in the literature is the discrepancy model, that is, the degree of match/mismatch between expectations for care and perceptions of care received. However, conceptual notions of the phenomenon are also implied by the content of the instruments themselves. The elements of these models vary based on their developer's orientation.

Linder-Pelz (1982) developed a model of patient satisfaction that suggested that patients' expectations of care, healthcare values, sense of entitlement, and interpersonal comparisons of care were antecedents of positive evaluations of care. However, when tested in a primary care setting, these variables explained only 8% of the variance in patient satisfaction levels. Greeneich (1993) proposed a model describing nurse, patient, and organizational characteristics that influence patient satisfaction. She also posited the notion of a critical nursing event, usually in relation to meeting or not meeting an important patient need, that has a lasting salient effect on a patient's satisfaction with care. This model has not been tested.

Comley and Beard (1998) attempted to derive a theory of patient satisfaction from various job satisfaction models and a review of factors reported in the literature that were found to influence patient satisfaction. They suggested that patient satisfaction, like job satisfaction, is a function of personal intrinsic factors and extrinsic organizational factors, and, thus, is not completely controllable by health care providers. Intrinsic factors include age, sex, socioeconomic status, ethnicity, occupation, diagnosis, and degree of illness. Extrinsic factors include type of nursing care delivery system, provider competence, promptness of service, comfort and cleanliness of the physical environment, and food quality. This model has not been empirically tested in a prospective study.

Pascoe (1983) described two models of consumer satisfaction based on the marketing literature. In the contrast model, clients compare service to previous experiences. Dissatisfaction results if there is a mismatch. In the assimilation model, clients attempt to resolve a sense of psychological dissonance created by the failure to have their expectations met by lowering those expectations. Thus, their satisfaction ratings are in relation to this lowered standard and are falsely high. Eriksen (1995) suggested that this model may account for the consistent findings of positively skewed patient satisfaction scores.

7.3 Approaches to Measurement of Patient Satisfaction with Nursing Care

The majority of patient satisfaction instruments in the literature are not based on theoretical models. However, the conceptualization of patient satisfaction is implied by the nature of the items in the questionnaires. Twenty-three instruments available in the nursing and health services literature were evaluated for their appropriateness as a nurse-sensitive outcome in this review. These instruments have varying degrees of reported psychometric data. The characteristics of these instruments are summarized in Table 7.1. For each measure, the title and author are identified, as well as the sample in which it was developed. The measurement domains, number of items, response format, and method of administration are also identified. Finally, evidence for the instrument's reliability and validity is reported. The details of the studies in which these instruments were used are presented in Table 7.2.

Several criteria were used to assess the relative value of these tools. First, the tool's comprehensiveness was assessed with regard to factors identified in the literature as determinants of patient satisfaction with nursing care quality. Also, based on recommendations in the literature that measures of patient satisfaction should reflect both nurse and patient perspectives, these tools were further evaluated to determine the extent to which quality indicators that patients identified in the literature were included. Comparisons of selected instruments using these two sets of criteria are shown in Table 7.3 and Table 7.4. In addition, the instruments were also evaluated in terms of availability of psychometric data, readability of items, length of the tool, ease of scoring, and sensitivity to actual nursing activities/responsibilities. Finally, the instruments were assessed to determine the extent to which the results of the responses to items on the questionnaire could be used by nursing administrators to improve the patient care process. Few of the instruments addressed all of the factors found in the literature.

Table 7.1. A Compendium of Selected Measures of Patient Satisfaction with Nursing Care Developed by Nursing and Health Services Researchers

Part A: Instruments Developed by Nursing Researchers

Instrument (author)	Target population	Domains (number of items and response format)	Method of administration	Reliability	Validity	Sensitivity to nursing care
Patient Satisfaction with Health Care Provider Scale (Marsh, 1999)	Patients of nurse practitioners and physicians	Access, humaneness, quality, and general satisfaction; 18 items rated on 5-point scale.	Self-administered	Cronbach's alpha reliability of .93 for total scale.	Content	No information available.
Patients' Perceptions of Quality Scale–Acute Care Version (Lynn & Moore, 1997)	Medical/surgical inpatients	Professional demeanor, treats me like an individual, mindfulness, and responsiveness; 54 items rated on a 5-point scale.	Self-administered	Cronbach's alpha reliabilities for the subscales of .80 to .94 (Lynn & Moore, 1997) and .62 to .96 (Moore et al., 1999).	Content	Percentage of RNs on unit and total nursing care hours per patient day were positive predictors of patient satisfaction (Moore et al., 1999).
Newcastle Satisfaction with Nursing Scale (McColl et al., 1996)	Inpatient hospital setting	Two scales: patient's experiences of nursing (manner, attentiveness, availability, reassurance, individual treatment, information, professionalism, knowledge, openness, informality) and satisfaction with that care (ward organization, ward environment); 45 items rated on 5- and 7-point scales.	Self-administered	No information available.	Content	No information available.
Patient Satisfaction Questionnaire (Forbes & Brown, 1995)	Outpatient surgery center	Caring, continuity of care, competence of nurses, and education of patients and family members; 21 items rated on a 5-point scale.	Self-administered	Cronbach's alpha reliability of .83; test-retest reliability assessed.	Content	No information available.
SERVQUAL for Patient Satisfaction with Nursing (Scardina, 1994)	Postoperative cardiothoracic patients	Expectations versus perceptions: domains include tangibles, reliability, responsiveness, assurance, and empathy; 44 items with 22 pairs of matching expectation/perception.	Self-administered	Cronbach's alpha reliabilities of .74 to .98 with the exception of the empathy perception (.40).	Content	No information available.

Table 7.1A (continued)

Instrument (author)	Target population	Domains (number of items and response format)	Method of administration	Reliability	Validity	Sensitivity to nursing care
Satisfaction with Nursing Care Questionnaire (Nash et al., 1994) *Adaptation of Eriksen's (1987) tool	Inpatient hospital setting	Particular concerns and rating scale for evaluation of care; 16 items rated on a 3-point scale.	Self-administered	No information available.	Content	No information available.
Quality of Multidisciplinary Care Scale (Blegen & Goode, 1993)	Maternity patients	Technical, communication, interpersonal, outcome, participation, general satisfaction, and maternity care; 31 items rated on a 5-point scale.	Self-administered	Cronbach's alpha reliabilities of .66 to .86 for subscales and .86 for total scale (Goode, 1995).	No information available.	Patient satisfaction with nursing care was significantly higher following implementation of a critical pathway system (Goode, 1995).
Care/Satisfaction Questionnaire (Larson & Ferketich, 1993)	Inpatient hospital setting	Nursing behaviors that denote caring to nurses and patients: accessibility, anticipation, comfort, trusting relationship, explaining and facilitating, and monitoring/following through. Domains include benign neglect, enabling, and assistive; 29 items rated by marking an "X" on a line indicating how much the patient agrees or disagrees (0 to 10).	Self-administered	Cronbach's alpha reliability of .94 for total scale.	Content, construct	No information available.
Critical Care Patient Satisfaction Survey (Megivern et al., 1992)	Critical care setting	Art of care, technical quality of care, physical environment, availability, continuity of care, efficacy/outcomes of care, recognition of individual qualities and needs, reassuring presence, promotion of patient autonomy, and patient/family education; 43 items rated on a 5-point scale with open-ended questions.	Self-administered	Inter-rater reliability.	Content	No information available.

Table 7.1A (continued)

Instrument (author)	Target population	Domains (number of items and response format)	Method of administration	Reliability	Validity	Sensitivity to nursing care
Patient Satisfaction with Nursing Care Questionnaire (Eriksen, 1987, 1995)	Inpatient hospital setting	Art of care, technical quality of care, physical environment, availability, continuity of care, and efficacy/outcomes of care; original 35 items, revised 34 items rated on a magnitude estimation scale.	Self-administered	No information available.	Construct, content	No information available.
La Monica-Oberst Patient Satisfaction Scale (La Monica et al., 1986); adapted by Munro et al. (1994). *Adaptation of Risser's (1975) tool	Oncology patients (La Monica et al., 1986); C-section, nononcologic hysterectomy patients; and women with gestational diabetes (Munro et al., 1994)	Patients' ratings of the extent to which they have experienced nurse behaviors during their hospital stay; domains include technical/professional, trusting relationship, education, dissatisfaction, interpersonal support, and good impression; original 41 items, revised to 28 by Munro et al.; 5- or 7-item scales.	Self-administered	Cronbach's alpha reliabilities of .92 to .97 for total scale; .80 to .96 for subscales.	Construct, content	Patient satisfaction with nursing care and patients' perceptions of organizational climate for service were each positively related to patients' perceptions of service quality (La Monica et al., 1986).
Patient Satisfaction Instrument (Hinshaw & Atwood, 1982) *Adaptation of Risser's (1975) tool	Medical/surgical inpatients and outpatients	Technical/professional, education, and trusting relationship; 25 items rated on a 5-point scale.	Self-administered	Cronbach's alpha reliabilities of .44 to .97 for subscales.	Construct, concurrent	Nursing care delivery model and patient length of time on the unit were significant predictors of patient satisfaction with nursing care (Kangas et al., 1999). Higher satisfaction score reported by patients cared for by the RNs working in a unit with shared governance, as opposed to units with traditional governance (Stumpf, 2001).

Table 7.1B (continued)

Instrument (author)	Target population	Domains (number of items and response format)	Method of administration	Reliability	Validity	Sensitivity to nursing care
Patient Satisfaction Scale (Risser, 1975)	Ambulatory care setting	Degree of congruency between patients' expectations of ideal nursing care and their perception of the real nursing care they receive; domains included technical/professional, education, and trusting relationship; 25 items rated on a 5-point scale.	Self-administered	Cronbach's alpha reliabilities of .91 for total scale; .63 to .89 for subscales.	Construct, content	Collaboration between RN/NA resulted in two areas of increased patient satisfaction, trust in the nurse, and feeling cared about by the nurse (Hayes, 1992).

Part B: Instruments Developed by Health Services Researchers

Instrument (author)	Target population	Domains (number of items and response format)	Method of administration	Reliability	Validity	Sensitivity to nursing care
Inpatient Nursing Service Quality (Koerner, 2000)	Inpatient hospital setting	Close relationships, uncertainty reduction, individualized care, compassion, and reliability; 14 items. Number of items vary for each subscale.	Self-administered	Cronbach's alpha reliabilities of .74 to .91 for subscales.	Content	No information available.
Press Ganey Satisfaction Measurement (Kaldenberg & Regrut, 1999)	Inpatient, emergency, and ambulatory care	Registration/access, lab/x-ray, nurses/staff, physicians, center/building; 26–32 items. Number of items vary for each subscale.	Self-administered	Cronbach's alpha reliabilities of .86 to .92 for subscales.	Content	A study reported in their own publications found a strong correlation between nurse job satisfaction and patient satisfaction when the Press Ganey inpatient satisfaction instrument was used.
Quality of Care Monitors (Carey & Seibert, 1993)	Inpatient, emergency, and ambulatory care	Different aspects of hospital experience: admission/billing, courtesy, nursing care, physician care, religious care, medical outcomes, food services, comfort and cleanliness, overall quality of care, and willingness to return and recommend; number of items varies. Response format 5-point Likert scale.	Self-administered	Cronbach's alpha reliabilities of .44 to .92 for subscales; test-retest reliability showed a kappa value of more than 60% (Charles et al., 1994).	Content, construct (Charles et al., 1994)	The nursing scale had the highest correlation with overall patient care ratings, with 59% of the variance in patient satisfaction explained by the Nursing Care Subscale, Courtesy Subscale, Comfort/Cleanliness Subscale, and Physician Care Subscale.

Table 7.1B (continued)

Instrument (author)	Target population	Domains (number of items and response format)	Method of administration	Reliability	Validity	Sensitivity to nursing care
Modified SERVQUAL (Babakus & Mangold, 1992)	Inpatient hospital setting	Reliability, responsiveness, assurance, empathy, and tangibles; 15 pairs of matching expectation/perception items rated on 5-point scales.	Self-administered	Cronbach's alpha reliabilities of .49 to .90 for subscales.	Construct, content	No information available.
Picker-Commonwealth Survey of Patient-Centered Care (Cleary et al., 1991)	Hospitals, ambulatory care	Respect for patients' values, preferences, and expressed needs; coordination of care and integration of services; information, communication, and education; physical comfort; emotional support and alleviation of fear and anxiety; involvement of family and friends; transition and continuity; item number varies.	Self-administered	Test-retest reliability assessed.	Content	A strong predictor of patient satisfaction with hospitalization was the inter-unit working relationships and hours per patient day (Sovie & Jawad, 2001).
Patient Judgments of Hospital Quality Questionnaire (Meterko et al., 1990)	Inpatient hospital setting	Nursing and daily care, hospital environment and ancillary staff, medical care, information, admissions, discharge and billing, overall quality of care and services, recommendations and intentions and overall health outcomes; 106 items used in pilot study; various forms available. Response format is 5-point Likert scale.	Self-administered	Cronbach's alpha reliabilities for subscales ranged from .66 to .94; test-retest reliability assessed.	Construct, content	Nursing subscale was the strongest predictor of overall rating of hospital quality and behavioral intentions (intention to return to the hospital if necessary and intention to recommend the hospital to others). Patients' perceptions of the overall quality of care were significantly related to the degree of emotional exhaustion nurses experienced (Leiter et al., 1998).

Table 7.1B (continued)

Instrument (author)	Target population	Domains (number of items and response format)	Method of administration	Reliability	Validity	Sensitivity to nursing care
Patient Satisfaction Questionnaire (Guzman et al., 1988)	Inpatient hospital setting	Nursing care, admission process, other hospital services, information-giving, and interpersonal skills; 30 items rated on a 3-point and a 5-point scale.	Self-administered	None reported.	None reported	No information available.
Patient Questionnaire (Abramowitz et al., 1987)	Inpatient hospital setting	Attribute satisfaction for 10 sets of services (admission, attending physicians, house staff, nurses, nurses' aides, housekeeping, food services, escort services, and other staff); 3 outcome measures: overall satisfaction, intent to return to hospital, and intent to recommend hospital to others; 37 items; Likert-response format.	Self-administered	Internal consistency reliability ranged from .51 to .95.	Construct, content	Patient satisfaction with nursing care was the only service related to overall satisfaction with hospital stay.

Table 7.2. Studies Investigating the Relationship between Nursing Variables and Patient Satisfaction

Author/date	Design of study	Characteristics of the sample, response rate, and setting	Patient satisfaction outcome	Intervention being evaluated/nursing variable being evaluated	Major results	Limitations
Abramowitz et al. (1987)	Descriptive correlational	841 patients from several units in a large New York teaching hospital ($RR = 91.3\%$).	Patient Questionnaire (Abramowitz et al., 1987)	Patient assessments of 10 services, including nursing	Patient satisfaction with nursing care was the only service related to overall satisfaction with hospital stay; satisfaction with nursing care and expectations for hospital care accounted for 24% of the variance in overall satisfaction; overall satisfaction strongly related to *paying attention to patients' concerns* ($r = .65$).	No limitations noted
Barkell et al. (2002)	Descriptive comparison	$n = 139$ prechange group; $n = 108$ posttest group; inpatient surgical unit in a Midwest community-based teaching hospital.	Parkside Patient Satisfaction Survey	Effects of a change in care delivery model (team nursing to total patient care) on patient satisfaction	No significant differences between the groups in overall patient satisfaction.	Cronbach's alpha reliabilities not reported
Charles et al. (1994)	Cross-sectional survey	Stratified random sample of 57 public acute-care hospitals in two provinces ($RR = 79\%$); 4,599 medical/surgical patients participated ($RR = 69\%$).	Modified version of the Picker Institute Patient Satisfaction Survey	Satisfaction with provider-patient communication, respect for preferences, attentiveness to physical needs, education, relationship between patient and physician, education and communication with family, pain management, and hospital discharge planning	61% of patients reported problems with 5 or fewer of 39 specific care processes evaluated; patients who were dissatisfied with the amount of time doctors and nurses spent discussing post-discharge activities reported significantly more problems.	No information on patient diagnosis or severity of illness for the episode of care

Table 7.2 (continued)

Author/date	Design of study	Characteristics of the sample, response rate, and setting	Patient satisfaction outcome	Intervention being evaluated/nursing variable being evaluated	Major results	Limitations
Doran et al. (2002)	Cross-sectional survey	372 patients (RR = 73%) and 254 nurses (RR = 35%) from 26 general medical-surgical and cardiac units in a southern Ontario tertiary hospital.	Patient Judgments of Hospital Quality–Nursing Subscale (Meterko et al., 1990)	The impact of nurse, unit, and patient structural variables on patient outcomes, and nurses' and patients' perceptions of nurses' role performance	Patient satisfaction with nursing care was higher on units where nurses reported good communication among the healthcare team members; patient satisfaction with nursing care was related to functional status, self-care ability, and emotional health at discharge.	Low nursing response rate (39%)
Goode (1995)	Experimental	Postpartum unit in a large acute-care tertiary, university-affiliated hospital in the Midwestern U.S.; overall RR = 69%. Experimental group: n = 107, data collection over 7.5 months; control group: n = 100, data collection over 6.5 months, no data collected during a 2-month phase-in period.	Quality of Multidisciplinary Care Scale (Blegan & Goode, 1993)	Evaluated impact of a multidisciplinary critical path with nurse case managers on patient satisfaction, staff job satisfaction, collaboration, and autonomy	Patients receiving care under the critical pathway system were significantly more satisfied than patients who received care under the old system (total patient care); *participation in decisions* was the only significantly different subscale between the two groups.	Cronbach's alpha reliabilities for subscales ranged from .66 to .86
Goodell & Van Ess Coeling (1994)	Pilot study	Random sample of 33 matched pairs of nurses/patients in an urban Midwest U.S. teaching hospital.	Patient Satisfaction Instrument (Hinshaw & Atwood, 1982)	Tested the relationship between patient satisfaction with nursing care and nurses' job satisfaction	Nurses' job satisfaction was not significantly related to patient satisfaction with nursing care.	Small sample size

Table 7.2 (continued)

Author/date	Design of study	Characteristics of the sample, response rate, and setting	Patient satisfaction outcome	Intervention being evaluated/nursing variable being evaluated	Major results	Limitations
Hayes (1992)	Experimental design; control and experimental groups on six general medical/surgical units; data collected at beginning, middle, and end of project	444 patients and 118 RNs from a large urban teaching center.	Patient Satisfaction with Nursing Care (Risser, 1975)	Evaluation of a professional practice model that included head nurses' involvement in restructuring the RN/NA working relationship, consistent assignments, clarification of the RN/NA relationship and responsibility, and team building.	Collaboration between RN/NA resulted in two areas of increased patient satisfaction: trust in the nurse and feeling cared about by the nurse; patient satisfaction decreased after two new head nurses were appointed, then increased to the previously high level, lending support to the influence of the head nurse.	No information on instrument or psychometric properties
Kaldenberg & Becker (1999)	Descriptive correlational; multi-site	36,078 patients from 275 ambulatory surgery centers across the U.S.	Press, Ganey Satisfaction Measurement (Kaldenberg & Regrut, 1999)	Patient satisfaction with nurses/staff, physicians, center/building, registration/access, and lab/x-ray.	Highest mean ratings to friendliness of the nurse (95%), nurses' concern for comfort (92.6%), and information given by nurses before surgery (92.7%); nurses/staff and building/center factors strongest predictors of the likelihood to recommend.	Cronbach's alpha not reported
Kangas et al. (1999)	Descriptive correlational; multi-site	Three hospitals, 92 nurses, and 90 patients from medical-surgical and ICU units.	Patient Satisfaction with Nursing Care (Hinshaw & Atwood, 1982)	RNs' job satisfaction, three nursing care delivery models (team nursing, case management, and primary nursing), organizational structures and culture, and controlling for patient characteristics.	Nursing care delivery model and patient length of time on the unit were significant predictors of patient satisfaction with nursing care ($R^2 = .10$); patients receiving care in the primary nursing delivery model were more satisfied.	Relatively small explained variance ($R^2 = 10\%$)

Table 7.2 (continued)

Author/date	Design of study	Characteristics of the sample, response rate, and setting	Patient satisfaction outcome	Intervention being evaluated/nursing variable being evaluated	Major results	Limitations
Larrabee et al. (1995)	Descriptive correlational; data collected at admission and discharge	Two medical-surgical units in a 455-bed urban hospital; 199 patients (RR = 71%).	Patient Judgments of Hospital Quality–Nursing Subscale (Meterko et al., 1990)	Testing a patient-focused model of quality by identifying predictors of patient perceptions of nursing care quality.	Pain severity at discharge and patient goal achievement were significant predictors of overall quality of care; nurses' perceptions of quality of care and goal achievement were not predictors of patient satisfaction.	No limitations noted
Lynn & McMillen (1999)	Descriptive	350 nurses and 448 patients from 40 medical-surgical units in seven hospitals in the southeastern U.S.	Patients' Perception of Quality Scale–Acute Care Version (PPQS-AV)	Evaluation of the extent of agreement between nurses and patients on the importance of various elements of quality nursing care.	Patients ranked the physical environment, psychological aspects of care, and professionalism higher; whereas nurses ranked trust, empathy, competence, examinations, and explanations higher.	No limitations noted
Lynn & Moore (1997)	Retrospective correlational; survey completed 24 hours prior to discharge	Patients and nurses from 16 medical-surgical units in an academic medical center in the southeastern U.S.	Patients' Perception of Quality Scale–Acute Care Version (PPQS-AV); Nurses' Perception of Quality Scale–Acute Care Version (NPQS-AV).	Relationship between the patients' perceptions of care received, the nurses' perceptions of care delivered, and traditional measures of nursing care quality (volume, acuity, and risk management indicators).	Neither patients' nor nurses' perceptions of care quality were strong predictors of "traditional" measures of patient care quality; of all possible subscale correlations, only those of the NPQS-ACV were significantly related to any of the traditional quality indicators.	Small sample size following data aggregation (16 units)

Table 7.2 (continued)

Author/date	Design of study	Characteristics of the sample, response rate, and setting	Patient satisfaction outcome	Intervention being evaluated/nursing variable being evaluated	Major results	Limitations
Moore et al. (1999)	Prospective and retrospective descriptive design	Patients and nurses from 16 medical-surgical units in a southeastern U.S. academic medical center.	Patient's Perception of Quality Scale–Acute Care Version	ANA Nursing Quality Indicators.	Percentage of RNs on the unit and total nursing care hours per patient day were predictors of patient satisfaction.	Small sample size following data aggregation (16 units)
Sovie & Jawad (2001)	Three-year longitudinal study; two acute-care adult inpatient units from 29 U.S. university teaching hospitals	n ranged from 12 to 26 per unit; *RR* not reported.	Combination of the Picker Institute and Press, Ganey Patient Satisfaction surveys	Three-year study of care restructuring collected data on nurse full-time equivalents (FTE), skill mix, and hours worked per patient day (HPPD).	Patient satisfaction increased to mid-80% range when HPPD increased from the 4–4.5-hour to the 5–6-hour range; inter-unit working relationships and HPPD were strong predictors of patient satisfaction with hospitalization; patient satisfaction with pain management was positively related to the HPPD and was influenced by physician-related factors on medical units and nurse-related factors on surgical units.	Data collected by different tools using different scales; efforts made to standardize the scores for comparable data; different methods used to complete questionnaires—mail, telephone, and interviews; Cronbach's alpha reliability estimates not reported
Stumpf (2001)	Ex-post-facto, correlational; five hospitals in southwestern Pennsylvania (three metropolitan, two rural)	16 units in five hospitals: 8 traditional/8 shared governance; $N = 120$ patients.	Patient's Opinion of Nursing Care (Hinshaw & Atwood, 1982)	Influence of unit governance type (shared governance vs. bureaucratic model) on culture, work satisfaction, nurse retention, and patient satisfaction.	Satisfaction with nursing care higher under shared governance model.	Statistical details not reported

Note:
LOS = length of stay
RR = sample response rate.

Table 7.3. Comparison of Seven Patient Satisfaction Instruments Using Quality Indicators Identified in the Literature

Identified Quality indicators	CARE/SAT (Larson & Ferketich, 1993)	Satisfaction with nursing care (Eriksen, 1995)	Lamonica-Oberst Patient Satisfaction Scale (Munro et al., 1994)	SERVQUAL for Patient Satisfaction with Nursing (Scardina, 1994)	Patient Judgments of Hospital Quality‡ (Meterko et al., 1990)	Picker-Commonwealth Survey of Patient-Centered Care‡ (Cleary et al., 1991)	Press Ganey Patient Satisfaction Survey‡ (Kaldenberg & Regrut, 1999)
Met expectations	*	****	****	**			
Caring style	**	****	*****	****	*		
Friendliness/courtesy	*	****	****	**	*	***	**
Attention to patient concerns	*******	*******	***	**	****	****	*
Information sharing	****	*	*******	*	***	****	**
Communication and interpersonal skills	****	*	***	**	**	***	*
Competence/skill	****	*	**	***	*	*	*
Goal achievement	**	****			**	***	*
Professional practice/care delivery models					*	**	

Table 7.3 (continued)

Identified Quality indicators	CARE/SAT (Larson & Ferketich, 1993)	Satisfaction with nursing care (Eriksen, 1995)	Lamonica-Oberst Patient Satisfaction Scale (Munro et al., 1994)	SERVQUAL for Patient Satisfaction with Nursing (Scardina, 1994)	Patient Judgments of Hospital Quality‡ (Meterko et al., 1990)	Picker-Commonwealth Survey of Patient-Centered Care‡ (Cleary et al., 1991)	Press Ganey Patient Satisfaction Survey‡ (Kaldenberg & Regrut, 1999)
Organizational factors				*****	**	*	**
Overall healthcare experience			*		*	**	*
Total items	29	34	28	22	28	30	11

Note:
*Each asterisk represents an item on the questionnaire
‡ = items relevant to nursing

263

Table 7.4. Comparison of Seven Patient Satisfaction Instruments Using Patient-Identified Quality Indicators

Identified Quality indicators	CARE/SAT (Larson & Ferketich, 1993)	Satisfaction with nursing care (Eriksen, 1995)	Lamonica-Oberst Patient Satisfaction Scale (Munro et al., 1994)	SERVQUAL for Patient Satisfaction with Nursing (Scardina, 1994)	Patient Judgments of Hospital Quality‡ (Meterko et al., 1990)	Picker-Commonwealth Survey of Patient-Centered Care‡ (Cleary et al., 1991)	Press Ganey Patient Satisfaction Survey‡ (Kaldenberg & Regrut, 1999)
Caring style	**	****	****	****	*		
Respectful manner	*	**	***	*	*	***	**
Attention to patient concerns	*******	*******	***	**	****	****	*
Participation in care	***	*	*		**	**	
Availability/timeliness of care	***	*	****	*****	**	****	*
Information sharing/interpretation of symptoms	****	*	******		***	****	**
Competence/skill	****	*	**	***	*	*	*
Pain control					*	**	
Physical care	*	*	**			*	

Table 7.4 (continued)

Identified Quality indicators	CARE/SAT (Larson & Ferketich, 1993)	Satisfaction with nursing care (Eriksen, 1995)	Lamonica-Oberst Patient Satisfaction Scale (Munro et al., 1994)	SERVQUAL for Patient Satisfaction with Nursing (Scardina, 1994)	Patient Judgments of Hospital Quality‡ (Meterko et al., 1990)	Picker-Commonwealth Survey of Patient-Centered Care‡ (Cleary et al., 1991)	Press Ganey Patient Satisfaction Survey‡ (Kaldenberg & Regrut, 1999)
Communication with other providers	**	*	*		**	***	
Education/preparation for discharge	*	*			**	****	*
Pleasant physical environment	*	*		****	*		*
Overall	*		*		*	**	*
Total items	29	34	28	22	28	30	11

Note:
*Each asterisk represents an item on the questionnaire

‡ = Items relevant to nursing

7.3.1 Instruments Developed by Nursing Researchers

Risser (1975), who was the first nurse researcher to implicitly propose a model of patient satisfaction, created a standardized measure of patient satisfaction by using a match between expectations and care received as a definition of satisfaction. Satisfaction consisted of three dimensions: (a) technical/professional behaviors (i.e., nursing knowledge and techniques required for competent nursing care); (b) a trusting relationship (i.e., communication and interpersonal skills required to create a healing climate); and (c) an educational relationship (i.e., information-sharing about patient condition and care processes). This measure has served as the basis for other instruments developed over the years by nurse researchers. Hinshaw and Atwood (1982) modified this tool to make it more suitable to inpatient settings, but they maintained the same underlying dimensions. In developing the La Monica-Oberst Patient Satisfaction Scale (LOPSS), La Monica, Oberst, Madea, and Wolf (1986) added items related to physical and comfort care, and obtained three categories of factors in an exploratory factor analysis: patient dissatisfaction, interpersonal support, and good impression. In La Monica et al.'s study, patient satisfaction with nursing care and patients' perceptions of the organizational climate for service were each positively related to patients' perceptions of service quality ($r = .74$, $p < .001$ and $r = .71$, $p < .001$, respectively). In 1994, Munro, Jacobsen, and Brooten modified the LOPSS and found two factors in a series of factor analyses: interpersonal support (14 items) and patient dissatisfaction (14 items).

In 1993, Larson and Ferketich developed the CARE/SAT, a 29-item measure of patient satisfaction with regard to nurses' caring behaviors. This tool was derived from the CARE-Q, a 50-item measure of nursing caring behaviors with well-established psychometric characteristics. The modified tool was designed to be easier to use in a clinical setting than the CARE-Q, in that it contained fewer items and employed a visual analogue for easy scoring by patients. The CARE/SAT total scale and subscales all had acceptable internal consistency and strong correlations with the Risser (1975) patient satisfaction measure ($r = .80$), providing evidence of construct validity.

Eriksen (1995) revised the Patient Satisfaction with Nursing Care Questionnaire following an extensive concept analysis and literature review. She deleted items pertaining to the technical quality of nursing care, based on the belief that patients are not sufficiently qualified to evaluate professional standards of care (Oberst, 1984). Besides re-wording items to more adequately reflect nursing care behaviors, she added new items, but no information is available in the published literature regarding their content. The revised instrument will require further testing to ascertain its psychometric properties. According to Pierce (1997), this tool is based on the clearest conceptualization of patient satisfaction available in the nursing literature. Nash et al. (1994) adapted this tool to evaluate the impact of a new professional practice model, shortening it to 16 items and converting the scale to a yes/no/not applicable format to facilitate patient use. No results or psychometric properties were reported. However, patients reported having difficulty using the original scaling format and preferred the three-category response format previously described.

More recently, Lynn and Moore (1997) sought to address criticisms in the literature that current patient satisfaction instruments reflected the provider's perspective to a greater extent than the patient's. Lynn and Sidani (1991) believed that any definition of patient satisfaction or description of quality must include the perspective of all parties involved in the care. Using both qualitative and quantitative methods, they elicited patients' perceptions of high-quality care in one-on-one interviews and developed a 54-item instrument, the Patient Perceptions of Quality Care–Acute Care Version (PPQC-ACV), to reflect attributes patients identified. Four factors were obtained in a factor analysis: professional demeanor, treating the patient like an individual, mindfulness, and responsiveness. They used a similar approach to create a 56-item tool to measure nurses' perceptions of the quality of care delivered to patients (Nurses' Perceptions of Quality Care–Acute Care Version [NPQS-ACV]). This tool consisted of five factors: developing a relationship, science of nursing, unit collaboration, the environment, and resources. Both tools were found to have good internal consistency and construct validity.

As the researchers predicted, neither the PPQC-ACV or the NPQS-ACV was a strong predictor of traditional measures of patient care quality (volume, acuity, and risk management indicators), which supported the authors' contention that the traditional outcome measures are not valid nurse-sensitive quality indicators. Of all possible subscale correlations, only those of the NPQS-ACV were significantly related to any of the traditional quality indicators. Interestingly, all NPQS-ACV subscales were related to volume indicators such as the number of admissions and number of patient days. That is, nurses' perceptions of patient care quality were negatively related to workload factors, which suggested that the increasingly higher volume of patients to care for with the same or fewer resources was perceived to have a negative impact on patient care quality. These new measures are of value since they represent patient and nurse perceptions of quality care elicited within the context of massive healthcare restructuring over the past five years. In a related study, Moore, Lynn, McMillen, and Evans (1999) examined the relationship between a modified version of the PPQC-ACV and the American Nurses Association Nursing Quality Indicators (American Nurses Association, 1996). Two structural quality indicators were significantly related to patient satisfaction with nursing care. The percentage of RNs on the unit was the most consistent predictor of patient satisfaction with nursing care, pain management, education, and overall care. The total number of nursing care hours provided per patient day was also a positive predictor of patient satisfaction with pain management and education. Internal consistency estimates for the factors ranged from 0.62 to 0.96. Work is ongoing to document the psychometric properties of the new instruments in a variety of patient populations and settings.

7.3.2 *Instruments Developed by Health Services Researchers*

In health services research, Ware, Davies-Avery, and Stewart (1978) were leaders in patient satisfaction research as part of their work to measure patient care quality outcomes. Ware et al.s' model, derived from interviews with both patients and providers, consisted of eight dimensions thought to be considered by patients when they evaluated their healthcare experience: the art of care, technical care quality, accessibility/convenience, payment method, physical environment, availability of providers, continuity of care, and efficacy/outcomes (Chang, 1997). The Patient Satisfaction Questionnaires I and II are used to operationalize components of the model. However, the tool is clearly oriented towards assessing aspects of medical care, not nursing care. Ware's model has been adapted by nurse researchers to develop taxonomies to analyze patient satisfaction with nursing care (Chang, 1997; Greeneich et al., 1992).

More recently, Ware and his associates developed another tool to operationalize a service quality evaluation model, the Patient Judgment of Hospital Quality Scale, or PJHQ (Rubin, Ware, & Hays, 1990). The model suggests that patients evaluate distinct categories of hospital care: (a) nursing and daily care, (b) hospital-environment and ancillary staff, (c) medical care, (d) information, (e) the admissions process, and (f) discharge and billing. This tool contains five specific items (nurses' skill and competence, nurses' attention to the patient's condition, nursing staff response to calls, nurses demonstrating a concerned and caring attitude, and information provided by nursing) evaluating nursing care that are included in the Nursing and Daily Care subscale. Nelson and Niederberger (1990) captured similar facets in their model: access to care, administrative management, clinical management, interpersonal management, continuity of care, and general satisfaction. A tool very similar to the PJHQ, the Patient Judgment Systems is used to operationalize this model. The PJHQ was found to have sound psychometric properties and has been used extensively in health services research. Demographic characteristics were found to have little effect on patient ratings. Interestingly, the nursing subscale was the strongest predictor of overall rating of hospital quality and behavioral intentions (intention to return to the hospital if necessary and intention to recommend the hospital to others). Atkins et al. (1996) found that two items—concern and caring attitude, and information provided by nurses—were strongly related to overall quality ($r = 0.69$ and $r = 0.71$, $p < 0.005$, respectively). In a study by Doran, Sidani, Keatings, and Doidge (2002), patients reported higher levels of satisfaction with nursing care on units where nurses reported good communication among the healthcare team members ($\beta = .14$). Patient satisfaction with nursing care was also related to functional status ($\beta = .11$), self-care ability ($\beta = .15$), and emotional health at discharge ($\beta = -.18$). Leiter et al. (1998) found that patients' perceptions of the overall quality of care were significantly related to the degree of emotional exhaustion nurses experienced. Patients on units where nurses found their work meaningful were more satisfied with all aspects of their hospital stay ($r = 0.79$, $p < 0.01$). Likewise, patients were less satisfied with their care on units where nursing staff more frequently expressed the intention to quit ($r = -0.53$, $p < 0.05$) and nurses expressed cynicism ($r = -0.53$, $p < 0.05$).

Parasuraman, Zeithaml, and Berry (1985) developed a marketing model of patient satisfaction from the business quality literature, using the SERVQUAL instrument to operationalize the model. The five general categories of quality include (a) assurance, or the knowledge and courtesy of employees and their ability to inspire confidence, including competence, communication, credibility, courtesy, and security; (b) reliability, or the ability to perform the promised service reliably and accurately; (c) empathy, or the provision of caring, individualized attention to customers; (d) responsiveness, or the willingness to help customers and provide prompt service; and (e) tangibles, or the physical environment, equipment, and appearance of personnel. This tool contains items tapping both patients' expectations of various aspects of care and patients' perceptions of the extent to which they received the care. However, support for this model in healthcare settings has been equivocal, raising questions about its generalizability and comprehensiveness for health care. The model has been criticized for its relative lack of attention to the emotional and interpersonal aspects of quality (Bowers et al., 1994; Gummesson, 1991; Koerner, 2000). It has also been criticized for its use of difference scores in operationalizing patient satisfaction, given the well-known reliability problems with such measures (Edwards, 1994; Nunnally & Bernstein, 1994). Babakus and Mangold (1992) established convergent validity of a modified version of this tool, which consisted only of perceived care received (SERPERF). They found strong correlations between this scale, a single-item measure of overall perceived quality, and a measure of intention to repeat use of the hospital's services if needed (.83 and .76, respectively). Niedz (1998) used the SERPERF and found that items tapping patient perceptions of actual care received were significantly related to overall patient perception of satisfaction with nursing care. In her study, expectation scores did not contribute to the prediction of these outcomes beyond that contributed by actual perceptions of care received. This finding is consistent with those of Taylor and Cronin (1994). Scardina (1994) adapted the SERVQUAL for use in evaluating nursing care. In a pilot study of 10 patients, the tool was found to have adequate content validity.

Others have suggested the need to use service-specific measures of quality in healthcare settings and to add other attributes, such as caring and communication (Bowers et al., 1994). In a well-designed mixed methods study, Koerner (2000) added items to the SERVQUAL to reflect aspects of compassionate care described in patient interviews. However, in her final analysis, very few of the original SERVQUAL items were found to have construct validity. As a result, the new tool, Inpatient Nursing Service Quality Scale (INSQS), was developed as a more valid measure of satisfaction with nursing care. The INSQS consists of five dimensions: compassion, individualized care, reliability, close relationships, and uncertainty reduction. Compassion and reliability were the strongest predictors of overall satisfaction with quality and intention to recommend the hospital to others.

The Parkside organization designed another market research-based tool, the Quality of Care Monitor, to measure both inpatient and outpatient perceptions of quality. This tool taps eight dimensions of patient care and contains nine items related to nursing care quality, including those nurse researchers have identified, such as competence, interpersonal relationships, and information sharing, among others. The nursing scale had high internal consistency (.88) and achieved the highest correlation with overall patient care ratings (Carey & Seibert, 1993). Carey and Seibert also found that 59% of the variance in patient satisfaction was explained by the Nursing Care Subscale, Courtesy Subscale, Comfort/Cleanliness Subscale, and Physician Care Subscale.

Other commercially available measures, such as those developed by the Picker Institute and Press Ganey Associates, are commonly used by hospitals as part of their measurement of patient care quality. The Picker instrument consists of seven categories: (a) patient preferences, (b) coordination of care, (c) information and education, (d) physical comfort, (e) emotional support, (f) involvement family and friends, and (g) continuity and transition. This instrument has been widely used in Canada. Charles et al. (1994) adapted this tool in a national survey of adult medical-surgical patients to identify common sources of patient satisfaction across 57 hospitals in six Canadian provinces. Over 90% of patients surveyed were satisfied with their relationship with their physician and with the degree of participation in decision-making. Problem areas identified were pain management, expectations for tests and procedures, knowledge of medications, and home management of their condition.

The Press Ganey tool includes items relating to comfort, pain management, patient explanations/education, promotions, caring relationships, and courtesy. This organization has recently acquired the Parkside group. In a study reported in their own publications (Kaldenberg & Regrut, 1999), a strong correlation was found between nurse job satisfaction and patient satisfaction when their inpatient satisfaction instrument was used ($r = .84$). It is difficult to ascertain from the brief report exactly how the analysis was conducted. However, since the highest correlations found were between nurses' satisfaction with variables commonly associated with empowering work environments and patient satisfaction, replication of this study seems warranted.

One of the positive attributes of these commercially available tools is that most were developed from data obtained in focus groups with both patients and providers, thereby overcoming some of the criticisms of earlier measures. In addition, these commercial enterprises provide data on the psychometric analyses conducted on these instruments and maintain large publicly accessible normative databases for various patient populations. However, many have been criticized for not tapping important aspects of nursing care and for being too global in nature. Thus, it is very important for nursing experts to be consulted in the process of choosing a tool for evaluating patient satisfaction with hospital care, in order to ensure that satisfaction with nursing care will be adequately evaluated.

7.4 Issues in Measuring Patient Satisfaction

Several issues are associated with the assessment of patient satisfaction. Despite the fact that patient satisfaction with nursing care has been shown to be the most critical determinant of patients' overall satisfaction with hospital care, Chang (1997) maintained that many instruments commonly used in large patient satisfaction surveys do not adequately capture important nursing activities, thereby limiting their utility as valid nurse-sensitive outcome measures. This is a problem when researchers attempt to link nursing activities and other factors, such as redesign of nursing care delivery systems (e.g., changes in staff mix and staffing ratios), to patient satisfaction. The wide range of healthcare personnel in hospital settings also makes it difficult for patients to differentiate nurses from non-nurses and, thus, threatens the reliability and validity of measurements of satisfaction with nursing care (Pascoe, 1983). Another issue relates to the positive skewness and lack of variability of most patient satisfaction ratings. These data characteristics create problems in determining the true effects of the phenomenon, and can have a negative impact on the statistical comparisons and relationships being studied. As a result, policy changes are difficult to justify based on empirical evidence. Finally, there is no standardization of measures of satisfaction with nursing care, making it impossible to compare across settings.

Lin (1996) summarized a variety of factors shown to have an influence on patient satisfaction ratings. Several relate to methodological issues, whereas others have to do with patient demographic characteristics and attitudes and nursing process variables. For instance, the timing of the survey has been found to affect patient satisfaction ratings. Although return rates tended to be better when patients were surveyed at discharge, the ratings were lower than when surveys were conducted several weeks post-discharge. Furthermore, ratings were higher when patients were surveyed several months post-discharge, in comparison to several weeks following discharge (Ley et al., 1976). Response rates were low (30%) when surveyed at several months post-discharge and several weeks following discharge. Opinions differ about the reasons for this. Ley et al. suggested that less-satisfied patients may be less likely to return questionnaires, whereas Ware, Snyder, Wright, and Allison (1983) argued that more-satisfied patients may be less likely to return questionnaires. More research is needed to address this issue if patient satisfaction data are to be of use to hospital administrators. Research has shown that using a response format that allows the patient to rate items on an excellent/poor rating scale (rather than agree/disagree), and including a neutral point on the scale both help to increase the variance of the score

(Ware & Hays, 1988). This scaling method helps to address the problem of skewed data typically obtained in patient satisfaction surveys.

Several patient demographic variables, such as gender, age, education, and race, have been inconsistently associated with patient satisfaction with nursing care. Pascoe (1983) found that older patients tended to report higher satisfaction with nursing care, whereas other studies have not supported this finding (Bader, 1988). Women have been found to be more satisfied with care than men in some studies (Pascoe, 1983; Ware et al., 1978), although other studies have found no gender effect (Doering, 1983; Hall & Dornan, 1990; Sitzia & Wood, 1997). Patient expectations also have been found to influence satisfaction ratings. Swan (1985) reported that patients with lower expectations and less knowledge of services available were more satisfied with their nursing care. In addition, patient health status has been shown to influence satisfaction ratings. That is, patients with good health status post-discharge report greater satisfaction than those with poor health status (Cleary et al., 1991; Cleary et al., 1989).

Finally, patients' perceptions of the nature of the nursing care process they experience during hospitalization have been shown to influence patient satisfaction ratings. Patients' perceptions of the competence of nurses caring for them and the manner in which care was delivered, including the nurses' interpersonal manner, communication skills, friendliness, and attentiveness to specific patient needs, have been associated with higher satisfaction (Cleary & McNeil, 1988; Sitzia & Wood, 1997).

Lin's (1996) review of the literature shows little evidence of measures derived from extant theoretical frameworks, inconsistent conceptualizations of the concept, limited reporting of validity information across studies, and a general lack of sensitivity of the measures due to highly positively skewed scores on rating scales. In addition, she found few examples of replicated studies or models attempting to explain mechanisms by which patient satisfaction is developed. Her conclusions are consistent with other reviews of patient satisfaction measures. Another problem noted by several researchers has to do with the difficulty that many patients had distinguishing among the different categories of nursing personnel in hospital settings (Abramowitz et al., 1987; Moritz, 1991). This problem raises issues about the reliability of measures of satisfaction with nursing care.

7.5   Discussion and Recommendations

The literature on patient satisfaction is indeed extensive and varied in both nursing and health services research. The empirical research linking antecedents and consequences of patient satisfaction is of varying levels of quality. The majority of the research reported is related to instrument development. Single-site studies with sampling problems are common, and the lack of consistent measurement of the concept across settings does not allow for comparisons. Much of the research has been correlational in nature and atheoretical. However, the growing body of work that identifies antecedents and consequences of patient satisfaction can be used as a basis for developing models to be tested. Researchers in both nursing and health services have recognized the need to develop conceptual frameworks that clarify the nature of the concept. There are a few systematic concept analyses of patient satisfaction in the literature. However, these models should be tested empirically.

There appears to be consensus in the literature that patient satisfaction is a multidimensional concept and that efforts should continue to clarify the concept to insure that it is measured accurately. In response to criticisms that many patient satisfaction measures tap primarily the provider's conception of aspects of quality that influence patient satisfaction, recent efforts have incorporated the patient's perspective in the concept's measurement. Several nursing researchers have shown that nurses' and patients' perceptions of what is satisfying in relation to patient care are different. Consistent pleas have arisen for the development and testing of sensitive instruments that are conceptually based and that have undergone extensive psychometric development and testing. Although many instruments exist in the literature, only recently have concerted efforts been made to assure adequate conceptualization, reliability, and validity. For example, several researchers have studied the impact of different methods of data collection on patient satisfaction ratings.

The most consistent substantive finding in the literature is that satisfaction with nursing care is the strongest predictor of overall satisfaction with the healthcare experience. The quality of interpersonal relationships between nurses and patients has been shown to be one of the most important aspects of nursing behavior that influences patient satisfaction. Although there is debate in the literature regarding the extent to which patients are capable of evaluating the competence of health professionals, such as nurses and physicians, patients' perceptions of their competence have nonetheless been linked to patients' satisfaction with their care in numerous studies. Patient satisfaction ratings are typically high, purportedly because of social desirability and feelings of vulnerability. This situation has resulted in a lack of sensitivity in statistical analyses.

Few controlled studies were found that examined patient satisfaction with nursing care as an outcome of specific nursing interventions. Patient satisfaction with nursing care was found to be significantly higher following implementation of a critical pathway system in a postpartum unit (Goode, 1995) and following a hospital restructuring process (Sovie & Jawad, 2001). Kangas et al. (1999) found that patients cared for in a primary nursing model reported higher satisfaction with nursing care than did those in traditional nursing care delivery modes, such as team nursing. Stumpf (2001) reported that patient satisfaction with nursing care was higher for patients cared for by nurses working in a unit with shared governance. Several studies reporting a significant impact of organizational interventions on patient satisfaction with nursing care did not specifically identify the instrument used to measure patient satisfaction. Many used their hospitals' existing patient satisfaction measures. Thus, information was insufficient to evaluate these studies. Other factors, such as nurses' job satisfaction, burnout, and staffing variables, appear to indirectly influence patient satisfaction with nursing care (Atkins et al., 1996; Kaldenberg & Regrut, 1999; Leiter et al., 1998; Moore et al., 1999).

The increased interest in patient satisfaction as a quality indicator in U.S. managed care environments has stimulated greater attention to developing standardized measures of the concept with adequate psychometric properties. With the change to a market orientation, healthcare marketers and consulting firms have become involved in the development and administration of patient satisfaction measures. These tools have been exported to Canada and other countries such as the United Kingdom and other European countries. Many of these measures have been developed without the input of healthcare professionals and have been criticized, in particular, for not capturing the essence of nursing activities related to patient care. However, more collaboration between nursing and health services researchers in the past decade has resulted in a mutual enrichment of the field. Several authors emphasized the importance of including nursing representatives in the process of selecting a commercially available patient satisfaction measure to assure that appropriate aspects of nursing care are contained in the instrument. Given the integral role of nursing services in the patient care experience and the consistent link between satisfaction with nursing care and overall patient satisfaction, this practice is crucial to obtaining meaningful data.

Based on this review of the literature relating to patient satisfaction with nursing care, several recommendations are offered:

- Continue efforts to clarify and define the nature of patient satisfaction. Develop and test theoretical models that articulate the mechanisms that affect changes in satisfaction over time. Ensure that both patients' and providers' viewpoints are represented. Use both qualitative and quantitative approaches to develop and validate these models.

- Develop and refine reliable and valid measures of satisfaction based on conceptually sound theoretical models. Avoid broad measures of patient satisfaction and develop multidimensional measures of quality that include both affective and instrumental components of satisfaction with nursing care. Use both closed- and open-ended items to maximize information. Test innovative approaches to measuring the concept in order to optimize sensitivity and usability of instruments (e.g., item design, scoring procedures).

- Develop and implement strong designs (e.g., multisite, longitudinal studies) to empirically test models of patient satisfaction. Employ sophisticated data analysis techniques to evaluate models of satisfaction (e.g., structural equation modelling, hierarchical linear modelling, time series analyses). Replicate studies to increase generalizability of findings.

- Publish information about patient satisfaction measures, including dimensions, sample items, and scoring procedures, as well as psychometric data and research results, in accessible sites, such as the World Wide Web, journals, etc.

- Increase collaboration between nurse researchers and health services researchers to further develop the body of knowledge related to patients' satisfaction with nursing care quality.

References

Abramowitz, S., Cote, A. A., & Berry, E. (1987). Analyzing patient satisfaction: A multianalytic approach. *Quality Review Bulletin, 13*, 122–130.

American Nurses Association. (1996). *Nursing quality indicators: A guide for implementation*. Washington, DC: American Nurses Publishing.

Andaleeb, S. S. (1998). Determinants of customer satisfaction with hospitals: A managerial model. *International Journal of Health Care Quality Assurance, 11*, 181–187.

Atkins, P. M., Marshall, B. S., & Javalgi, R. G. (1996). Happy employees lead to loyal patients. *Journal of Health Care Marketing, 16*(4), 15–23.

Babakus, E., & Mangold, W. G. (1992). Adapting the SERVQUAL scale to hospital services: An empirical investigation. *Health Services Research, 26*, 767–786.

Bader, M. M. (1988). Nursing care behaviours that predict patient satisfaction. *Journal of Nursing Quality Assurance, 2*, 11–17.

Baradell, J. G. (1995). Clinical outcomes and satisfaction of patients of clinical nurse specialists in psychiatric-mental health nursing. *Archives of Psychiatric Nursing, 9*, 240–250.

Barkell, N. P., Killinger, K. A., & Schultz, S. D. (2002). The relationship between nurse staffing models and patient outcomes: A descriptive study. *Outcomes Management, 6*(1), 27–33.

Batalden, P. B., & Nelson, E. C. (1990). Hospital quality: Patient, physician, and employee judgments. *International Journal of Health Care Quality Assurance, 3*, 7–17.

Blegen, M. A., & Goode, C. J. (1993). *Measuring the quality of multidisciplinary care*. Paper presented at the ANA Council of Nurse Researchers meeting, Washington, DC.

Bond, S., & Thomas, L. (1992). Measuring patients' satisfaction with nursing care. *Journal of Advanced Nursing, 17*, 52–63.

Bowers, M. R., Swan, J. E., & Koehler, W. F. (1994). What attributes determine quality and satisfaction with health care delivery? *Health Care Manager Review, 19*(4), 49–55.

Bowling, A. (1992). Assessing health needs and measuring patient satisfaction. *Nursing Times, 88*(31), 31–33.

Carey, R. G., & Posavac, E. J. (1982). Using patient information to identify areas for service improvement. *Healthcare Management Review, 7*(2), 43–48.

Carey, R. G., & Seibert, J. H. (1993). A patient survey system to measure quality improvement questionnaire reliability and validity. *Medical Care, 31*, 834–845.

Chang, B. L., Uman, G. C., Lawrence, L. S., Ware, J. E., & Kane, R. L. (1984). The effect of systematically varying components of nursing care satisfaction in elderly ambulatory women. *Western Journal of Nursing Research, 6*, 366–379.

Chang, K. (1997). Dimensions and indicators of patients' perceived nursing care quality in the hospital setting. *Journal of Nursing Care Quality, 11*(6), 26–37.

Charles, C., Gauld, M., Chambers, L., O'Brien, B., Haynes, B., & LaBelle, R. (1994). How was your hospital stay? Patients' reports about their care in Canadian hospitals. *Canadian Medical Association Journal, 150*, 1813–1822.

Cleary, P. D., & McNeil, B. J. (1988). Patient satisfaction as an indicator of quality care. *Inquiry, 25*, 25–36.

Cleary, P. D., Keroy, L., Karapanos, G., & McMullen, W. (1989). Patient assessments of hospital care. *Quality Review Bulletin, 15*, 172–179.

Cleary, P. D., Edgman-Levitan, S., Roberts, M., Moloney, T. W., McMullen, W., Walker, J. D., et al. (1991). Patients evaluate their hospital care: A national survey. *Health Affairs, 10*, 254–267.

Comley, A. L., & Beard, M. T. (1998). Toward a derived theory of patient satisfaction. *The Journal of Theory Construction and Testing, 2*(2), 44–50.

Conbere, P. C., McGovern, P., Kochevar, L., & Widtfeldt, A. (1992). Measuring satisfaction with medical case management: A quality improvement tool. *American Association of Occupational Health Nurses Journal, 40*, 333–341, 358–360.

Cottle, D. W. (1989). *Client-centred service: How to keep them coming back for more.* New York: John Wiley.

Cronin, J. J., & Taylor, S. A. (1992). Measuring service quality: A reexamination and extension. *Journal of Marketing, 56*(3), 55.

Davidow, W. A., & Uttal, B. (1989). *Total customer service.* New York: Harper & Row.

Denton, D. K. (1989). *Quality service.* Houston, TX: Gulf Publishing.

Doering, E. R. (1983). Factors influencing inpatient satisfaction with care. *Quality Review Bulletin, 9*, 291–299.

Donabedian, A. (1988). Quality assessment and assurance: Unity of purpose, diversity of means. *Inquiry, 25*, 173–219.

Doran, D. M., Sidani, S., Keatings, M., & Doidge, D. (2002). An empirical test of the Nursing Role Effectiveness Model. *Journal of Advanced Nursing, 38*, 29–39.

Edwards, J. R. (1994). The study of congruence in organizational behavior research: Critique and a proposed alternative. *Organizational Behavior and Human Decision Processes, 58*, 51–100 (erratum, 58, 323–325).

Eriksen, L. R. (1987). Patient satisfaction: An indicator of nursing care quality? *Nursing Management, 18*(7), 31–35.

Eriksen, L. R. (1995). Patient satisfaction with nursing care: Concept satisfaction. *Journal of Nursing Measurement, 3*, 59–76.

Farrell, G. A. (1991). How accurately do nurses perceive patients' needs? A comparison of general and psychiatric settings. *Journal of Advanced Nursing, 16*, 1062–1070.

Forbes, D. A. (1996). Clarification of the constructs of satisfaction and dissatisfaction with home care. *Public Health Nursing, 13*, 377–385.

Forbes, M. L., & Brown, H. N. (1995). Developing an instrument for measuring patient satisfaction. *Association of Operating Room Nurses Journal, 61*, 737–743.

Fosbinder, D. (1994). Patient perceptions of nursing care: An emerging theory of interpersonal competence. *Journal of Advanced Nursing, 20*, 1085–1093.

Goode, C. J. (1995). Impact of a Care Map and case management on patient satisfaction and staff satisfaction, collaboration and autonomy. *Nursing Economics, 13*, 337–348.

Goodell, T., & Van Ess Coeling, H. (1994). Outcomes of nurses' satisfaction. *Journal of Nursing Administration, 24*(11), 36–41.

Graveley, E., & Littlefield, J. (1992). A cost-effectiveness analysis of three staffing models for the delivery of low-risk prenatal care. *American Journal of Public Health, 82*, 180–184.

Greeneich, D. (1993). The link between new and return business and quality of care: Patient satisfaction. *Advances in Nursing Science, 16*, 62–67.

Greeneich, D. S., Long, C. O., & Miller, B. K. (1992). Patient satisfaction update: Research applied to practice. *Applied Nursing Research, 5*(1), 43–48.

Gummesson, E. (1991). Service quality: A holistic view. In S. W. Brown, E. Gummesson, B. B. Edvardsson, & B. Gustavsson (Eds.), *Service quality: Multidisciplinary and multinational perspectives* (pp. 3–22). Lexington, MA: Lexington Books.

Guzman, P. M., Sliepcevich, E. M., Lacey, E. P., Vitello, E. M., Matten, M. R., Woehlke, P. L., et al. (1988). Tapping patient satisfaction: A strategy for quality assessment. *Patient Education and Counseling, 12*, 225–233.

Hall, J. A., & Dornan, M. C. (1990). Patient sociodemographic characteristics as predictors of satisfaction with medical care: A meta-analysis. *Social Science & Medicine, 30*, 811–818.

Hanan, M., & Karp, P. (1989). *Customer satisfaction*. New York: American Management Association.

Hayes, P. (1992). Evaluation of a professional practice model. *Nursing Administration Quarterly, 16*(4), 57–64.

Hays, R. D., Nelson, E. C., Rubin, H. R., Ware, J. E., & Meterko, M. (1990). Further evaluations of the PJHQ scales. *Medical Care, 28*(Suppl. 9), S29–S39.

Heinemann, D., Lengacher, C. A., van Cott, M. L., Mabe, P., & Swymer, S. (1996). Partners in patient care: Measuring the effects on patient satisfaction and other quality indicators. *Nursing Economics, 14*, 276–285.

Hill, J. (1997). Patient satisfaction in a nurse-led rheumatology clinic. *Journal of Advanced Nursing, 25*, 347–354.

Hinshaw, A., & Atwood, J. (1982). A patient satisfaction instrument: Precision by replication. *Nursing Research, 31*, 170–175.

Kaldenberg, D. O., & Becker, B. W. (1999). Evaluations of care by ambulatory surgery patients. *Health Care Management Review, 24*(3), 73–81.

Kaldenberg, D. O., & Regrut, B. A. (1999). Do satisfied patients depend on satisfied employees? Or, do satisfied employees depend on satisfied patients? In *The Satisfaction Report Newsletter: Vol. 3* (pp. 1–4). South Bend, IN: Press, Ganey Associates.

Kangas, S., Kee, C. C., & McKee-Waddle, R. (1999). Organizational factors, nurses' job satisfaction, and patient satisfaction with nursing care. *Journal of Nursing Administration, 29,* 32–42.

Knaus, V. L., Felten, S., Burton, S., Fobes, P., & Davis, K. (1997). The use of nurse practitioners in the acute care setting. *Journal of Nursing Administration, 27*(2), 20–27.

Koerner, M. M. (2000). The conceptual domain of service quality for inpatient nursing services. *Journal of Business Research, 48,* 267–283.

Kovner, C. (1989). Nurse-patient agreement and outcomes after surgery. *Western Journal of Nursing Research, 11,* 7–17.

Krouse, H., & Roberts, S. (1989). Nurse-patient interactive styles: Power, control and satisfaction. *Western Journal of Nursing Research, 11,* 717–725.

La Monica, E. L., Oberst, M. T., Madea, A. R., & Wolf, R. M. (1986). Development of patient satisfaction scale. *Research in nursing & health, 9,* 43–50.

Larrabee, J. H., Engle, V. F., & Tolley, E. A. (1995). Predictors of patient-perceived quality. *Scandinavian Journal of Caring Science, 9,* 153–164.

Larson, P. J. (1987). Comparison of cancer patients' and professional nurses' perceptions of important nurse caring behaviors. *Heart & Lung, 16,* 187–193.

Larson, P. J., & Ferketich, S. L. (1993). Patients' satisfaction with nurses' caring during hospitalization. *Western Journal of Nursing Research, 15,* 690–707.

Leiter, M. P., Harvie, P., & Frizzel, C. (1998). The correspondence of patient satisfaction and nurse burnout. *Social Science & Medicine, 47,* 1611–1617.

Lewis, K., & Woodside, R. (1992). Patient satisfaction with care in the emergency department. *Journal of Advanced Nursing, 17,* 959–964.

Ley, P. J., Kinsey, S. T., & Atherton, B. (1976). Increasing patients' satisfaction with communication. *British Journal of Social and Clinical Psychology, 15,* 403–413.

Lin, C. (1996). Patient satisfaction with nursing care as an outcome variable: Dilemmas for nursing evaluation researchers. *Journal of Professional Nursing, 12,* 207–216.

Linder-Pelz, S. (1982). Toward a theory of patient satisfaction. *Social Science & Medicine, 16,* 577–582.

Ludwig-Beymer, P., Ryan, C. J., Johnson, N. J., Hennessey, K. A., Gattuso, M. C., & Epsom, R. (1993). Using patient perceptions to improve quality care. *Journal of Nursing Care Quality, 7*(2), 42–51.

Lynn, M. R., & Sidani, S. (1991). *The next step: The patient's perception of quality scale.* Paper presented at the 24th Annual WSRN Communicating Nursing Research Conference, Albuquerque, NM.

Lynn, M. R., & Moore, K. (1997). Relationship between traditional quality indicators and perceptions of care. *Seminars for Nurse Managers, 5,* 187–193.

Lynn, M. R., & McMillen, B. J. (1999). Do nurses know what patients think is important in nursing care? *Journal of Nursing Care Quality, 13*(5), 65–74.

Mahon, P. Y. (1996). An analysis of the concept *patient satisfaction* as it relates to contemporary nursing. *Journal of Advanced Nursing, 24,* 1241–1248.

Marsh, G. W. (1999). Measuring patient satisfaction outcomes across provider disciplines. *Journal of Nursing Measurement, 7*(1), 47–62.

McColl, E., Thomas, L., & Bond, S. (1996). A study to determine patient satisfaction with nursing care. *Nursing Standard, 10,* 34–38.

Megivern, K., Halm, M. A., & Jones, G. (1992). Measuring patient satisfaction as an outcome of nursing care. *Journal of Nursing Care Quality, 6*(4), 9–24.

Meterko, M., Nelson, E. C., Rubin, H. R., Batalden, P., Berwick, D. M., Hays, R. D., et al. (1990). Patients' judgment of hospital quality: A report on a pilot study. *Medical Care, 28*(Supplement), S1–S56.

Moore, K., Lynn, M. R., McMillen, B. J., & Evans, S. (1999). Implementation of the ANA Report Card. *Journal of Nursing Administration, 29*(6), 48–54.

Moritz, P. (1991). Innovative nursing practice models and patient outcomes. *Nursing Outlook, 39,* 111–114.

Munro, B., Jacobsen, B. S., & Brooten, D. A. (1994). Re-examination of the psychometric characteristics of the La Monica-Oberst Patient Satisfaction Scale. *Research in Nursing and Health, 17,* 119–125.

Nash, M. G., Blackwood, D., Boone, E. B., Klar, R., Lewis, E., MacInnis, K., et al. (1994). Managing expectations between patient and nurse. *Journal of Nursing Administration, 24*(11), 49–55.

Nelson, C. W., & Niederberger, J. (1990). Patient satisfaction surveys: An opportunity for total quality improvement. *Hospital and Health Services Administration, 35,* 409–427.

Niedz, B.A. (1998). Correlates of hospitalized patients' perceptions of service quality. *Research in Nursing & Health, 21,* 339–349.

Nunally, J. C., & Bernstein, I. H. (1994). *Psychometric theory* (3rd ed.). New York: McGraw-Hill.

Oberst, M. T. (1984). Patient's perceptions of care. *Cancer, 53,* 2366–2375.

Parasuraman, A., Zeithaml, V., & Berry, L. (1985). A conceptual model of service quality and its implications for future research. *Journal of Marketing, 49,* 41–50.

Pascoe, G. C. (1983). Patient satisfaction in primary health care: A literature review and analysis. *Evaluation and Program Planning, 6,* 185–210.

Petersen, M. (1988). Measuring patient satisfaction: Collecting useful data. *Journal of Nursing Quality Assurance, 2*(3), 25–35.

Pierce, S. F. (1997). Nurse-sensitive health care outcomes in acute care settings: An integrative analysis of the literature. *Journal of Nursing Care Quality, 11*(4), 60–72.

Risser, N. (1975). Development of an instrument to measure patient satisfaction with nurses and nursing care in primary care settings. *Nursing Research, 24,* 45–52.

Rubin, H. R., Gandeck, B., Rogers, W. H., Kosinski, M., McHorney, C. A., & Ware, J. E. (1988). Patients' ratings of outpatient visits in different practice settings: Results from the medical outcomes study. *Journal of the American Medical Association, 270,* 835–840.

Rubin, H. R., Ware, J. E., & Hays, R. D. (1990). The PJHQ questionnaire: Exploratory factor analysis and empirical scale construction. *Medical Care, 28*(Suppl. 9), S22–S29.

Scardina, S. A. (1994). SERVQUAL: A tool for evaluating patient satisfaction with nursing care. *Journal of Nursing Care Quality, 8*(2), 38–46.

Sitzia, J., & Wood, N. (1997). Patient satisfaction: A review of issues and concepts. *Social Science & Medicine, 45*, 1829–1843.

Sovie, M. D., & Jawad, A. F. (2001). Hospital restructuring and its impact on outcomes: Nursing staff regulations are premature. *Journal of Nursing Administration, 31*, 588–600.

Stumpf, L. R. (2001). A comparison of governance types and patient satisfaction outcomes. *Journal of Nursing Administration, 31*, 196–202.

Swan, J. (1985). Deepening the understanding of hospital patient satisfaction: Fulfillment and equity of effects. *Journal of Health Care Marketing, 5*(3), 14.

Swan, J. E., & Carroll, M. G. (1980). Patient satisfaction and overview of research—1965 to 1978. In H. K. Hunt & R. L. Day (Eds.), *Refining concepts and measures of consumer satisfaction and complaining behavior* (pp. 112–118). Bloomington: Indiana University, Foundation for the School of Business.

Taylor, S. A. (1994). Distinguishing service quality from patient satisfaction in developing health care marketing strategies. *Hospital and Health Services Administration, 39*, 221–236.

Taylor, S., & Cronin, J. (1994). Modeling patient satisfaction and service quality. *Journal of Health Care Marketing, 14*(1), 34.

Thomas, L. H., & Bond, S. (1996). Measuring patients' satisfaction with nursing: 1990–1994. *Journal of Advanced Nursing, 23*, 747–756.

Thompson, D. A., Yarnold, P. R., Williams, D. R., & Adams, S. L. (1996). Effects of actual waiting time, perceived waiting time, information delivery and expressive quality on patient satisfaction in the emergency department. *Annals of Emergency Medicine, 28*, 657–665.

Twardon, C., & Gartner, M. (1991). Empowering nurses: Patient satisfaction with primary nursing in home health. *Journal of Nursing Administration, 21*(11), 39–43.

von Essen, L., & Sjoden, P. O. (1991). Patient and staff perceptions of caring: Review and replication. *Journal of Advanced Nursing, 16*, 1363–1374.

von Essen, L., & Sjoden, P. (1995). Perceived occurrence and importance of caring behaviours among patients and staff in psychiatric, medical, and surgical care. *Journal of Advanced Nursing, 21*, 266–276.

Ware, J., Jr., Davies-Avery, A., & Stewart, A. (1978). The measurement and meaning of patient satisfaction. *Health & Medical Care Services Review, 1*, 1.

Ware, J. E., & Hays, R. D. (1988). Methods for measuring patient satisfaction with specific medical encounters. *Medical Care, 26*, 393–401.

Ware, J. E., Snyder, M. K., Wright, W. R., & Allison, R. D. (1983). Defining and measuring patient satisfaction with medical care. *Evaluation and Program Planning, 6*, 247–263.

Webb, C., & Hope, K. (1995). What kind of nurses do patients want? *Journal of Clinical Nursing, 4*, 101–108.

Weisman, C. S., & Nathason, C. A. (1985). Professional satisfaction and client outcomes: A comparative organizational analysis. *Medical Care, 23*, 1179–1192.

Williams, B. (1994). Patient satisfaction: A valid concept? *Social Science & Medicine, 38*, 509–516.

Woodside, A. G., Frey, L. L., & Daly, R. T. (1989). Linking service quality, customer satisfaction, and behavioral intention. *Journal of Health Care Marketing, 9*(4), 5–17.

Young, W. B., Minnick, A. F., & Marcantonio, R. (1996). How wide is the gap in defining quality care? Comparison of patient and nurse perceptions of important aspects of patient care. *Journal of Nursing Administration, 26*, 15–20.

8

Nursing Outcome:
Nurses' Job Satisfaction

Linda McGillis Hall, RN, PhD

Assistant Professor

Faculty of Nursing, University of Toronto &

New Investigator, Canadian Institutes of Health Research

8.1 Introduction

Job satisfaction, or the extent to which employees like their work, is one of the most studied concepts in organizational research (Agho, 1993). Much of the work in this area emerges out of research from the 1960s, although interest in nursing job satisfaction has been evident since 1940 (Nahm, 1940). Substantial research has been done to identify the determinants of job satisfaction, as well as its effects on job performance and on individual employee behavior in the work setting (e.g., organizational commitment, absenteeism, and turnover).

Within the discipline of nursing, attention has been focused on examining nursing job satisfaction and how it relates to nurse behaviours such as turnover (Blegen & Mueller, 1987; Davidson et al., 1997; Irvine & Evans, 1995; Lum et al., 1998; Price & Mueller, 1981, 1986; Shader et al., 2001; Weisman et al.,

1981), and intention to quit (Davidson et al., 1997; Eberhardt et al., 1995). To a lesser extent, the research has also examined behaviours associated with nursing job stress (Blegen, 1993; Bratt et al., 2000) and organizational commitment (Blegen, 1993; Lum et al., 1998; McGillis Hall et al., 2002; McNeese-Smith, 1995). A meta-analysis has demonstrated that behavioral intentions and turnover, job satisfaction and behavioral intentions, and job satisfaction and turnover were related (Irvine & Evans, 1995). Research also indicates that nurses' job satisfaction is associated with several organizational and contextual characteristics such as salary, kinship, communication, social integration, justice, promotion, participation, education, opportunity, and routine (Cavanagh, 1992). Few studies have examined the relationship between nursing job satisfaction and patient outcomes. However, the job satisfaction of nurses is of central importance when examining the effect of nursing interventions on patient outcomes.

This chapter:

- Proposes a conceptual definition of nursing job satisfaction based on the literature

- Presents the theoretical underpinnings of job satisfaction research

- Examines the way in which nursing job satisfaction has been conceptualized, primarily relating to antecedent factors that influence job satisfaction

- Critically examines the empirical evidence linking nursing job satisfaction to specific interventions, focusing particularly on studies that relate nursing job satisfaction to patient outcomes

- Discusses issues with the assessment of nursing job satisfaction

- Reviews the approaches to measuring nursing job satisfaction, giving consideration to the reliability, validity, and sensitivity of the nursing job satisfaction instruments

- Recommends instruments to measure nursing job satisfaction, based on the research literature

- Identifies gaps in the literature and future research needs.

This review examined literature relating to theoretical and empirical work in the broad field of job satisfaction and the specific field of nursing job satisfaction, using the methodology outlined in Chapter 1. The search yielded a total of 321 relevant sources, of which 116 met the criteria for inclusion in this chapter.

8.2 Definition of the Concept of Job Satisfaction

Job satisfaction has been defined as "the feelings a worker has about his or her job or job experiences in relation to previous experiences, current expectations, or available alternatives" (Balzar, et al., 1990). Price & Mueller (1986) define job satisfaction as the degree of positive affective orientation towards employment. Within the field of nursing, Atwood & Hinshaw (1977) conceptualize job satisfaction as the perception of nursing staff's subjective feelings about their job and work situation. Similarly, Stamps (1997) describes satisfaction as how people feel about their jobs.

8.3 Theoretical Underpinnings of Nursing Job Satisfaction

Job satisfaction is a key component in most theories of work motivation and work behavior (Balzar et al., 1990). Some theories describe satisfaction as a direct "cause" of specific work behaviors, while others see it as a "consequence." A number of theoretical models, which can be categorized as content or process theories, have been used to explain the nature of job satisfaction (Campbell et al., 1970). "Content" theories include Maslow's Hierarchy of Need Theory (1970) and Herzberg's Motivation-Hygiene Theory (1966), which attempt to specify needs that must be met if an individual is to be satisfied at work. "Process" theories, such as Porter & Lawler's (1968) Expectancy Model of Motivation and the Dawis & Lofquist (1984) Theory of Work Adjustment, attempt to account for the way expectations, needs, and values interact with the characteristics or tasks of the job, the worker, and the work environment to produce job satisfaction. Most instruments developed to measure nursing job satisfaction have theoretical links to these works.

8.4 Factors that Influence Nursing Job Satisfaction

According to the nursing literature, a number of factors influence nursing job satisfaction, including antecedent variables that are perceived by the individual nurse in response to the work itself, and variables associated with the work environment. This conceptualization is consistent with Hackman and Oldham's (1976) theory, which suggests that individual and contextual work environment characteristics can influence job satisfaction, and with Blegen's (1993) meta-analysis of variables associated with nurses' job satisfaction. The antecedent variables include autonomy and control over practice, intent to leave and turnover, job stress, organizational commitment, relationships with peers and supervisors, organizational climate, and changes in the structure of care delivery.

8.4.1 Autonomy and Control Over Practice

Control over nursing practice and autonomy (Blegen & Mueller, 1987; Fung-kam, 1998; Hinshaw et al., 1987; Johnston, 1991; Kennerly, 2000; McCloskey, 1990; McGillis Hall et al., 2002; Mottaz, 1988; Williams, 1990; Wyckoff Lancero & Gerber, 1995), as well as locus of control (Blegen, 1993; Mueller & McCloskey, 1990), have been widely studied in relation to job satisfaction in nurses, with conflicting results. Blegen & Mueller (1987) used causal modeling to determine variables related to nurses' job satisfaction and found that job satisfaction was not affected by autonomy. Fung-kam (1998) conducted a cross-sectional survey of 365 registered nurses in Hong Kong and determined that, although not significantly related to job satisfaction, autonomy was valued by nurses in the study.

In contrast, Hinshaw et al. (1987) used causal modeling to explore turnover in nursing in a study of 1,597 nurses from 15 U.S. hospitals, and found that organizational job satisfaction was influenced by control over practice. Johnston (1991) conducted a descriptive study of 385 western U. S. nurses and reported that one of the variables ranked as most important and likely to influence nurses' job satisfaction was autonomy. McCloskey (1990) used regression analysis in a study that determined that nurses with low job satisfaction also had lower autonomy, social integration, work motivation, and poor commitment and intent to stay with the organization. Wyckoff Lancero and Gerber (1995) used multiple regression to determine that work satisfaction was positively predicted by control over nursing practice. In a correlational study conducted in a New York hospital, significant positive relationships were also reported between nurses' job satisfaction and empowerment (Radice, 1994).

8.4.2 Intent to Leave and Turnover

In a study of 281 nurses from 26 nursing homes in Florida, the significant predictors of job satisfaction used in the regression model were intent to leave and the length of time that nurses had intended to stay in their position (Coward et al., 1995). A study of 327 nurses from three U.S. hospitals reported a negative relationship between job satisfaction and turnover intention, with nurses' job satisfaction accounting for 24% of the variance in turnover intention (Eberhardt et al., 1995). Research examining the impact of pay policies on the turnover intent of nurses in a Canadian pediatric setting used causal modeling and found that organizational commitment had a direct influence on intention to quit, while job satisfaction had only an indirect effect (Lum et al., 1998). In a longitudinal study of nurses in an eastern U.S. hospital, the nurses' perceptions of limited promotional opportunities, high routinization in their work, low decision-making latitude, and poor communication were predictive of intent to leave; while fewer years on the job, expressed intent to leave, and not enough time to do the job well were predictive of turnover in the regression model (Davidson et al., 1997).

8.4.3 Job Stress

Job stress was negatively correlated with organizational work satisfaction and professional job satisfaction using regression analysis in a study involving almost 2,000 pediatric critical-care nurses in 65 hospitals in the U.S. and Canada (Bratt et al., 2000). In a study across 15 U.S. hospitals using causal modeling, job satisfaction was found to buffer job stress (Hinshaw et al., 1987). Work satisfaction, job stress, group cohesion, and weekend overtime were predictive in a regression analysis of anticipated turnover in nurses in a southeastern U.S. hospital (Shader et al., 2001). In a meta-analysis of 48 studies, nurses' job satisfaction was most highly related to stress (Blegen, 1993).

8.4.4 Organizational Commitment

In a correlational study of nurses in the western U.S., specific nursing leadership behaviors related to challenging processes, enabling others to act, and inspiring a shared vision were predictive of organizational commitment (McNeese-Smith, 1995). Nurses who reported high levels of satisfaction with scheduling, interaction opportunities, praise/recognition, professional opportunities, and control/responsibility also had high levels of organizational commitment in a study conducted by McGillis Hall et al. (2002). In a meta-analysis conducted by Blegen (1993), organizational commitment was highly related to job satisfaction.

8.4.5 Relationships with Peers and Supervisors

Several authors have noted that relationships with coworkers and supervisors can influence job satisfaction (Blegen, 1993; Coward et al., 1995; Decker, 1997; Lynch, 1994; Mottaz, 1988; Sorrentino, 1992). The perception that supervisors are interested in nurses' career aspirations was found to be a significant predictor in a regression analysis of the job satisfaction of nurses in long-term care settings (Coward et al., 1995). Perceived relationship with the unit manager, coworkers, physicians, other units/departments, unit tenure, and job/non-job conflict were also important predictors of job satisfaction (Decker, 1997).

A correlational study of a sample of nurses from hospitals across two western U.S. states reported a significant positive relationship between leadership behaviors and nurses' job satisfaction, productivity, and commitment (McNeese-

Smith, 1995). Nurses who were mentored reported higher levels of job satisfaction than those who did not experience a mentoring relationship in a study conducted by Ecklund (1998). Work environment relationship variables, such as involvement, peer cohesion, and supervisor support, accounted for significant differences in nurses' job satisfaction as did systems maintenance and change variables, such as task clarity, control, innovation, and physical comfort (Tumulty et al., 1994). A study of nurses from four southeastern U.S. hospitals found a significant relationship between management style on the unit and nurses' job satisfaction, with management style explaining 36.6% of the variance in job satisfaction scores (Lucas, 1991). In a study involving over 1,000 nurses from 19 teaching hospitals in Canada, hierarchical linear modeling determined that nursing leadership had a significant positive influence on nurses' perceptions of job satisfaction (McGillis Hall et al., 2001).

8.4.6 Organizational Climate

Nurses from four units of a U.S. teaching hospital who described their organizational climate as high in responsibility, warmth, support, and identity had high levels of job satisfaction (Gillies et al., 1990). Dimensions of organizational climate were also related to job satisfaction in a study of pediatric nurses in California (Urden, 1999). Organizational structure, support, standards, and professional status were reported to be significant correlates of job satisfaction and organizational climate in a regression model employed by Keuter, Byrne, Voell, & Larson (2000). In a study of community nurses in Texas, nurses' satisfaction with the quality of care provided to patients was positively related to competence, physical work environment, staffing, and patient outcome (Boswell, 1992). In a study of three community hospitals in Canada, repeated measures multivariate analysis of variance was used to explore a change in the job satisfaction of nurses following downsizing (Armstrong-Stassen et al., 1996). Overall job satisfaction was not affected by hospital downsizing, although a significant deterioration in satisfaction with career future, hospital identification, supervision, and co-workers was found following downsizing (Armstrong-Stassen et al., 1996).

8.4.7 Changes in Structure of Care Delivery

A recent study of nurses at a university hospital in the mid-Atlantic region of the U.S. found a relationship between job satisfaction and structural components of the organization, professional recognition, and working relationships (Keuter et al., 2000). Among nurses in 37 New Jersey hospitals, changes in the work environment, such as the implementation of case management, shared governance, reorganization of care delivery models, and education aimed at improving the recruitment and retention of nurses, contributed to higher levels of nurse satisfaction in the regression analysis (Kovner et al., 1994). A change in the nursing practice model was found to have a significant effect on nurses' job satisfaction in a study at a Florida teaching hospital (Lengacher et al., 1994). Organizational job satisfaction and professional job satisfaction of nurses in a South Carolina hospital improved significantly following implementation of shared governance in a comparative study conducted by Jones, Stasiowski, Simons, Boyd, & Lucas (1993). In a sample of 409 nurses in a southeastern U.S. hospital, role clarity was found to be a predictor of job satisfaction (Kroposki et al., 1999).

Analysis of covariance was used in a study that compared two units undergoing a change in care delivery (Song et al., 1997). Nurses on a special care unit characterized by shared governance and case management experienced higher job satisfaction and lower absenteeism than nurses on a traditional intensive care unit (Song et al., 1997). A study of 731 nurses across 22 Florida hospitals found that hospital size was a significant predictor of job satisfaction in the regression model, although job-specific characteristics were much more powerful predictors of nursing job satisfaction (Coward et al., 1992). Routinization of work, promotional opportunities, distributive justice, age, day shift, workload, kinship responsibility, and opportunity for jobs outside the employing hospital were found to be significant variables in a causal model of nursing job satisfaction (Blegen, 1993).

In summary, these studies identify the broad range of factors in the work environment that influence nurses' job satisfaction. They also highlight the need for measures that capture the complex interactions that occur within nursing work, as well as the multiple facets of the nursing role.

8.5 Linking Nursing Job Satisfaction to Patient Outcome Achievement

Ten empirical studies were identified and reviewed in Table 8.1. All of these studies evaluated patient outcomes in which nursing job satisfaction was an outcome measure. Eight of these studies were conducted in an acute-care hospital setting, one in a community setting, and one in a long-term care setting. As Table 8.1 demonstrates, few studies have explored the relationship between nursing job satisfaction and patient outcomes, and most efforts to measure patient outcomes have focused primarily on patient satisfaction. In addition, the results of these studies are somewhat inconsistent.

More than two decades ago, Atwood & Hinshaw (1977) identified the need for research studies with multiple indicators, which can account for the effects of interventions on both the nurse and the patient. The authors theorized that interventions could have a direct impact on nursing job satisfaction, which could in turn indirectly influence patient outcomes through the care delivered. In testing this model, researchers noted that nursing job satisfaction improved following the implementation of an intervention that resulted in a staffing change from an RN/Licensed Practical Nurse (LPN) model to an all-RN staff; however, patient satisfaction with the technical skills and trusting aspects of nursing declined (Atwood & Hinshaw, 1977). Subsequent reports indicated that patient satisfaction with education and technical care declined during the middle phase of the study, when nurse staffing was moving towards an all-RN model (Hinshaw et al., 1981). By the time the full change had occurred and an all-RN staff was in place, patient satisfaction was equal to or better than at baseline.

Weisman and Nathanson (1985) identified that staff satisfaction had not been linked to outcomes associated with clients in their study exploring the relationship between nurses' job satisfaction and patient satisfaction with the level of service received in a clinic setting. Using a longitudinal approach and causal modeling, the researchers explored patient satisfaction, as well as compliance with treatment. The level of nurses' job satisfaction was found to be a strong determinant of patient satisfaction with the service provided (Weisman & Nathanson, 1985). Because the rate of patient compliance with the treatment regimen was predicted by patient satisfaction, this in turn had an effect on patient outcomes. This study is one of the first studies to examine nurses' contribution to patient care outcomes as evidenced through treatment compliance.

In a long-term care setting, nurses' job satisfaction was significantly related to exposure to aggressive patient behaviors (Dougherty et al., 1992). Data from self-reports and semi-structured interviews formed the description of aggressive patient behaviors, while surveys were conducted for nurses' job satisfaction. Although aggressive behavior is not articulated as a patient outcome, it is theoretically plausible that nursing interventions can have an impact on patient behaviors. Regression analysis indicated that exposure to aggressive patient behavior was a better predictor of nurses' job satisfaction than any other demographic variable or job factor in the study (Dougherty et al., 1992).

A correlational study conducted in a midwestern U.S. teaching hospital found no significant relationships among nurses' job satisfaction, the quality of nursing care provided, and patient satisfaction with nursing care (Goodell & Coeling, 1994). The authors noted that inherent difficulties exist in trying to establish relationships between job satisfaction and patient outcomes. Specifically, there is a need for diverse samples across more than one hospital to more adequately capture the relationships between nurses' job satisfaction and the quality of care, or patient satisfaction (Goodell & Coeling, 1994).

In a study examining the impact of a new model of professional practice for critical care units, Cone, McGovern, Barnard, and Riegel (1995) explored nurses' job satisfaction and patient satisfaction with nursing care. The researchers used paired t tests to compare data from nurses in the study unit and the control unit, and unpaired *t* tests to compare patient satisfaction with care. Nurse satisfaction with coworkers and supervisors increased significantly on the unit that implemented the new model of professional practice, which included critical care assistants (CCAs) providing direct patient care under the direction of registered nurses. When researchers compared data prior to and eight months after implementation of the new practice model, they found no changes in patient satisfaction with the quality of nursing care. This led the researchers to suggest that patient satisfaction with the quality of care didn't change with the introduction of CCAs to the critical care team (Cone et al., 1995).

Grindel, Peterson, Kinneman, and Turner (1996) suggest that many factors affect patient care delivery, efficiency, and effectiveness in clinical practice environments. This reinforces the need to gain perceptions from patients, nurses, and physicians. In a cross-sectional study of 730 nurses and 250 patients from across 44 patient care units in U.S. hospitals, nurses reported a fair degree of job satisfaction related to work perceptions and working conditions, autonomy, and relationships with coworkers and management, while patients reported a high degree of satisfaction with nursing care (Grindel et al., 1996).

A study across three U.S. hospitals explored the relationships between nurses' job satisfaction, patient satisfaction with nursing care, nursing care delivery models, organizational structure, and organizational culture (Kangas et al., 1999), and found that a supportive work environment and working in a critical care unit were significant predictors of nurses' job satisfaction in the regression analysis. Predictors of patient satisfaction included a primary care delivery model and length of time on the unit (Kangas et al., 1999).

McNeese-Smith (1999) examined the relationship between nurses' job satisfaction and patient satisfaction in a 500-bed U.S. hospital. There were no significant relationships between nurses' job satisfaction and patient satisfaction. However, when the influence of managers was introduced into the analysis, correlations were found. Specifically, managerial motivation for achievement was positively related to nurses' job satisfaction and to patient satisfaction.

McGillis Hall et al. (2001) examined the impact of different nursing staff mix models on nurse, patient, and system outcomes in the Canadian healthcare environment. Patient outcomes included functional health outcomes, pain intensity, and perceptions of the quality of nursing care. Nurse outcomes included nurses' job satisfaction, job stress, role tension, and perceptions of the effectiveness of care provided to patients. While some nurse staffing variables had an impact on patient outcomes in this study, researchers found no relationship between nurses' job satisfaction and patient functional health and pain outcomes using hierarchical linear analysis. The effectiveness of communication on the unit was a significant predictor of patient satisfaction, although this effect disappeared when nurse job satisfaction was included in the regression model, which suggests that nursing job satisfaction has a direct effect on patient satisfaction (McGillis Hall et al., 2001).

Table 8.1. Studies Investigating the Relationship between Nurses' Job Satisfaction and Patient Outcomes: Study Findings

Author/date published	Design of study	Characteristics of the sample and response rate (RR) and the setting	Nurse job satisfaction outcome: definition of the outcome concept	Intervention being evaluated/nursing variables tested	Results/findings	Limitations
Atwood & Hinshaw (1977)	Descriptive, Pretest-Posttest	Southwestern U.S. hospital; $N = 2$ populations: nurses (phase 1, $N = 18$; phase 2, $N = 15$), and patients (phase 1, $N = 17$; phase 2, $N = 21$).	Job satisfaction (Brayfield & Rothe, 1951) modified by adding seven items (total 25 items).	Change in nursing staff patterns (shift from an RN and non-RN staff to an all-RN staff). Patient satisfaction (Risser, 1975).	After staffing change, job satisfaction higher for the staff as a whole ($t = -6.50$, $df = 31$, $p < 0.00$) and for RNs involved in both phases of the study ($t = -3.97$, $N = 9$, $p < 0.00$). Patients' satisfaction with nursing care post-staffing change indicated lowered satisfaction in technical skill and trust ($t = 4.20$, $df = 29$, $p < 0.00$; $t = 3.42$, $df = 30$, $p = 0.002$).	Small sample size of nurses and patients.
Cone et al. (1995)	Descriptive, Pretest-Posttest with comparison	Two convenience samples from population of critical care nurses. Sample $N = 52$ nurses before implementation; at follow-up 8 months later, $n = 16$ nurses worked in the program, $n = 36$ nurses worked in the comparison unit. Representative sample: $N = 11$ critical care nurses, $n = 4$ full-time in program, $n = 3$ in comparison, $n = 4$ worked both units during the study period when staffing had been opened in model program.	Defined as the morale and well-being experienced by the nurse at work. Job descriptive index-revised (Smith et al., 1969); nurse job satisfaction scale (Torres, 1988).	Professional practice model: implementation of critical care assistants (CCAs) under supervision of nurses to provide patient care in a critical care unit; increase in nurse-patient ratio; self-scheduling and elimination of hierarchical relationships.	Job satisfaction did not change significantly over time in those participating in the program. Initial work satisfaction was higher among nurses participating in the program compared to those in the comparison unit ($t = 2.05$, $P = 0.05$). Satisfaction with supervision ($P = 0.09$) and coworkers ($P = 0.001$) in program increased significantly over time; no change in control unit; nurses who had worked in the program were more satisfied than dissatisfied; workload was primary factor for dissatisfaction.	Authors perceive nurse satisfaction instruments to be "dated" (e.g., fail to capture aspects such as workload); & potential Hawthorne effect from special attention received during study.

Table 8.1 (continued)

293

Author/date published	Design of study	Characteristics of the sample and response rate (RR) and the setting	Nurse job satisfaction outcome: definition of the outcome concept	Intervention being evaluated/nursing variables tested	Results/findings	Limitations
Dougherty et al. (1992)	Descriptive Questionnaire; interview	US geriatric long-term care hospital; sample: $N = 28$ ($n = 8$ men, $n = 20$ women); participants: mental health workers ($n = 16$, LPNs: $n = 7$, RNs: $n = 5$).	Index of work satisfaction; questionnaire (Stamps & Piedmonte, 1986) revised by adding three statements, rewording four statements, and deleting nine statements.	Aggressive behavior: defined as physical, verbal, or generally disruptive behavior.	Verbally aggressive behavior related to job satisfaction ($r = -0.766$) with similar strength as physical aggression ($r = -0.622$). Job satisfaction significantly correlated with overall exposure to aggressive behavior ($r = -0.777$); results of regression analysis indicate exposure to aggressive behavior was a better predictor of job satisfaction ($R^2 = 0.594$, $F(1, 24) = 35.04$, $p < 0.001$) than any other intrinsic or extrinsic job factor or demographic variable (with the exception of education, which added significantly to the overall variance ($R^2 = 0.669$, $F(2, 23) = 23.21$, $p = 0.0001$).	More discriminating measures of constructs needed; attitudes towards these patients should also be considered; education may influence responses.
Goodell & Coeling (1994)	Correlational	Urban midwestern U.S. teaching hospital; nursing job satisfaction scale: $n = 130$ RNs & LPNs on four units ($RR = 52\%$); quality of care study: $n = 9$ inpatient units with two groups defined—two highest quality units (group 1), two lowest quality units (group 2); patient satisfaction scale: $n = 33$ RN & LPNs, $n = 168$ patients; definition of elements of job satisfaction: $n = 301$ RNs & LPNs ($RR = 50\%$).	Index of work satisfaction (Slavitt et al., 1978).	Quality of nursing care and patient satisfaction with nursing care—Patient satisfaction instrument (Risser, 1975).	Significant difference in job satisfaction between groups 1 and 2 on professional status subscale of the IWS ($t = -2.33$, $p = 0.029$). Pay ranked by RNs as most important component of job satisfaction, followed by professional status, autonomy, interaction, task requirements, and organizational policies.	Larger, more diverse sample, beyond one hospital, needed to determine relationships; response rate somewhat low.

Table 8.1 (continued)

Author/date published	Design of study	Characteristics of the sample and response rate (RR) and the setting	Nurse job satisfaction outcome: definition of the outcome concept	Intervention being evaluated/nursing variables tested	Results/findings	Limitations
Grindel et al. (1996)	Descriptive	Sample: nursing personnel $N = 1{,}728$; $n = 44$ units, $n = 12$ administrative & specialty groups; $RR = 42.24\%$. RNs: 82.7%, LPNs: 3.2%, unit clerks: 5.5%, RNAs: 1.9%.	Nurse job satisfaction scale (Torres, 1992).	Autonomy (subscale of job characteristics inventory by Sims et al., 1976); work perception; work conditions; relationship with coworkers and management.	Nurses reported a fair degree of job satisfaction supported by scores in work perceptions, work conditions, autonomy, and relationship with coworkers and management. Development and recognition scores were lower. Nurses perceived their degree of autonomy in practice as good.	Challenges with an evaluation approach described—labor intensive, length of process.
Hinshaw et al. (1981)	Longitudinal: T^1 = one month prior to staffing change, T^2 = three months after change, T^3 = nine months after change	Southwestern U.S. university hospital; $N = 1$ inpatient medical unit; random sample of English-speaking, medically alert patients.	Index of job satisfaction (Brayfield & Rothe, 1951).	Change in staffing pattern from a mixed staff (non-RN & RN) to an all-RN staff.	Job satisfaction was significantly higher in T^2 and remained higher in T^3 than it had been prior to the change ($F = 26.10$, $p < 0.001$).	Single-site sample.
Kangas et al. (1999)	Descriptive, correlational	Setting: $N = 3$ hospitals with different nursing care delivery models (team, primary, and case management). Sample: $N = 102$ nurses, $N = 102$ patients; $RR = 90\%$ nurses, $RR = 88\%$ patients.	Demographic data form; Nurse job satisfaction scale (Torres, 1988).	Nursing care delivery model; organizational culture (organizational culture index by Wallach, 1983); personal background and demographic factors.	Perceiving environment as supportive and working in critical care unit were significant predictors of nurses' job satisfaction scores. The two variables together predicted 55% of variance in job satisfaction ($\beta = -0.709$ for support and -0.305 for type of unit, $P = 0.003$).	Nurse responses not matched with data from patients they cared for—unable to do individual comparisons.

Table 8.1 (continued)

Author/date published	Design of study	Characteristics of the sample and response rate (RR) and the setting	Nurse job satisfaction outcome: definition of the outcome concept	Intervention being evaluated/nursing variables tested	Results/findings	Limitations
McGillis Hall et al. (2001)	Descriptive repeated measures design. Data was collected through interviews, administrative records, questionnaires, and chart abstraction.	19 urban teaching hospitals in Ontario, Canada. Sample: $N = 1,116$ nurses, $N = 2,046$ patients.	Job Descriptive Index (JDI) (Ironson et al., 1989). This scale is comprised of 18 items related to general job satisfaction.	Functional Independence Measure (FIM) (Hamilton et al., 1987), and the Medical Outcome Study SF-36 (Stewart & Kamberg, 1992); the FIM consists of 18 items measuring activities of daily living, sphincter control, transfers, and locomotion. The SF-36 (acute form) is a 36-item scale measuring eight health domains: physical functioning, role limitations due to physical health, role limitations due to emotional problems, social functioning, bodily pain, mental health, and general health perceptions. Brief Pain Inventory-Short Form (BPI-SF) (Cleeland, 1991); the BPI-SF measures the severity of pain and its impact on the patient's functioning. Patient Judgement of Hospital Quality	Nursing leadership was found to have a statistically significant positive influence on nurses' perceptions of job satisfaction ($t = 4.88$, $p < 0.0001$). The lower the average complexity of patients, the higher nursing job satisfaction ($t = -3.17$, $p = 0.003$). On units where there was a lower proportion of RNs/RPNs, there was a higher number of medication errors. Similarly, units with a lower proportion of RNs/RPNs and a less-experienced staff had higher rates of wound infection. The proportion of regulated staff on the unit was associated with better FIM scores and better social function scores at hospital discharge. In addition, a mix of staff that involved RNs and unregulated workers was associated with better pain outcomes at discharge than a mix that involved RNs/RPNs and unregulated workers. Patients were more satisfied with their obstetrical nursing care on units where there was a higher proportion of regulated staff (RNs/RPNs).	Generalizability limited to adult, acute care settings; conducted in teaching hospitals only.

Table 8.1 (continued)

Author/date published	Design of study	Characteristics of the sample and response rate (RR) and the setting	Nurse job satisfaction outcome: definition of the outcome concept	Intervention being evaluated/nursing variables tested	Results/findings	Limitations
[McGillis Hall et al. (2001) continued]				Questionnaire (PJHQ) (Rubin et al., 1990); the nursing care quality subscale of PJHQ consists of five items in which patients are asked to rate on a five-point scale the quality of care received from nurses during their hospital stay. Secondary outcomes: unit-level data were collected on patient falls, medication errors, wound infections, and urinary tract infections.		
McNeese-Smith (1999)	Ex-post facto, correlational study	Large Los Angeles County university hospital. Sample: $N = 15$ nurse managers, $N = 285$ full-time nurses ($RR = 77.5\%$, $N = 221$), $N = 299$ patients.	Job-in-general scale (JIG) (Smith et al., 1989): measures overall job satisfaction and consists of 18 one- to three-word adjectives describing the employee's feelings about the job in general.	Patient Judgements of Hospital Quality (Meterko et al., 1990) consists of 100 questions to measure patient evaluations of hospital care. Questions are presented on a five-point Likert-type scale. Power motivation questions: used for measuring the motivation of the manager.	Managerial motivation for power showed negative relationship to nurse job satisfaction ($r = -0.13$, $p = 0.06$); manager motivation for achievement was positively correlated to nurse job satisfaction ($r = 0.25$, $p = 0.0002$); there was a positive relationship between the manager's motivation for achievement and the patient satisfaction mean score ($r = 0.19$, $p = 0.004$).	Unable to do nurse and patient comparisons at level of individual; generalizability limited due to setting.

Table 8.1 (continued)

Author/date published	Design of study	Characteristics of the sample and response rate (RR) and the setting	Nurse job satisfaction outcome: definition of the outcome concept	Intervention being evaluated/nursing variables tested	Results/findings	Limitations
Weisman & Nathanson (1985)	Longitudinal study; baseline interviews, follow-up telephone interviews; three measurement times: baseline, six-month follow-up, and twelve-month follow-up.	$N = 78$ county health department family planning clinics (rural and urban) in the U.S.; $n = 344$ family planning and community health nurses, all RNs ($RR = 86\%$); $n = 2900$ clients (baseline $RR = 80\%$, follow-up $RR = 76\%$ of baseline).	Job satisfaction measured with a 15-item multifacet measure.	Client compliance measured with telephone interviews; client satisfaction measured in personal interviews.	Higher clinic staff job satisfaction levels predict higher client satisfaction levels ($r = + 0.24$, $\beta = + 0.32$); staff job satisfaction is the strongest predictor of client satisfaction. Higher levels of nursing influence on clinic policies and activities produce lower levels of client satisfaction ($\beta = -0.23$, $P < 0.10$). Aggregate job satisfaction level of nursing staff is the strongest determinant among the variables studied on the aggregate satisfaction level of teenage clients. Client satisfaction level predicts the rate of clients' subsequent contraceptive compliance.	Relationships between nurse and client satisfaction may be spurious: may not have captured the variable that influenced them.

In summary, limited research has explored the linkages between nursing job satisfaction and patient outcomes. Most of these studies examine a management or organizational intervention, such as a change in nurse staffing or in a care delivery model, rather than specific nursing interventions. This may be appropriate, given that the literature review demonstrated that a substantial number of the factors that influence nurses' job satisfaction emerge from the work environment.

The majority of studies reported in this chapter described the development and/or testing of a nursing job satisfaction instrument. While a few of the studies have used regression analysis or hierarchical linear modeling, the majority of studies have employed correlational techniques. The strength of the literature linking nurses' job satisfaction to patient outcomes is quite limited at this time.

The challenge remains to examine ways to link nursing job satisfaction to patient outcomes that go beyond the traditional measure of patient satisfaction with nursing care. Specifically, researchers should conduct studies that compare and contrast nursing job satisfaction with the results of nursing interventions (e.g., nurses' satisfaction with the level of functional status reported by patients on discharge, as a result of the nursing interventions provided). These nurse-sensitive patient outcomes or results of nursing care can be conceptually linked to the knowledge and practice of professionally prepared nurses.

8.6 Issues in the Assessment of Nursing Job Satisfaction

The literature review identified several issues in the assessment of nursing job satisfaction, including: 1) a theoretical measure to meet the needs of the practice environment, and 2) the desired scope of the measure of nursing job satisfaction.

8.6.1 Can a Theoretical Measure Meet the Needs of the Practice Environment?

The literature identified a number of nursing-specific instruments (Hinshaw & Atwood, 1985; Mueller & McCloskey, 1990; Stamps & Piedmonte, 1986), as well as instruments developed in the management sciences (Smith et al., 1969; Weiss et al., 1967), which are used to measure nursing job satisfaction. Some nursing job satisfaction instruments are theoretically based (Mueller & McCloskey, 1990), while others have identified some challenges related to maintaining such theoretical linkages (Stamps, 1997). For example, Stamps & Piedmonte (1986) devote a chapter to discussing theories of work satisfaction, suggesting that their instrument is influenced by need fulfillment theory and social reference group theory through "inclusion of questions comparing peer groups' attitudes." A decade later, the author suggests that, although a nurse satisfaction questionnaire examining satisfying components of a job is "theoretically important," it is of less "practical" value because the satisfying components of the job may be outside the scope of the organization's control (Stamps, 1997). This illustrates the gap that often occurs when integrating theory into practice, and highlights the challenges in linking nurses' job satisfaction to the outcomes of nursing interventions.

8.6.2 *What Is the Desired Scope of the Measure of Nursing Job Satisfaction?*

A great deal of attention has been paid to the merits of measuring different aspects of job satisfaction (Rice et al., 1991). For example, "global" measures of job satisfaction may predict important employee behaviors. While these global measures provide general impressions from employees about satisfaction with their work, employees can feel differently about specific aspects of that work (Smith et al., 1969). Thus, "facet" scales can be used to differentiate specific areas of job satisfaction, and to diagnose strengths and weaknesses in various sections of an organization (Ironson et al., 1989). Given the complex set of factors that influence nurses' job satisfaction, it is important for researchers to assess whether global measures capture the scope of what they are trying to measure in satisfaction studies.

Within the field of nursing, some authors suggest that there are different kinds of satisfaction, such as organizational work satisfaction, that differ from professional occupational satisfaction (Hinshaw & Atwood, 1985). Specifically, "organizational satisfaction" is conceptualized as a staff member's positive or negative opinion of her or his job in terms of pay or reward, nursing administration, professional status accorded, and interaction with colleagues (Hinshaw & Atwood, 1985; Slavitt et al., 1978). Thus, organizational satisfaction is a multidimensional construct that relates to the performance of nursing work within the larger organization. In contrast, "professional satisfaction" refers to nursing staff's opinion of the quality of care that nurses deliver, the time to conduct care activities, and general enjoyment of their work (Brayfield & Rothe, 1951; Hinshaw & Atwood, 1985). Within the current work environment, where a nursing shortage exists and is likely to continue, it is important for healthcare administrators and leaders to have a broad understanding of nursing job satisfaction. Measures that assess both the professional and the organizational aspects of nursing work may be needed. Theoretically, professional satisfaction is most congruent with the assessment of nurse-sensitive patient outcomes.

One of the most important considerations in identifying a measure of nursing job satisfaction is determining which dimensions of job satisfaction to capture. For example, some measures tap dimensions related to the professional components of nursing work, such as quality of care, enjoyment, and time to do one's job (Hinshaw & Atwood, 1985). In contrast, others capture the domains of nursing work in the work environment, such as extrinsic rewards, scheduling, family/work balance, co-workers, interaction, professional opportunities, praise and recognition, and control and responsibility (Mueller & McCloskey, 1990).

When examining specific instruments, it is important to consider these issues and to use them as criteria in selecting appropriate research measures.

8.7 Evidence Concerning Approaches to Measuring Nursing Job Satisfaction

The literature identified a number of instruments that have been used to measure job satisfaction, but only those used with nurses are included in this review. Although many job satisfaction instruments might be relevant in assessing nurses' perceptions of job satisfaction, they require further evaluation in studies with nurses to determine their sensitivity to the nursing population. Eight instruments measuring nursing job satisfaction were identified in the empirical nursing literature, and their characteristics are summarized in Table 8.2, by author and instrument name. Another three general job satisfaction instruments that have been used in the nursing environment are also presented.

8.8 Nursing Measures of Job Satisfaction

8.8.1 Index of Work Satisfaction (IWS)

The Index of Work Satisfaction (IWS) (Stamps & Piedmonte, 1986; Stamps et al., 1978; Slavitt et al., 1978) is the most widely used measure of nurses' job satisfaction found in the literature. The IWS includes subscales that measure professional status, task requirement, autonomy, interactions with other nurses, and pay. It has been used extensively in the United States in a variety of teaching, rural, and community settings, including acute care, long-term care, critical care, psychiatry, medicine, surgery, and pediatrics. It has also been used in Japan and Hong Kong.

Comments that scoring is too difficult have resulted in many researchers using the Likert-type section of the scale only, and the IWS is frequently not computed (Stamps, 1997). Less than one-third of the studies examined used both components of the study scale (Ecklund, 1998; Fung-kam, 1998; Goodell & Coeling, 1994; Johnston, 1991; Kovner et al., 1994; Prothero et al., 1999; Radice, 1994). Few of these studies reported Cronbach's alpha scale reliabilities for the individual scale components. Most reported scale reliability for the entire scale (Gillies et al., 1990; Muus et al., 1993; Urden, 1999; Wyckoff Lancero &

Table 8.2. Instruments Measuring Job Satisfaction

A: Nursing Measures of job Satisfaction

Instrument (author)	Target population	Domains, number of items, and response format	Method of administration	Reliability	Validity
Index of Work Satisfaction (Slavitt et al., 1978)	Hospital and home nursing staff	Domains: professional status, task requirement, autonomy, interactions with other nurses, pay. 48 items, 5-point Likert-type scale.	Self-administered	—Internal consistency for subscales, 0.35 to 0.70 (Coward et al., 1995). —Reliability of 0.82 for entire scale (Ecklund, 1998). —Internal consistency for subscales, 0.35 to 0.70 (Francis-Felsen, 1996). —Reliability of 0.82 for the whole scale and 0.52 to 0.81 for the subscales (Fung-kam, 1998). —Cronbach's alpha of 0.91 (Gillies et al., 1990). —Internal consistency of 0.89 (Hayes, 1994). —Cronbach's alphas of 0.52 to 0.81 for subscales, with a total alpha of 0.82003 (Johnston, 1991). —Reliability of 0.85 (Keuter et al., 2000). —Reliabilities of subscales from 0.44 to 0.84 (Kovner et al., 1994). — Subscale reliabilities from 0.70 to 0.90, with an overall coefficient of 0.80 to 0.90 (Lengacher et al., 1994). —Reliability for total satisfaction of 0.89 (Muus et al., 1993). —Reliability of 0.80 to 0.90 (Prothero et al., 1999). —Total alpha of 0.82 (Radice, 1994). —Reliability for total satisfaction of 0.89 (Stratton et al., 1995).	—Content validity (Durkin et al., 1992; Stamps & Piedmonte, 1986; Stratton et al., 1995; Kovner et al., 1994). —Construct validity (Yamashita, 1995; Lengacher et al, 1994; Johnston, 1991)

Table 8.2A (continued)

Instrument (author)	Target population	Domains, number of items, and response format	Method of administration	Reliability	Validity
[Index of Work Satisfaction (Slavitt et al., 1978) continued]				—Cronbach's alpha of 0.86 (Stamps & Piedmont, 1986). —Overall reliability of 0.88 (Urden, 1999). —Cronbach's alpha of 0.82, with subscale reliabilities of 0.81 to 0.82 (Yamashita, 1995). —Subscale reliabilities from 0.514 to 0.859 (Durkin et al., 1992). —Overall reliability of 0.82, with subscale reliabilities from 0.59 to 0.80 (Shader et al., 2001).	
McCloskey & Mueller Satisfaction Scale (McCloskey & Mueller, 1990)	Hospital nursing staff	Domains: extrinsic rewards, scheduling satisfaction, family/work balance, co-workers, interactions, professional opportunities, praise/recognition, and control/responsibility. 30 items, 5-point scale.	Self-administered	—Reliability of 0.90 (Chaboyer et al., 1999). —Cronbach's alpha of 0.89 (Krugman & Preheim, 1999). —Reliability of 0.89 (Ajamieh et al., 1996). —Internal consistency of 0.89 and test-retest reliability of 0.63 (McCloskey & Mueller, 1990). —Cronbach's alpha of 0.91 for the global scale (Cumbey & Alexander, 1998).	—Criterion-related validity (Misener et al., 1996).

Table 8.2A (continued)

Instrument (author)	Target population	Domains, number of items, and response format	Method of administration	Reliability	Validity
Nursing Job Satisfaction Scale (Hinshaw & Atwood, 1985)	Hospital nursing staff	Domains: quality of care, enjoyment on the job, and time to do one's job. 23 items, 5-point Likert scale.	Self-administered	—Cronbach's alpha of 0.86; subscales ranging from 0.62 to 0.78 (Bratt et al., 2000). —Cronbach's alphas of 0.70 to 0.91 (Davidson et al., 1997). —Reliabilities of 0.76 to 0.86 for the subscales and 0.88 overall (Atwood & Hinshaw, 1984). —Reliabilities of 0.72 to 0.88 (Hinshaw et al., 1981). —Reliability of 0.90 (Atwood & Hinshaw, 1986).	—Discriminant validity (Atwood & Hinshaw, 1977). —Convergent validity (Atwood & Hinshaw, 1977). —Construct validity (Atwood & Hinshaw, 1984). —Construct, convergent, and discriminant validity (Hinshaw et al., 1981).
Nurse Job Satisfaction Scale (Torres, 1988)	Hospital nursing staff	Domains: autonomy, ability to be creative, work load, morale, and opportunity for advancement. 36 items, 5-point Likert scale.	Self-administered	—Reliability of 0.83 (Grindel et al., 1996). —Cronbach's alpha of 0.85 (Kangas et al., 1999).	—Content validity (Grindel et al., 1996).
Job Satisfaction (Munson & Heda, 1974)	Hospital nursing staff	Domains: extrinsic satisfaction (security, financial rewards); interpersonal satisfaction (belongingness needs); involvement satisfaction (ego needs); and intrinsic task satisfaction (self-actualizing needs). 13 items, 7-point Likert scale. Overall job satisfaction score is a mean of the responses.	Self-administered	—Reliability of 0.89 (Lucas, 1991).	No information available.

Table 8.2A (continued)

Instrument (author)	Target population	Domains, number of items, and response format	Method of administration	Reliability	Validity
The Measure of Job Satisfaction (Traynor & Wade, 1993)	Staff nurses	Domains: personal satisfaction, satisfaction with workload, with professional support, with training, and with pay and prospects. 40 items, 5-point scale. Overall job satisfaction is the sum of subscale scores.	Self-administered	—Overall reliability of 0.93, with subscale reliabilities of 0.84 to 0.88. Test-retest reliabilities of 0.86-0.93 (Molassiotis & Haberman, 1996). —Overall reliability of 0.93, overall test-retest reliability of 0.89. Subscale reliabilities of 0.84 to 0.88, with subscale test-retest reliabilities of 0.76 to 0.91 (Wade, 1993).	—Concurrent and discriminant validity (Traynor & Wade, 1993). —Overall concurrent validity (Wade, 1993).
Work Quality Index (Whitley & Putzier, 1994)	Hospital nursing staff	Domains: staff's perception and satisfaction with the quality of their work and work environment. 38 items, 7-point scale.	Self-administered	—Reliability of 0.9565 (Ling, 1996).	No information available.

B. General Job Satisfaction Measures

Instrument (author)	Target population	Domains, number of items, and response format	Method of administration	Reliability	Validity
Job Descriptive Index (Smith et al., 1969)	Hospital nursing staff	Domains: satisfaction with work, opportunities for promotion, relationship with coworkers, satisfaction with pay, and relationship with supervisors. Number of items 72. Response format "Yes," "No," "Not sure."	Self-administered	—Reliabilities of $\beta = 67$ at Time 1 and $\alpha = 66$ at Time 2, and test-retest reliability of 0.71 (Bateman & Strasser, 1983). —Reliability of 0.93 (Cone et al., 1995). —Test-retest reliability demonstrated to be above 75% (Robinson et al., 1969; Smith, 1974). —Domain reliabilities from 0.69 to 0.82 (Kiyak et al., 1997). —Average internal consistency of 0.88 across six samples (Balzar et al., 1990).	—Concurrent validity (Cone et al., 1995) —Construct validity (Cone et al., 1995)

Table 8.2B (continued)

Instrument (author)	Target population	Domains, number of items, and response format	Method of administration	Reliability	Validity
[Job Descriptive Index (Smith et al., 1969) continued]				—Domain reliabilities of 0.79 to 0.89, with overall reliability of 0.93 (Westaway et al., 1996). —Subscale reliabilities of 0.85 to 0.91 (Judge, 1993). —Subscale reliabilities of 0.63 to 0.88 (Bussing, 1992).	
Job Satisfaction Inventory (Brayfield & Rothe, 1951)	Hospital nursing staff	Global indication of job satisfaction measured. 18 items, 5-point Likert scale.	Self-administered	—Reliability of 0.90 (Agho, 1993). —Reliability of 0.88 (Guppy & Gutteridge, 1991).	No information available.
Minnesota Satisfaction Questionnaire (Weiss et al., 1967)	Hospital nursing staff	Domains: intrinsic (job content factors such as work type, achievement, ability utilization); extrinsic (job context factors such as working conditions, supervision, co-workers); and total job satisfaction. 20 items, 5-point scale.	Self-administered	—Reliability of 0.87 (Armstrong-Stassen et al., 1996). —Reliabilities vary from 0.84 to 0.91. Test-retest reliability of the general scale varies from 0.70 over the period of a year to 0.89 over a period of a week (Bester et al., 1997). —Internal consistency of 0.86 (Cameron et al., 1994).	—Content validity (Weiss et al., 1967). —Criterion/concurrent (Weiss et al., 1967). —Construct validity (Weiss et al., 1967).

Gerber, 1995). This is important because at least three studies cited by the scale developer in her recent text identified that the "professional status" component of the scale demonstrated low reliabilities of between .29 and .49 (Stamps, 1997). Further examination of the literature indicates similar concerns. Kovner et al. (1994) and Juhl, Dunkin, Stratton, Geller, & Ludtke (1993) reported a Cronbach's alpha of .44 and .40, respectively, for the professional status scale, while another research team (Francis-Felsen et al., 1996) reported an alpha of .55 on this subscale.

Questions about the direction of the scoring for some scale items have caused some investigators to modify the scale in their research (Stamps, 1997). A review of the literature found several additional studies in which changes to the instrument had been made (Burnard et al., 1999; Coward et al., 1995; Dougherty et al., 1992; Francis-Felsen et al., 1996; Gillies et al., 1990; Hayes, 1994; Juhl et al., 1993; Kroposki et al., 1999; Muus et al., 1993; Stratton et al., 1995; Wyckoff Lancero & Gerber, 1995; Yamashita, 1995). Some researchers have eliminated component scales such as the "pay subscale" (Dougherty et al., 1992; Kroposki et al., 1999; Wyckoff Lancero & Gerber, 1995) and the "physician interaction subscale" (Coward et al., 1995). Other researchers do not specifically indicate which subscales or items have been deleted (Gillies et al., 1990; Muus et al., 1993; Stratton et al., 1995). However, in those studies in which both components of the instrument have been used, participants have consistently identified pay as one of the top three areas of importance (Coward et al., 1995; Fung-kam, 1998; Johnston, 1991; Kovner et al., 1994). Some researchers have also changed the 7-point Likert scale to a 5-point scale (Dougherty et al., 1992; Hayes, 1994; Juhl et al., 1993; Muus et al., 1993; Stratton et al., 1995; Yamashita, 1995). Other studies used the Likert-type questions only (Keuter et al., 2000; Lengacher et al., 1994).

8.8.2 *McCloskey/Mueller Satisfaction Scale (MMSS)*

The McCloskey/Mueller Satisfaction Scale (MMSS) (Mueller & McCloskey, 1990), a well-recognized measure of nursing job satisfaction, includes the dimensions of extrinsic rewards, scheduling, family/work balance, co-workers, interaction, professional opportunities, praise and recognition, and control and responsibility. In recent nursing literature, several studies have used the MMSS in a variety of settings, including hospital, community, public health, and home health (Ajamieh et al., 1996; Anderko et al., 1999; Chaboyer et al., 1999; Crose, 1999; Cumbey & Alexander, 1998; Hastings & Waltz, 1995; Krugman & Preheim, 1999; Lynch, 1994; McGillis Hall et al., 2002; Misener et al., 1996). However, only three provided information on scale reliability for their studies, both of which were very high (Chaboyer et al., 1999; Cumbey & Alexander, 1998; McGillis Hall et al., 2002). None of the researchers identified any concerns related to administering the instrument. The developers indicate that this instrument was designed to meet the need for an easy-to-use, reliable, and valid measure of nursing job satisfaction, given the complex scoring procedures associated with the IWS (Mueller & McCloskey, 1990). In an effort to identify it as an international measure of nursing job satisfaction, this instrument has had some testing in an international population (Misener et al., 1996).

8.8.3 Nursing Job Satisfaction Scale (NJS)

The Nursing Job Satisfaction Scale (NJS) was adapted for use in nursing from the Brayfield & Rothe (1951) scale by Hinshaw & Atwood (1985), by including items more specific to the nursing work situation, such as the quality of care provided, enjoyment on the job, and time to do one's job. In the recent nursing literature, several studies use the NJS in a variety of settings, including hospital and community (Boswell, 1992; Davidson et al., 1997; Jones et al., 1993; Laffrey et al., 1997; Pizer et al., 1992). Only one provided information on scale reliability, which ranged from .70 to .91 (Davidson et al., 1997). Researchers identified no concerns related to administering the instrument.

8.8.4 Nursing Job Satisfaction Scale (NJSS)

A nurse job satisfaction scale, emerging from Maslow's Hierarchy of Needs (1970) and Herzberg's Motivation-Hygiene (1966) theories, was developed and tested by Torres (1992). The instrument contains items related to decision-making power, variety of work, complexity, and recognition. Few studies could be found in the literature using this instrument (Cone et al., 1995; Grindel et al., 1996; Kangas et al., 1999), and only one reported Cronbach's alpha reliability (Kangas et al., 1999).

8.8.5 Measure of Nursing Job Satisfaction (MNJS)

A measure of nursing job satisfaction based on Maslow's Hierarchy of Needs (1970) was adapted from Porter & Lawler (1968) by Munson & Heda (1974). The instrument contains items related to intrinsic task satisfaction, involvement satisfaction, interpersonal satisfaction, and extrinsic satisfaction. Few studies were found in the literature that used this instrument (Lucas, 1991; Nakata & Saylor, 1994), and only one reported a scale reliability of 0.90 (Lucas, 1991).

8.8.6 *Measure of Job Satisfaction (MJS)*

The Measure of Job Satisfaction (MJS) was developed to examine nurses' job satisfaction in the community nursing work environment. It contains items related to personal satisfaction, satisfaction with workload, professional support, training, pay, and work prospects (Traynor & Wade, 1993; Wade, 1993). Only one study found in the literature used this instrument, and it did not report scale reliability (Molassiotis & Haberman, 1996).

8.8.7 *Work Quality Index (WQI)*

This instrument was developed to measure nurses' satisfaction with the quality of their work and work environment. It includes scales that measure work environment, autonomy, work worth, relationships, role enactment, and benefits (Whitley & Putzier, 1994). The authors attribute the validation of these scale themes to the work of earlier researchers, such as Mueller & McCloskey (1990). Very little use of this instrument can be found in the literature. One author identified that the power of her study was questionable because the sample size was not achieved (Ling, 1996), and a second author used only five of the six scales that comprise the instrument (Urden, 1999).

8.8.8 *Job Satisfaction Survey (Price & Mueller, 1981, 1986)*

Limited use of this instrument was found in recent literature, perhaps due to the fact that job satisfaction was only one component in the original instrument, which was used to measure turnover in nursing, and that, until the recent nursing shortage, the concept of turnover has been of little interest to researchers. Although a few studies used the 1981 turnover model, all of the components in the model were not assessed (Agho, 1993; Cavanagh, 1992). Agho examined seven domains of the turnover model reporting Cronbach's alpha scale reliability of .90, while Cavanagh examined 11. Blegen & Mueller (1987) applied the model in a study of nurses' job satisfaction, reporting Cronbach's alpha scores for the individual scales ranging from .43 to .93, and a job satisfaction scale alpha of .88.

8.9 General Job Satisfaction Measures

8.9.1 *Job Descriptive Index (JDI)*

Although not developed specifically for nursing, the Job Descriptive Index (JDI) is the most widely used measure of job satisfaction in existence in the management sciences (Zedeck, 1987). It examines five facets: satisfaction with work, opportunities for promotion, relationships with coworkers, satisfaction with pay, and relationships with supervisors. The instrument is easy to use and takes approximately five minutes to complete. It has repeatedly been found to be a reliable and valid measure of job satisfaction (Parsons & Hulin, 1982; Smith et al., 1969). The nursing literature documents several applications of this instrument to the nursing environment (Bateman & Strasser, 1983; Bechtold et al., 1980; Cone et al., 1995; Judge, 1993; Kiyak et al., 1997; Knoop, 1995; McGillis Hall et al., 2001; McNeese-Smith, 1995; Ndiwane, 1999; Roedel & Nystrom, 1988; Westaway et al., 1996). It has been used in nursing in Canada, the United States, and Africa, in settings ranging from acute care and critical care to the community. Scale reliabilities reported in these nursing studies were consistently high, ranging from .69 to .93 (Cone et al., 1995; Judge, 1993; Kiyak et al., 1997; Westaway et al., 1996). Researchers identified no concerns related to administering the instrument.

8.9.2 *Brayfield and Rothe Satisfaction Scale*

Brayfield & Rothe (1951) developed a general measure of job satisfaction that assumes that an individual's job satisfaction can be inferred from his or her attitude towards work. The measure has good reliability, and both face and criterion validity have been confirmed. Although few studies were found that used this instrument in the nursing context (Agho et al., 1992; Guppy & Gutteridge, 1991; Kennerly, 2000), the first two reported high scale reliability for its use.

8.9.3 *Minnesota Satisfaction Questionnaire (MSQ)*

The Minnesota Satisfaction Questionnaire (MSQ) is a measure of job satisfaction with established reliability and construct validity. At least one author has expressed concern that some scale items appear to be identical, which can lead to high reports of internal consistency on the scales (Guion, 1978). For example, "the chance to be of service to others" is quite similar to "the chance to be of service to people." While some evidence exists that the MSQ—particularly the short-form version—has been used in the nursing environment, its use has been fairly limited (Armstrong-Stassen et al., 1996; Bester et al., 1997; Cameron et al., 1994; Keil et al., 2000; Mitchell, 1994; Smith & Tziner, 1998; Sorrentino, 1992). These studies have occurred primarily in hospitals in Canada and the United States. One report from outside North America was found.

8.10 Recommendations and Directions for Future Research

Nurses' job satisfaction is an important concept to consider when studying nursing interventions related to patient outcomes. This systematic review of the nursing literature provides evidence that several approaches to measuring nursing job satisfaction may be useful tools in future studies that examine nursing job satisfaction in relation to nurse-sensitive outcomes.

Throughout the nursing research literature, there has been moderate use of at least four job satisfaction instruments: the Index of Work Satisfaction (Stamps & Piedmonte, 1986); the Job Descriptive Index (Smith et al., 1969); the Nursing Job Satisfaction scale (Hinshaw & Atwood, 1985); and the McCloskey/Mueller Satisfaction Scale (Mueller & McCloskey, 1990). Each of these instruments appears to have been carefully developed with appropriate attention to construct validity, and most have been applied broadly across a number of demographic groups within nursing. Most have had reliability assessed on an ongoing basis through multiple applications of the instruments in a variety of settings and countries. However, for the most part, little or no attention has been paid to any ongoing assessment of their validity. This makes selection of one measure for use in the nursing environment problematic. Nunnally (1978) suggests that measures should be kept under constant surveillance to see if they are behaving as they should.

Several other instruments have had limited application in the nursing literature (Munson & Heda, 1974; Torres, 1992; Whitley & Putzier, 1994), although preliminary research reports are promising. While occupation-specific measures do not allow comparisons across other worker groups, they may be more effective in delineating components of satisfaction that are most relevant to the particular occupation they were designed to measure (Mueller & McCloskey, 1990). A number of acceptable job satisfaction measures exist in the literature; however, they have not been widely applied in the nursing environment.

Based on this literature and instrument review, the Hinshaw & Atwood (1985) Nursing Job Satisfaction Scale and the McCloskey/Mueller Satisfaction Scale (Mueller & McCloskey, 1990) should be tested in future research studies of the relationship between nursing job satisfaction and nursing care interventions. In addition, from the perspective of general job satisfaction instruments, the Job Descriptive Index also warrants further study in nursing environments. The reliability and validity of these instruments are well established, and study reports of their use are positive. The Index of Work Satisfaction (Stamps & Piedmonte, 1986; Stamps et al, 1978; Slavitt et al., 1978) holds promise if the concerns related to the lack of standardization in administration and subscales are addressed.

From a theoretical perspective, the instruments recommended all capture some dimensions that can be conceptually linked to nurse-sensitive outcomes, such as functional status and symptom control. For example, the NJS explores nurses' perceptions of the quality of patient care provided.

As the conceptual definitions of job satisfaction suggest, nursing job satisfaction measures have focused primarily on nurses' job or work situations. This presents a challenge for researchers interested in capturing the effectiveness of nursing practice as it relates to nursing interventions. In the future, as the field of nurse-sensitive patient outcomes evolves, there will be a need to develop job satisfaction instruments that relate directly and indirectly to the practice processes of nursing in relation to patient outcomes.

References

Agho, A. (1993). The moderating effects of dispositional affectivity on relationships between job characteristics and nurses' job satisfaction. *Research in Nursing and Health, 16*, 451–458.

Agho, A., Price, J. L., & Mueller, C. W. (1992). Discriminant validity of measures of job satisfaction, positive affectivity and negative affectivity. *Journal of Occupational and Organizational Psychology, 65*, 185–196.

Ajamieh, A. R. A., Misener, T., Haddock, K. S., & Gleaton, J. U. (1996). Job satisfaction correlates among Palestinian nurses in the West Bank. *International Journal of Nursing Studies, 33*, 422–432.

Anderko, L., Robertson, J., & Lewis, P. (1999). Job satisfaction in a rural differentiated-practice setting. *Nursing Connections, 12*(1), 49–58.

Armstrong-Stassen, M., Cameron, S. J., & Horsburgh, M. E. (1996). The impact of organizational downsizing on the job satisfaction of nurses. *Canadian Journal of Nursing Administration, 9*(4), 8–32.

Atwood, J. R., & Hinshaw, A. S. (1977). Multiple indicators of nurse and patient outcomes as a method for evaluating a change in staffing patterns. *Communicating Nursing Research, 10*, 235–255.

Atwood, J. R., & Hinshaw, A. S. (1986). Professional/occupational nurse job satisfaction scale. In *Anticipated turnover among nursing staff.* Final Report Contract No. 1 R01 NU00908). Washington, DC: Department of Health and Human Services. Pg. 298.

Balzar, W. K., Smith, P. C., Kravitz, D. A., Lovell, S. E., Paul, K. B., Reilly, B. A., & Reilly, C. E. (1990). *Users' manual for the Job Descriptive Index (JDI) and the Job in General (JIG) scales.* Bowling Green, Ohio: Bowling Green State University.

Bateman, T. S., & Strasser, S. (1983). A cross-lagged regression test of the relationships between job tension and employee satisfaction. *Journal of Applied Psychology, 68,* 439–445.

Bechtold, S. E., Szilagyi, A. D., & Sims, H. P. (1980). Antecedents of employee satisfaction in a hospital environment. *Health Care Management Review, 5*(1), 77–88.

Bester, C. L., Richter, E. C., & Boshoff, A. B. (1997). Prediction of nurses' job satisfaction level. *Curationis, 20*(4), 59–63.

Blegen, M. A. (1993). Nurses' job satisfaction: A meta-analysis of related variables. *Nursing Research, 42,* 36–41.

Blegen, M.A., & Mueller, C.W. (1987). Nurses' job satisfaction: A longitudinal analysis. *Research in Nursing and Health, 10,* 227–237.

Boswell, C. A. (1992). Work stress and job satisfaction for the community health nurse. *Journal of Community Health Nursing, 9*(4), 221–227.

Bratt, M. M., Broome, M., Kelber, S., & Lostocco, L. (2000). Influence of stress and nursing leadership on job satisfaction of pediatric intensive care unit nurses. *American Journal of Critical Care, 9*(5), 307–317.

Brayfield, A., & Rothe, H. (1951). An index of job satisfaction. *Journal of Applied Psychology, 35*(5), 307–311.

Burnard, P., Morrison, P., & Phillips, C. (1999). Job satisfaction amongst nurses in an interim secure forensic unit in Wales. *Australian and New Zealand Journal of Mental Health Nursing, 8,* 9–18.

Bussing, A. (1992) A dynamic view of job satisfaction in psychiatric nurses in Germany. *Work and Stress, 6*(3), 239–259.

Cameron, S. J., Horsburgh, M. E., & Armstrong-Stassen, M. (1994). Job satisfaction, propensity to leave and burnout in RNs and RNAs: A multivariate perspective. *Canadian Journal of Nursing Administration, 7*(3), 43–64.

Campbell, J. P., Dunnette, M. D., Lawler, E. E., & Weick, K. E. (1970). *Managerial Behaviour, Performance and Effectiveness.* New York: McGraw-Hill.

Cavanagh, S. J. (1992). Job satisfaction of nursing staff working in hospitals. *Journal of Advanced Nursing, 17,* 704–711.

Chaboyer, W., Williams, G., Corkill, W., & Creamer, J. (1999). Predictors of job satisfaction in remote hospital nursing. *CJNL, 12*(2), 30–40.

Cleeland, C. C. (1991). Pain Assessment in cancer. In D. Obosa (Ed.). *Effects of cancer on quality of life.* Boca Raton, FL: CRC Press. (pp. 293–305).

Cone, M., McGovern, C. C., Barnard, B., & Riegel, B. (1995). Satisfaction with a model of professional practice in critical care. *Critical Care Nursing Quarterly, 18*(3), 67–74.

Coward, R. T., Hogan, T. L., Duncan, R. P., Horne, C. H., Hilker, M. A., & Felsen, L. M. (1995). Job satisfaction of nurses employed in rural and urban long-term care facilities. *Research in Nursing & Health, 18,* 271–284.

Coward, R. T., Horne, C., Duncan, R. P., & Dwyer, J.W. (1992). Job satisfaction among hospital nurses: facility size and location comparisons. *The Journal of Rural Health, 8*(4), 255–267.

Crose, P. S. (1999). Job characteristics related to job satisfaction in rehabilitation nursing. *Rehabilitation Nursing, 24*(3), 95–102.

Cumbey, D. A., & Alexander, J. W. (1998). The relationship of job satisfaction with organizational variables in public health nursing. *Journal of Nursing Administration, 28*(5), 39–46.

Davidson, H., Folcarelli, P. H., Crawford, S., Duprat, L., & Clifford, J. C. (1997). The effects of health care reforms on job satisfaction and voluntary turnover among hospital-based nurses. *Medical Care, 35*, 634–645.

Dawis, R. V., & Lofquist, L. H. (1984). *A Psychological Theory of Work Adjustment.* Minneapolis, MN: University of Minnesota Press.

Decker, F. H. (1997). Occupational and nonoccupational factors in job satisfaction and psychological distress among nurses. *Research in Nursing and Health, 20*, 453–464.

Dougherty, L. M., Bolger, J. P., Preston, D. G., Jones, S. S., & Payne, H. C. (1992). Effects of exposure to aggressive behavior on job satisfaction of health care staff. *Journal of Applied Gerontology, 11*(2), 160–172.

Dunkin, J., Juhl, N., Stratton, T., Geller, J., & Ludtke, R. (1992). Job satisfaction and retention of rural community health nurses in North Dakota. *The Journal of Rural Health, 8*(4), 268–275.

Eberhardt, B. J., Pooyan, A., & Moser, S. B. (1995). Moderators of the relationship between job satisfaction and nurses' intention to quit. *The International Journal of Organizational Analysis, 3*(4), 394–406.

Ecklund, M. M. (1998). The relationship of mentoring to job satisfaction of critical care nurses. *Journal of the New York State Nurses Association, 29*(2), 13–15.

Francis-Felsen, L. C., Coward, R. T., Hogan, T. L., Duncan, R. P., Hilker, A. M., & Horne, C. (1996). Factors influencing intentions of nursing personnel to leave employment in long-term care settings. *Journal of Applied Gerontology, 15*, 450–470.

Fung-kam, Le. (1998). Job satisfaction and autonomy of Hong Kong registered nurses. *Journal of Advanced Nursing, 27*, 355–363.

Gillies, D. A., Franklin, M., & Child, D. A. (1990). Relationship between organizational climate and job satisfaction of nursing personnel. *Nursing Administration Quarterly, 14*(4), 15–22.

Goodell, T. T., & Coeling, H. V. E. (1994). Outcomes of nurses' job satisfaction. *Journal of Nursing Administration, 24*(11), 36–41.

Grindel, C. G., Peterson, K., Kinneman, M., & Turner, T. L. (1996). The practice environment project: A process of outcome evaluation. *Journal of Nursing Administration, 26*(5), 43–51.

Guion, R. M. (1978). Review. In O. K. Buros, *The Eighth Mental Measurements Yearbook, Volume II.* New Jersey: The Gryphon Press (pp. 1677–1680).

Guppy, A., & Gutteridge, T. (1991). Job satisfaction and occupational stress in UK general hospital nursing staff. *Work and Stress, 5*(4), 315–323.

Hackman, J. R., & Oldham, G. R. (1976). Motivation through the design of work: Test of a theory. *Organizational Behaviour and Human Performance, 16*, 250–279.

Hamilton, B. B., Granger, C. V., Sherwin, F. S., Zielezny, M., & Tashman, J. S. (1987). A uniform national data system for medical rehabilitation. In M. J. Fuhrer (Ed.) *Rehabilitation outcomes: Analysis and measurement.* Baltimore: Paul H. Brooks Publishing Company (pp. 135–147).

Hastings, C., & Waltz, C. (1995). Assessing the outcomes of professional practice redesign: Impact on staff nurse perceptions. *Journal of Nursing Administration, 25*(3), 34–42.

Hayes, P. M. (1994). Non-nursing functions: time for them to go. *Nursing Economics, 12,* 120–125.

Herzberg, F. (1966). *Work and the Nature of Man.* New York: World Publishing Co.

Hinshaw, A. S. & Atwood, J. R. (1985). *Anticipated Turnover Among Nursing Staff Study.* Final Report. (1R01NU00908). The University of Arizona, Tucson.

Hinshaw, A. S., Scofield, R., & Atwood, J. R. (1981). Staff, patient and cost outcomes of all registered nurse staffing. *Journal of Nursing Administration, 11*(11–12), 30–36.

Hinshaw, A. S., Smeltzer, C. H., & Atwood, J. R. (1987). Innovative retention strategies for nursing staff. *Journal of Nursing Administration, 17*(6), 8–16.

Ironson, G. H., Smith, P. C., Brannick, M. T., Gibson, W. M., & Paul, K. B. (1989). Construction of a job in general scale: A comparison of global, composite, and specific measures. *Journal of Applied Psychology, 74,* 193–200.

Irvine, D. M., & Evans, M. G. (1995). Job satisfaction and turnover among nurses: Integrating research findings across studies. *Nursing Research, 44,* 246–252.

Johnston, C. L. (1991). Sources of work satisfaction/dissatisfaction for hospital registered nurses. *Western Journal of Nursing Research, 13,* 503–513.

Jones, C. B., Stasiowski, S., Simons, B. J., Boyd, N. J., & Lucas, M. D. (1993). Shared governance and the nursing practice environment. *Nursing Economics, 11,* 208–214.

Judge, T. A. (1993). Does affective disposition moderate the relationship between job satisfaction and voluntary turnover? *Journal of Applied Psychology, 78,* 395–401.

Juhl, N., Dunkin, J. W., Stratton, T., Geller, J., & Ludtke, R. (1993). Job satisfaction of rural public and home health nurses. *Public Health Nursing, 10*(1), 42–47.

Kangas, S., Kee, C. C., & McKee-Waddle, R. (1999). Organizational factors, nurses' job satisfaction, and patient satisfaction with nursing care. *Journal of Nursing Administration, 29*(1), 32–42.

Keil, J. M., Armstrong-Stassen, M., Cameron, S., & Horsburgh, M. E. (2000). Part-time nurses: The effect of work status congruency on job attitudes. *Applied Psychology: An International Review. 49*(2), 227–236.

Kennerly, S. (2000). Perceived worker autonomy: The foundation for shared governance. *Journal of Nursing Administration, 30*(12), 611–617.

Keuter, K., Byrne, E., Voell, J., & Larson, E. (2000). Nurses' job satisfaction and organizational climate in a dynamic work environment. *Applied Nursing Research, 13*(1), 46–49.

Kiyak, H. S., Namazi, K. H., & Kahana, E. F. (1997). Job commitment and turnover among women working in facilities serving older persons. *Research on Aging, 19*(2), 223–246.

Knoop, R. (1995). Relationships among job involvement, job satisfaction, and organizational commitment for nurses. *Journal of Psychology, 129*, 643–649.

Kovner, C. T., Hendrickson, G., Knickman, J. R., & Finkler, S. A. (1994). Nursing care delivery models and nurse satisfaction. *Nursing Administration Quarterly, 19*(1), 74–85.

Kroposki, M., Murdaugh, C. L., Tavakoli, A. S., & Parsons, M. (1999). Role clarity, organizational commitment, and job satisfaction during hospital reengineering. *Nursing Connections, 12*(1), 27–34.

Krugman, M., & Preheim, G. (1999). Longitudinal evaluation of professional nursing practice redesign. *Journal of Nursing Administration, 29*(5), 10–20.

Laffrey, S. C., Dickenson, D., & Diem, E. (1997). Role identity and job satisfaction of community health nurses. *International Journal of Nursing Practice, 3*, 178–187.

Lengacher, C. A., Kent, K., Mabe, P. R., Heinemann, D., VanCott, M. L., & Bowling, C. D. (1994). Effects of the partners in care practice model on nursing outcomes. *Nursing Economics, 12*, 300–308.

Ling, C. W. (1996). Performance of a self-directed work team in a home healthcare agency. *Journal of Nursing Administration, 26*(9), 36–40.

Lucas, M. D. (1991). Management style and staff nurse job satisfaction. *Journal of Professional Nursing, 7*(2), 119–125.

Lum, L., Kervin, J., Clark, K., Reid, F., & Sirola, W. (1998). Explaining nursing turnover intent: Job satisfaction, pay satisfaction, or organizational commitment? *Journal of Organizational Behaviour, 19*, 305–320.

Lynch, S. A. (1994). Job satisfaction of home health nurses. *Home Healthcare Nurse, 12*(5), 21–28.

Maslow, A. H. (1970). *Motivation and Personality* (Second Edition). New York: Harper & Row.

McCloskey, J. C. (1990). Two requirements for job contentment: Autonomy and social integration. *Image: The Journal of Nursing Scholarship, 22*(3), 140–143.

McGillis Hall, L., Irvine, D., Baker, G. R., Pink, G., Sidani, S., O'Brien Pallas, L., & Donner, G. (2001). *A Study of the Impact of Nursing Staff Mix Models & Organizational Change Strategies on Patient, System & Nurse Outcomes*. Toronto, ON: Faculty of Nursing, University of Toronto and Canadian Health Services Research Foundation/Ontario Council of Teaching Hospitals.

McGillis Hall, L., Waddell, J., Donner, G. J., & Wheeler, M. (2002). Outcomes of a Career Development Program for Registered Nurses. Final Report. Toronto: Faculty of Nursing, University of Toronto.

McNeese-Smith, D. (1995). Job satisfaction, productivity, and organizational commitment: The result of leadership. *Journal of Nursing Administration, 25*(9), 17–26.

McNeese-Smith, D. (1999). A content analysis of staff nurse descriptions of job satisfaction and dissatisfaction. *Journal of Advanced Nursing, 29*(6), 1332–1341.

Meterko, M., Nelson, E. C., Rubin, H. R., Batalden, P., Berwick, D. M., Hays, R. D., & Ware, J. E. (1990). Patients' judgment of hospital quality: A report on a pilot study. *Medical Care, 28*(supp.), S1–S56.

Misener, T. R., Haddock, S., Gleaton, J. U., & Ajamieh, A. R. A. (1996). Toward an international measure of job satisfaction. *Nursing Research, 45*(2), 87–91.

Mitchell, M. B. (1994). The effect of work role values on job satisfaction. *Journal of Advanced Nursing, 20,* 958–963.

Molassiotis, A., & Haberman, M. (1996). Evaluation of burnout and job satisfaction in marrow transplant nurses. *Cancer Nursing, 19*(5), 360–367.

Mottaz, C. J. (1988). Work satisfaction among hospital nurses. *Hospital and Health Services Administration, 33*(1), 57–74.

Mueller, C. W., & McCloskey, J. C. (1990). Nurses' job satisfaction: A proposed measure. *Nursing Research, 39,* 113–117.

Munson, F. C., & Heda, S. S. (1974). An instrument for measuring nursing satisfaction. *Nursing Research, 23*(2), 159–166.

Muus, K. J., Stratton, T. D., Dunkin, J. W., & Juhl, N. (1993). Retaining registered nurses in rural community hospitals. *Journal of Nursing Administration, 23*(3), 38–43.

Nahm, H. (1940). Job satisfaction in nursing. *The American Journal of Nursing, 40,* 1389–1392.

Nakata, J. A., & Saylor, C. (1994). Management style and staff nurse satisfaction in a changing environment. *Nursing Adminsitration Quarterly, 18*(3), 51–57.

Ndiwane, A. (1999). Factors that influence job satisfaction of nurses in urban and rural community health centers in Cameroon: Implications for policy. *Clinical Excellence for Nurse Practitioners, 3*(3), 172–180.

Nunnally, J. C. (1978). *Psychometric Theory.* New York: McGraw-Hill.

Parson, C. K., & Hulin, C. L. (1982). An empirical comparison of item response theory and hierarchical factor analysis in applications to the measurement of job satisfaction. *Journal of Applied Psychology, 67*(6), 826–834.

Pizer, C. M., Collard, A. F., James, S. M., & Bonaparte, B. H. (1992). Nurses' job satisfaction: Are there differences between foreign and U.S. educated nurses? *Image: The Journal of Nursing Scholarship, 24,* 301–306.

Porter, L. W., & Lawler, E. E. (1968). *Managerial Attitudes and Performance.* Homewood, IL: Dorsey Press.

Price, J. L., & Mueller, C. W. (1981). *Professional Turnover: The Case of Nurses.* New York: SP Medical and Scientific Books.

Price, J. L., & Mueller, C. W. (1986). *Absenteeism and Turnover of Hospital Employees.* Greenwich, CT: JAI Press.

Prothero, M. M., Marshall, E. S., & Fosbinder, D. M. (1999). Implementing differentiated practice: Personal values and work satisfaction among hospital staff nurses. *Journal for Nurses in Staff Development, 15*(5), 185–192.

Radice, B. (1994). The relationship between nurse empowerment in the hospital work environment and job satisfaction: A pilot study. *Journal of the New York State Nurses Association, 25*(2), 14–17.

Rice, R. W., Gentile, D. A., & McFarlin, D. B. (1991). Facet importance and job satisfaction. *Journal of Applied Psychology, 76,* 31–39.

Robinson, J. P. R., Athanasiou, K. B., & Head. (1969). *Measures of Occupational Attitudes.* Ann Arbor, MI: Institute for Social Research.

Roedel, R. R., & Nystrom, P. C. (1988). Nursing jobs and satisfaction. *Nursing Management, 19*(2), 34–38.

Rubin, H., Ware, J. E., & Hayes, R. D. (1990). The PJHQ Questionnaire. *Medical Care, 28*(9), 22–43.

Shader, K., Broome, M. E., Broome, C. D., West, M. E., & Nash, M. (2001). Factors influencing satisfaction and anticipated turnover for nurses in an academic medical center. *Journal of Nursing Administration, 31*(4), 210–216.

Sims, H. P., Szilagyi, A. D., & Keller, R. T. (1976). The measurement of job characteristics. *Academy of Management Journal, 19*, 195–212.

Slavitt, D. B., Stamps, P. L., Piedmonte, E. B., & Haase, A. M. B. (1978). Nurses' satisfaction with their work situation. *Nursing Research, 27*, 114–120.

Smith, D., & Tziner, A. (1998). Moderating effects of affective disposition and social support on the relationship between person-environment fit and strain. *Psychological Reports, 82*, 963–983.

Smith, P., Ironson, G. H., Brannick, M. T., et al. (1989). Construction of a job in general scale: A comparison of global, composite, and specific measures. *Journal of Applied Psychology, 74*(2), 1–8.

Smith, P. C., Kendall, L. M., & Hulin, C. L. (1969). *The measurement of satisfaction in work and retirement: A strategy for the study of attitudes.* Chicago: Rand McNally & Company.

Smith, P. C., Smith, O. W., & Rollo, L. (1974). Factor structure for blacks and whites of the Job Descriptive Index and its discrimination of job satisfaction. *Journal of Applied Psychology, 59*, 99–100.

Song, R., Daly, B. J., Rudy, E. B., Douglas, S., & Dyer, M. A. (1997). Nurses' job satisfaction, absenteeism, and turnover after implementing a special care unit practice model. *Research in Nursing and Health, 20*, 443–452.

Sorrentino, E. A. (1992). The effect of head nurse behaviours on nurse job satisfaction and performance. *Hospital and Health Services Administration, 37*(1), 103–113.

Stamps, P. L. (1997). *Nurses and work satisfaction: An index for measurement* (Second Edition). Chicago: Health Administration Press.

Stamps, P. L., & Piedmonte, E. B. (1986). *Nurses and work satisfaction: An index for measurement.* Ann Arbor, Michigan: Heath Administration Press Perspectives.

Stamps, P. L., Piedmonte, E. B., Slavitt, D. B., & Haase, A. M. (1978). Measurement of work satisfaction among health professionals. *Medical Care, 16*, 337–351.

Stewart, A. L., Kamberg, C. J. (1992). Physical functioning measures. In A. L. Stewart & J. E. Ware, Jr. (Eds.). *Measuring functing and well-being: The medical outcomes study approach.* Durham, NC: Duke University Press. (pp. 86–101).

Stratton, T. D., Dunkin, J. W., Juhl, N., & Geller, J. M. (1995). Retainment incentives in three rural practice settings: Variations in job satisfaction among staff registered nurses. *Applied Nursing Research, 8*(2), 73–80.

Torres, G. (1992). A reassessment of instruments for use in a multivariate evaluation of a collaborative practice project. In Strickland, O. L., Waltz, C. F., Eds., *Measurement of Nursing Outcomes, Vol 2: Measuring Nursing Performance.* New York: Springer Publishing Company, 381–391.

Traynor, M., & Wade, B. (1993). The development of a measure of job satisfaction for use in monitoring the morale of community nurses in four trusts. *Journal of Advanced Nursing, 18,* 127–136.

Tumulty, G., Jernigan, I. E., & Kohut, G. F. (1994). The impact of perceived work environment on job satisfaction of hospital staff nurses. *Applied Nursing Research, 7*(2), 84–90.

Urden, L. D. (1999). The impact of organizational climate on nurse satisfaction: Management implications. *Nursing Leadership Forum, 4*(2), 44–48.

Wade, B. E. (1993). The job satisfaction of health visitors, district nurses and practice nurses working in areas served by four trusts: Year 1. *Journal of Advanced Nursing, 18,* 992–1004.

Wallach, E. J. (1983). Individuals and organizations: The cultural match. *Training Development Journal, Feb.,* 29–36.

Weisman, C. S., Alexander, C. S., & Chase, G. A. (1981). Determinants of hospital staff nurse turnover. *Medical Care, 19*(4), 431–443.

Weisman, C. S., & Nathanson, C. A. (1985). Professional satisfaction and client outcomes. *Medical Care, 23,* 1179–1192.

Weiss, D. J., Dawis, R. V., England, G. W., & Lofquist, L. H. (1967). *Manual for the Minnesota Satisfaction Questionnaire.* Minneapolis: University of Minnesota Industrial Relations Center.

Westaway, M. S., Wessie, G. M., Viljoen, E., Booysen, U., & Wolmarans, L. (1996). Job satisfaction and self-esteem of South African nurses. *Curationis, 19*(3), 17–20.

Whitley, M. P., & Putzier, D. J. (1994). Measuring nurses' satisfaction with the quality of their work environment. *Journal of Nursing Care Quality, 8*(3), 43–51.

Williams, C. (1990). Job satisfaction: comparing CC and med/surg nurses. *Nursing Management, 21,* 104A–104H.

Wyckoff Lancero, A., & Gerber, R. M. (1995). Comparing work satisfaction in two case management models. *Nursing Management, 26*(11), 45–48.

Yamashita, M. (1995). Job satisfaction in Japanese nurses. *Journal of Advanced Nursing, 22,* 158–164.

Zedeck, S. (1987). *Satisfaction in Union Members and Their Spouses.* Paper presented at the Job Satisfaction: Advances in Research and Practice Conference, Bowling Green, Ohio.

9

Nursing Minimum Data Sets

Claire Mallette, RN, MSc, PhD (cand.)

Chief Nursing Officer, Workplace Safety & Insurance Board

9.1 Introduction

Healthcare providers, as well as policy- and decision-makers, have identified the need for outcome data to evaluate the effectiveness and efficiency of healthcare systems (Canadian Nurses Association, 2000). A number of healthcare databases have now been developed to record information about patients'/clients' healthcare utilization and health outcomes. These databases extract and record data such as length of stay, healthcare costs, admission and discharge dates, primary and secondary medical diagnoses, adverse occurrences, mortality, activities of daily living, and case mix (Delaney & Moorhead, 1995). This information can then be used to plan and evaluate services at the system level, develop report cards for accountability and benchmarking, and, ultimately, develop an accountability framework. The quality and validity of these databases is important because the information contained within them is used by local, regional, and national policy-makers to make important decisions about our healthcare systems (Prophet & Delaney, 1998).

Unfortunately, much of the data needed to measure and evaluate nurses' contribution to patient care is largely absent from existing healthcare databases (Goossen et al., 1998). As a result, nurses' contributions to patient outcomes and health care remains, for the most part, invisible (Goossen et al., 1998). To rectify this absence of meaningful information for evaluating nurses' contributions to health care, the healthcare system requires consistent data collection methods using standardized language in order to be able to aggregate and compare data across programs, sectors, and jurisdictions (Blewitt & Jones, 1996).

A literature search identified databases that attempt to gather that type of information. Four that are nursing-specific databases or nursing minimum data sets (NMDS) will be discussed, while two are more generic, multidisciplinary databases (i.e., the Resident Assessment Instrument (RAI) Series, used in nursing homes, and the Outcome and Assessment Information Set (OASIS) database, used in home health care).

This chapter reviews these databases, and for each one:

- Identifies its origin

- Identifies and defines its essential elements

- Describes how the database was evaluated for data quality and validity (where such testing has been undertaken)

- Discusses its strengths and limitations.

This chapter also discusses the classification systems most commonly used in nursing minimum data sets (NMDS) to classify patient issues, nursing interventions, and nursing outcomes.

The review of literature on relevant databases involved a search of articles in CINHAL, Medline, Health Star, Science Citation Index, and Proquest. The key words used to search the literature were "nursing minimum data set" (NMDS), "minimum data set" (MDS), "North American Nursing Diagnosis Association" (NANDA), "Iowa Nursing Interventions Classification" (NIC), "Nursing Outcomes Classification" (NOC), "Resident Assessment Instruments" (RAI), and "Outcome and Assessment Information Set" (OASIS). Articles deemed appropriate for review met the following criteria: nursing-related, involved empirical research using minimum database information, described an outcome measurement related to nursing and quality care, and included reliability and validity of database tools and instruments. Articles that commented on the development and utilization of the nursing minimum data set were also reviewed.

9.2 Nursing Minimum Data Sets

The concept of a Uniform Minimum Health Data Set (UMHDS) was first developed in 1969 by the U.S. Health Information Policy Council to identify national health data standards and guidelines in the United States (Ryan & Delaney, 1995). The UMHDS has been defined as a minimum data set of items with uniform definitions and categories for specific aspects of the healthcare system (Coenen & Schoneman, 1995). The goal of the UMHDS is to meet the essential needs of multiple data users. As a result of the UMHDS, three patient-focused health data sets were developed: the Uniform Hospital Discharge Set, the Long-Term Care Minimum Data Set, and the Uniform Ambulatory Medical Care Minimum Data Set (Ryan & Delaney, 1995). However, none of these data sets include essential nursing data.

A nursing minimum data set is a minimum set of essential elements specific to nursing (Coenen & Schoneman, 1995). Goossen et al. (1998) have identified five essential steps to developing a nursing minimum data set:

- Identify appropriate data items as variables

- Accurately define the variables

- Specify the range of possible values or terminology for each variable

- Document the actual patient data in the patient file using the appropriate terminology for the particular variables

- Code the patient data from the individual patient files and aggregate it into databases for different purposes, such as healthcare evaluation, policy, and research.

9.2.1 The Nursing Minimum Data Set (NMDS)

The first nursing minimum data set (NMDS) was developed in the United States in 1985, in response to the absence of nursing information in healthcare information databases (Anderson & Hannah, 1993; Coenen & Schoneman, 1995). It was designed to facilitate the extraction of essential, core minimum data elements to describe nursing practice (Clark, 1998a). The NMDS, which was developed and derived from the concept of the Uniform Minimum Health Data Set (UMHDS), was developed by six task force groups from a national group of 64 experts at an NMDS invitational conference (Goossen et al., 2000). The Postconference Task Force refined the NMDS items and recommended them as the content for the U.S. NMDS (Goossen et al., 2000). The purposes of the NMDS were to:

1. Establish comparability of nursing data across clinical populations, settings, geographic areas, and time.

2. Describe the nursing care of clients and their families in a variety of settings, including institutional and non-institutional.

3. Demonstrate or project trends regarding nursing care provided and allocation of nursing resources to clients according to their health problems and nursing diagnoses.

4. Promote nursing research through links to other databases and other healthcare information systems.

5. Provide data related to nursing care to facilitate and influence clinical administrative and health policy decision-making (Coenen & Schoneman, 1995).

The U.S. NMDS is a minimum set of essential elements organized into three broad categories:

- Nursing care elements, such as nursing diagnosis, nursing intervention, nursing outcome, and intensity of nursing care.

- Patient demographic elements, such as personal identification, date of birth, sex, race and ethnicity, and residence.

- Service elements, such as a unique facility or service agency number, a unique health number for the patient, a unique number of the primary nurse provider, episode admission or encounter date, discharge or termination date, disposition of patient, and expected payer for the services (O'Brien Pallas et al., 1995; Coenen & Schoneman, 1995).

9.2.2 Community Nursing Minimum Data Set Australia (CNMDSA)

In Australia, the development of the Community Nursing Minimum Data Set Australia (CNMDSA) began in 1990. Goossen et al. (2000) report that the CNMDSA was developed to compare the performance of institutions, allocate resources, monitor and compare the health status of the population, and deliver information to decision-makers and policy-makers. Although the CNMDSA is used nationally, it is limited to community care settings. The indicators/items for the CNMDSA were identified based on consultations with: 300 nurses working in the areas of field/community nursing, and middle and senior management; non-nurses with an interest in the CNMDSA; and nurses from hospitals, education, and other work settings. The consultations identified 66 possible items considered necessary for the practice of community nursing in Australia. A Delphi approach was used to prioritize the items, and a focus group was then conducted to determine the specific items and their operational definitions. The result was the 17-item CNMDSA. The nursing care data elements explored include nursing diagnosis, goals of nursing care, nursing intervention, client dependency, and discharge. As no known reports of CNMDSA field-testing have been published, it is not possible to comment on its validity and reliability in collecting data on nursing outcomes in the community setting.

9.2.3 Health Information: Nursing Components (HI:NC)

In Canada, the first step in developing a nursing minimum data set occurred in 1993 at the NMDS conference sponsored by the Canadian Nurses Association (CNA, 2000). Leaders in the fields of information management, nursing research, and nursing classification systems participated in the conference. The overall objective was to develop an NMDS to ensure the availability and accessibility of nursing data in a standardized form. At the conclusion of the conference, participants proposed nursing-specific elements for inclusion in a national health data set (CNA, 2000). The NMDS was given the name Health Information: Nursing Components (HI:NC) to reflect a focus on the patient and the patient's needs and outcomes, rather than on individual healthcare professions (Hannah & Anderson, 1994). The HI:NC can be used nationally and in all settings (Goossen et al., 1998).

The HI:NC includes:

- Eight patient demographic items

- Medical care items, such as medical diagnosis, procedures, and whether the patient is alive or dead at the time of classification

- Nursing care elements, which describe the client status, nursing interventions, client outcomes, and nursing intensity

- Service elements, such as provincial/institutional chart number, doctor identifier, consultant identifier, nurse identifier, and principal nurse provider

- Episode items, such as admission date and hour, discharge date and hour, and length of stay

- Other related data, such as the institution, main point of service, and payer (CNA, 2000; Goossen et al., 1998).

The next stage in the development of the HI:NC was to identify an existing classification system that includes relevant data elements. The Alberta Association of Registered Nurses (AARN) examined eight classification systems that had been developed internationally and describe client status, nursing interventions, and client outcomes (CNA, 2000). Although the AARN Working Group determined that none of these classification systems was suitable for the purpose of the HI:NC, it concluded that the International Classification of Nursing Practice (ICNP) appeared to hold the most promise.

In 1999, the Canadian Nurses Association supported in principle the ICNP as the most universal, generic, and comprehensive classification system for nursing. They concluded that the ICNP provides a detailed integration of the principal international classification systems and begins to describe and compare nursing practices across healthcare settings, client populations, and geographical regions. As a result, the ICNP was recommended as the foundational classification system for Canadian nursing practice (CNA, 2000).

9.2.4 *International Classification Of Nursing Practice (ICNP)*

The International Classification of Nursing Practice (ICNP) is the International Council of Nurses' (ICN) endeavor to develop a standardized international nursing language (Cruz et al., 2000). The purposes of the ICNP are to:

1. Identify feasibility of nursing data collection and comparison of nursing practices internationally

2. Make visible what nurses do

3. Collect and provide nursing data related to nursing practice to influence nursing education, health policy, and research (Goossen et al., 1998).

The scope of the ICNP is multinational and can be applied to all practice settings (Goossen et al., 1998). The ICNP's three primary elements are nursing phenomena (the focus of nursing, also called nursing diagnoses), nursing interventions, and clinical outcomes (CNA, 2000).

The Alpha version of the ICNP was released in 1996 (Ruland, 2001). Its goals were to provide a vocabulary and a new classification system for nursing, as well as a framework into which existing vocabularies and classifications can be cross-mapped (Clark, 1998a, 1998b). This version consisted of the diagnosis and intervention components of nursing practice, and was translated into 15 languages (CNA, 2000).

The Beta version was released in 1999 and is a refinement based on feedback and lessons learned from field testing the Alpha version (CNA, 2000). The Beta version is designed so that nursing phenomena and nursing intervention classifications are multiaxial and hierarchical (Ruland, 2001). This allows for different concepts in clinical practice to be expressed as combinations of concepts from different axes or hierarchies of the ICNP (Ruland, 2001). For example, the complex concept of impaired mobility can be broken down into separate axes, such as mobility and impaired. This allows for the terms in different axes to be combined in various ways, and increases the richness and flexibility of the data (Clark, 1998a). Ruland (2001) describes the axes in the nursing phenomenon component as being focus, judgment, frequency, duration, body site, topology, likelihood, and distribution. The intervention classification consists of action type, target, means, time, location, topology, routes, and beneficiary. The Beta version is presently being tested in clinical practice settings.

9.2.5 Comparisions Of NMDS Systems

Goossen et al. (1998) examined the differences and similarities of national and international NMDS systems. Common features include nursing diagnosis, nursing interventions, nursing outcome, and demographic data about the patient, nurse, and institution. The number of data elements varies: 27 in the HI:NC, 17 in the CNMDSA, and 16 in both the ICNP and U.S. NMDS.

Reports describing the implementation and testing of the ICNP and CNDMSA are limited. The CNDMSA has not been described in peer-reviewed literature. Testing of the ICNP is underway, with reporting occurring primarily in reports from the International Council of Nurses and conferences. One reported study by Ruland (2001) evaluated the ICNP Beta version for domain completeness, applicability of axial structure, and utility in clinical practice. A subset of terms describing the areas of circulation and elimination were examined from 30 nursing records of a cardiac intensive care unit and 60 records in a nursing home. Composite phrases were analyzed and the various nouns, adjectives, and verbs in the data set were organized according to the axial structure of the nursing phenomena and intervention sections of the ICNP. Although the two trained coders were expert nurses in the field and coded terms were compared and inspected for agreement, the study reports no inter-rater reliability. Only 27% to 35% of the abstracted intervention terms could be classified within the ICNP. In contrast, 47% to 69% of nursing phenomena terms could be classified (Ruland, 2001). The research team also had difficulty coding terms that expressed patients' perspectives, preferences, behaviors, experiences, and signs and symptoms within the ICNP. The findings from this data set indicated that the nursing phenomena (nursing diagnoses) classification is better developed than the nursing intervention classification.

In contrast, elements of the U.S. NMDS have been widely tested. Results of these studies have been reported in peer-reviewed literature (Goossen et al., 1998). Ryan and Delaney (1995) reviewed NMDS research from the United States and reported that the NMDS has been used in hospital studies to create demographic profiles of patients with specific nursing diagnoses. Findings from these studies indicated significant associations between nursing diagnoses and patient characteristics such as sex, race, age, medical diagnoses, and length of stay. These results provide evidence of the construct validity of the nursing diagnosis categories.

9.3   Classification Systems

Standardized nursing data supports the study of health problems across populations, settings, and caregivers, which can increase knowledge of nursing and quality outcomes (Bowles & Naylor, 1996). To ensure consistency and comparability, an NMDS must use standardized nursing language. Without a standardized language, the data are essentially useless in predicting trends or comparing trends across practice settings (Delaney & Moorhead, 1995).

Nursing classification systems are a sub-component of nursing minimum databases. They are designed to label, classify, and operationally define the elements in the database. Three major types of classification systems have been developed for nursing: those that classify patient problems/nursing diagnoses; those that classify nursing interventions; and those that classify nursing outcomes. Some of the most widely used classification systems are the North American Nursing Diagnoses Association (NANDA), Nursing Interventions Classification (NIC), Home Health Care Classification (HHCC), the Omaha Classification System (OCS), and Nursing Outcomes Classification (NOC). According to the literature, these classification systems provide standard data and are acceptable for the documentation of nursing practice.

The four NMDS discussed in this chapter utilize these classification systems. For example, the U.S. NMDS utilizes the NANDA, NIC, NOC, HHCC, and OCS classification systems. CNMDSA uses only NANDA at this time. The HI:NC uses NANDA, NIC, NOC, and OCS, and is investigating the HHCC (Goossen et al., 1998). The ICNP maps data elements from the existing nursing classification systems. Four of the recognized American Nurses Association classification systems have been mapped to the ICNP: NANDA, NIC, HHCC, and OCS (Bakken Henry et al., 1998).

9.3.1   Nursing Diagnoses

Nursing diagnoses provide a standardized language for identifying patient issues and an initial basis against which to measure nursing interventions and outcomes (Delaney & Moorhead, 1995). Nursing diagnoses originated approximately 30 years ago and are being used in diverse practice settings (Delaney et al., 2000).

The North American Nursing Diagnosis Association (NANDA) defines nursing diagnoses as "a clinical judgment about individual family or community responses to actual or potential health problems/life processes. Nursing diagnoses provide the basis for selection of nursing interventions to achieve outcomes for which the nurse is accountable" (Saba, 1993). At the current time, there are approximately 155 nursing diagnoses that describe patients' actual and potential health problems. A nursing diagnosis includes a comprehensive description of the problem, its etiology, and related signs and symptoms (Van Achterberg et al., 2002).

Advocates for the use of nursing diagnoses, such as Rantz (2001), state that the use of nursing diagnoses is a way for nurses to communicate with one another. Using nursing diagnoses helps standardize nursing issues, and provides the ability to computerize nursing documentation, compare data across practice settings, and evaluate outcomes of care. The use of nursing diagnoses is also considered an essential step in developing a common language to describe patient situations for which nursing has a responsibility and guiding professional practice (Smith Higuchi et al., 1999).

Some issues have also been identified in the use of nursing diagnoses. Some nurses believe that the use of nursing diagnoses is isolating and does not have meaning for other health care providers, patients, and their families (Maas & Wilkinson, 2000). Beyea and Wilkinson (1999) argue that in today's healthcare environment, most patient problems are managed in a collaborative, multidisciplinary fashion, so insulating each profession through practices such as the utilization of nursing diagnoses is no longer realistic or appropriate.

The use of nursing diagnoses in clinical practice has also been identified as an issue. While nursing diagnoses are adopted in nursing textbooks and curricula, the use of nursing diagnoses in hospital documentation is inconsistent. Smith Higuchi et al. (1999) describe one study that examined a randomized sample of patient records from four hospitals that had respiratory care units for the use of nursing diagnoses. Two of the hospitals were large teaching facilities, while the others were smaller community institutions. According to the findings, evidence of nursing diagnosis documentation ranged from 26% to 94%. The use of nursing diagnoses in clinical practice documentation was enhanced in organizations that had formal educational programs and computer-generated care plans.

While it is important to use standardized language and classification, translation of the classification systems to different languages at the international level has not been an easy process (Clark, 1998). Even within the English language there are issues. In England, the NANDA taxonomy was chosen as the standardized language in the Hospital Information Classification System. However, even though the English language was being used, the context of some terminology was not transferable. For example, terms such as "regimen" and "unilateral neglect" were not used in England and had to be changed to more appropriate language for British health care providers (Clark, 1998a). When nursing diagnoses terminology is used internationally, it must be adapted to reflect cultural and language diversity.

The CINHAL database was searched for the past five years using the limits of English and research articles. Approximately 88 studies were identified that included nursing diagnoses. The research focused on examining and utilizing nursing diagnoses to explore patient needs in a variety of healthcare settings, workload intensity, and the reliability and validity of the use of nursing diagnoses. Of these articles, over 50% appeared in the Nursing Diagnosis Journal, which was first published in 1990. The journal provides an avenue for the publication of research on nursing diagnoses and articles describing the implementation of this research (Whitley, 1999).

Whitley (1999) reviewed the processes and methodologies for research validation of nursing diagnoses over the past 25 years and found that, while a great deal of research and validation of nursing diagnoses have been implemented, there continues to be a need for conceptual clarity. Small sample sizes are also a limitation of much of the nursing diagnosis research, which means that most of the evaluation has been limited to descriptive studies. Studies with larger sample sizes would enable multivariate analysis of interrelationships among variables as necessary in construct validation work (Whitley, 1999).

9.3.2 *OMAHA Classification System (OCS)*

The Visiting Nurses Association of Omaha began to develop the Omaha Classification (OCS) System in 1970 (Bowles & Naylor, 1996). This classification system was the first to include standardized language for nursing interventions, and was developed to meet the minimum data needs of community health nurses (Delaney & Moorhead, 1995). The purpose of the OCS is to provide a precise comprehensive method for care planning and documentation, and to serve as a system for feedback on outcome achievement (Bowles & Naylor, 1996). Based on 15 years of research and development undertaken by the Visiting Nurses Association of Omaha and the Division of Nursing, Public Health Services, U.S. Department of Health and Human Services, the OCS has primarily been used by community-focused healthcare providers, although more recently it has undergone testing in acute-care settings (Martin, 1999).

The OCS consists of terms and codes catalogued from general to specific (Martin, 1999). Bowles and Naylor (1996) describe the three components of the OCS: the Problem Classification Scheme, the Problem Rating Scale for Outcomes, and the Intervention Scheme. The Problem Classification Scheme provides a method for the user to assess the client and family, and to identify essential data and patterns (Martin, 1999). The Problem Classification Scheme consists of four levels. The first level has four domains—environmental, psychosocial, physiological and health-related behaviors—that provide an organizational structure for the data. The second level includes 40 nursing diagnoses that identify, name, and organize patient issues. The third level has two modifiers, which identify whether the problem is an individual or family issue and whether it is health promotion or a potential or actual problem, and is used in conjunction with the client problems (Martin, 1999). The fourth level includes clusters of signs and symptoms specific to each problem.

The Problem Rating Scale for Outcomes provides nurses with a systematic method to measure client change. The three concepts of knowledge, behavior and status are scored on a five-point ordinal scale from the most negative to the most positive state of the issue on admission, at regularly scheduled intervals, and at discharge from home care (Bowles & Naylor, 1996). The initial assessment provides a baseline that can be compared with data gathered at later dates. The information can be used to assess the client's progress in relation to the effectiveness of interventions and to identify the plan of care (Martin, 1999).

The Intervention Scheme is designed to help the health care provider identify and document plans of care and interventions for the client's specific nursing diagnoses (Martin, 1999). It has three levels. The first level consists of four broad categories—health teaching, guidance and counseling, treatments and procedures, and surveillance—one or more of which are used to develop, describe, and document a client-specific intervention (Martin, 1999). The second level consists of 62 targets, which describe problem-specific intervention categories and are defined as objects of health-related activities that the nurse can use to guide the nursing interventions (Martin, 1999). The third level comprises client-specific information and allows narrative information to be included in the client record (Bowles & Naylor, 1996; Martin, 1999).

A major strength of the OCS is its potential to link patient issues to nursing interventions and outcomes. The OCS has been translated into Danish and Japanese (Martin, 1999). It has been used in approximately 41 states and in over 200 community-focused practice settings and, as a result, has undergone extensive field-testing and revision since its development. Staff nurses who used the OCS reported that the Intervention Scheme was a valuable tool for planning and documenting nursing activities (Martin & Scheet, 1992). An inter-rater agreement of 80% or higher was obtained for eight out of 12 records (Martin & Scheet, 1992).

Bowles (1999) evaluated the ability of the OCS to be used in acute-care settings. In her study, 30 patient records were randomly chosen and coded using content analysis. Signs, symptoms, problem interventions, and targets of those interventions were matched to OCS terms. Inter-rater reliability was reported at >.79 for the Kappa scores. The researcher found the four domains in the Problem Classification Scheme broad, holistic, and abstract enough that the majority of the problems, interventions, and targets from the hospital record could be coded within the OCS. While this initial study demonstrated that the OCS is relevant to an acute-care setting, the sample size was small, the study was limited to one hospital, and no empirical results were reported. Further testing is required in acute-care settings with larger sample sizes and diverse patient populations in order to support expansion of the OCS into acute-care settings.

The OCS is a comprehensive classification system for nursing practice in the community. It has served as a model for standardized language, and is written in a language that has clear meaning that can easily be interpreted by multidisciplinary healthcare teams (Bowles & Naylor, 1996). Continued research is required to validate the relationship between nursing practice and the outcome indicators identified in the OCS, to expand its use to acute-care settings, and to promote the development of the OCS nationally and internationally.

9.3.3 The Home Health Care Classification (HHCC)

The Home Health Care Classification (HHCC), developed from a study funded by the Health Care Financing Administration (Saba, 2001b), assesses and classifies care for home health Medicare patients, including measuring the outcomes of their care (Saba, 2001a). Its development was based on data collected on actual resource use that could be objectively measured and used to predict resource requirements. A national sample of 646 home health agencies was used. The home health agencies were randomly stratified by staff size, type of ownership, and geographic location (Bowles & Naylor, 1996). Data collected from 8,961 newly discharged cases represented each patient's entire healthcare experience from admission to discharge (Saba, 2001a). Data on the nursing diagnoses and nursing interventions provided during the time the client received home health care were collected by home health care nurses using two open-ended narrative statements. The narrative statements for the first 1,000 clients were entered into a computer database to identify common terminology (Bowles & Naylor, 1996). The terms for nursing diagnoses and interventions were sorted separately, and matched together by patient. Based on this analysis, two vocabularies were developed, tested, refined, and used to code the 40,361 narrative nursing diagnoses and 80,283 nursing intervention statements (Saba, 2001a). They became the HHCC of Nursing Diagnoses and HHCC of Nursing Intervention vocabularies (Saba, 2001b). There is no report of validity or reliability testing during development of the system.

The HHCC of Nursing Diagnoses includes 145 diagnostic labels based on the NANDA taxonomy and other home health conditions. Each nursing diagnosis also uses one of three modifiers—stabilized, improved, or deteriorated—to describe the expected and actual outcomes of care (Saba, 2001b). The HHCC of Nursing Interventions includes 160 activities, each of which can be described by one of four modifiers—assess, care, teach, and/or refer—to identify the type of action of the intervention (Saba, 2001b).

The two vocabularies are further categorized according to 20 care components that represent functional, health behavioral, physiological, and psychological patterns of care. The 20 care components serve as a standard framework for mapping and linking the two inter-related HHCC taxonomies to each other, and to other health-related classifications (Saba, 2001a). They are used to classify the types of care provided to clients over time, settings, population groups, and geographical locations (Saba, 2001a).

The American Nursing Association has identified the HHCC vocabularies as acceptable for documenting nursing practice using standard data. They have been translated into Portuguese, Dutch, Korean, and Spanish. They are also used for collecting nursing data in Switzerland, Argentina, the Netherlands, and Belgium. However, the research on the HHCC reported in the literature is limited to instrument development research. A literature search of the HHCC conducted on the CINHAL database identified 339 articles, but all but 12 were home health classifications of nursing diagnoses and interventions by Saba (1994). None of the 12 articles reported research on the use and testing of the HHCC for assessing, documenting, or evaluating home health and ambulatory care. More research is required to determine whether the variables identified reflect a linkage between nursing diagnoses, interventions, and outcomes, and to test the HHCC application in clinical practice (Bowles & Naylor, 1996).

9.3.4 Iowa Nursing Intervention Classification (NIC)

The Nursing Intervention Classification System (NIC), established in 1987, is a research-based standardized language developed by the Iowa Interventions Project (CNA, 2000; LaDuke, 2000). McCloskey and Bulechek (1999) define an intervention as "any treatment, based upon clinical judgment and knowledge, that a nurse performs to enhance patient/client outcomes." The NIC is the only information system that attempts to capture all interventions provided by nurses, regardless of the setting and specialty (Delaney & Moorhead, 1995), including independent and collaborative interventions as well as basic and complex interventions (Iowa Intervention Project, 1995). The primary purpose of the classification system is to standardize nursing intervention terms and articulate the range of activities in nursing practice (Bowker et al., 2001; Bowles & Naylor, 1996).

The NIC was developed from information extracted from nursing textbooks, care-planning guides, and information systems. The first edition was published in 1992 and the third edition in 2000 (Anonymous, 2001). The system includes seven domains, 30 classes of care, and 486 interventions that represent both general and specialty nursing practice (Anonymous, 2001). The interventions form a template to guide patient care and documentation (LaDuke, 2000). While some activities are collaborative, most emphasize the independent nature and value of nursing practice. However, the language used is common to all healthcare professionals (Bowles & Naylor, 1996; LaDuke, 2000). The interventions are coded in a three-level taxonomic structure (McCloskey & Bulechek,

1999). The first level is the most abstract and consists of six domains that explore physiological (both basic and complex), behavioral, safety, family, and health systems. The second level includes 27 classes organized within the six domains. The third level consists of the interventions grouped according to class and domain (McCloskey & Bulechek, 1999).

Multiple research methods were used to develop the NIC system, including content analysis and focus group review (Anonymous, 2001). To assess face and content validity of the NIC, a two-round Delphi questionnaire was administered to advanced practice nurses in specialty areas (Bowles & Naylor, 1996). Nearly 300 members of the Midwest Nursing Research Society were also surveyed to assess the validity of the NIC taxonomy. Similarity analysis, hierarchical clustering, and multidimensional scaling were performed to construct the NIC taxonomy. The NIC was also field tested in five clinical sites in a variety of clinical care settings, such as a university hospital, a long-term care facility, and a community hospital. Because the NIC was designed to capture all interventions provided by nurses, regardless of the setting and specialty, the field testing was undertaken to test its generalizability (Bowles & Naylor, 1996). More than 1,000 individuals and approximately 50 professional associations provided input into the NIC's development (Anonymous, 2001).

According to McCloskey and Bulechek (1999), the NIC facilitates the promotion of clinical documentation, communication of care across settings, aggregation of data across systems and settings, outcome and productivity research, and curriculum design. The NIC interventions have been linked with NANDA, OCS, the Nursing Outcomes Classification, the Resident Assessment Protocols for long-term care, and the Outcomes and Assessment Information Set (Anonymous, 2001). Over 300 clinical agencies located in 46 states and 20 countries are using the NIC to document nursing interventions (Anonymous, 2001), and the NIC has been translated or is in the process of being translated into Chinese, Dutch, French, German, Icelandic, Japanese, Korean, Portuguese, and Spanish (Anonymous, 2001).

Published research on the implementation of the NIC system is limited. One area of research focused on the use of the NIC system to determine the cost of nursing care. A study published anonymously in Nursing Economics (2001) described how nurse experts assessed 433 interventions in the NIC second edition, using the 27 classes of the organizing taxonomic structure. The nurse experts were asked to identify an average time for implementing the nursing interventions that could be used to determine reimbursement rates, by selecting one of five possible time estimates ranging from 15 minutes or less to over one hour. Each group of raters worked together to rate the classes of interventions. The findings indicated that of the 4,333 interventions, 54% were rated as taking 30 minutes or less of nursing time. The greatest number of interventions were estimated to take 16 to 30 minutes (Anonymous, 2001). There are limitations in the reporting of this study. It does not include the number of nurse experts who rated the NIC interventions, or the criteria used to identify them as nurse experts. No reliability or validity results are reported. The times assigned to each intervention are the nurse experts' estimations based on their knowledge. If the purpose of assigning times to interventions were to estimate nursing costs, it would be important to validate these ratings within clinical practice settings. However, studying each intervention through work sampling methods is resource- and time-intensive, as well as costly. McCloskey and Bulechek (1999) argue that estimates of time for nursing interventions done by nurses who implement the interventions are an accurate and efficient method of identifying time values.

While the NIC system standardizes nursing intervention terms, more research is needed to test the system's utility in clinical settings, and to study the link between nursing diagnoses, the NIC interventions, and outcomes.

9.3.5 *Nursing Outcome Classification System*

With the increased focus on healthcare costs and quality of care, healthcare professionals are being held accountable for demonstrating quality outcomes as a result of their practice (Daly et al., 1997; Maas et al., 1996). The emphasis on effectiveness and patient outcome research has resulted in the need for valid ways to identify, standardize, and measure patient outcomes that are sensitive to nursing care (Maas et al., 1996). Standardized patient outcome documentation is also necessary to develop computerized healthcare information systems and to access information related to nursing practice (Daly et al., 1997).

The Nursing Outcomes Classification (NOC) is a comprehensive classification of patient outcomes that are responsive to nursing interventions. It is the first comprehensive standardized language and measurement for nursing-sensitive patient outcomes (Prophet & Delaney, 1998).

With the NANDA and the NIC, it completes the NMDS nursing process elements (Daly et al., 1997). The NOC has also been linked to Gordon's functional patterns, the Omaha Problem system, Resident Admission Protocols used in nursing homes, and the OASIS system (University of Iowa, 2002).

The NOC defines an outcome as a measurable individual, family, or community state or behavior that is sensitive to nursing perceptions and is measured along a continuum (Johnson, 1998). The NOC (Second Edition) has 260 outcomes, including 247 individual-, seven-family, and six community-level outcomes (University of Iowa, 2002). Each NOC outcome consists of a definition, a list of indicators that assist in evaluating the patient status, a five-point Likert measurement scale to measure patient status, and a short list of references used in the development of the outcome (Johnson, 1998). The 260 outcomes are categorized into 29 classes and seven domains. To facilitate the entry and extraction of information from a computer database, a unique code is assigned to each outcome. As the outcomes are generalizable to all settings, they can be used across the healthcare continuum. Patient outcomes can be examined throughout the illness episode or over an extended period of care (University of Iowa, 2002).

A research team at the University of Iowa College of Nursing began developing the NOC (Johnson et al., 1996). The team devised a methodology for developing an outcome-based nursing classification system in 1991 (Johnson & Maas, 1998; Johnson et al., 1996). They identified that diagnoses refer to patient issues, interventions to nursing actions, and outcomes to patient responses to nursing care (Johnson et al., 1996). They also emphasized that nurses are only one component of the healthcare team that may influence patient outcomes (Johnson et al., 1996).

To develop the NOC, the research team asked key questions, such as:

- Who is the patient?

- What do the patient outcomes describe?

- At what levels of abstraction should outcomes be developed?

- How should the outcomes be stated?

- What are the nursing-sensitive patient outcomes?

- Are nursing-sensitive patient outcomes the resolution of nursing diagnoses?

- When should patient outcomes be measured? (Maas et al., 1996).

The initial outcomes were developed from textbooks, standardized care plans, critical pathways, nursing information systems, outcome studies, research instruments, and standards of practice (Johnson et al., 1996). Literature sources were selected based on the following criteria: presented clear statements that described specific states or behaviors of patients or family members; included a comprehensive list of outcome statements; presented outcome statements that were measurable; and presented outcome statements that were designed to evaluate nursing interventions (Maas et al., 1996). The sources were chosen to represent healthcare issues and settings across the lifespan. Health promotion and illness management were also included in the review (Maas et al., 1996).

Inductive, deductive, qualitative, and quantitative strategies were used to develop outcome statements (Johnson & Maas, 1998). The research team initially generated over 4,500 outcomes, but reduced them to 282 outcome labels using grouping exercises (Johnson & Maas, 1998). They used the Medical Outcomes Study framework to develop a framework for analyzing the 282 outcome labels and identifying the following eight broad outcome categories: family caregiver status; health attitudes, knowledge, and behavior; perceived well-being; physical functional status; physiological status; psychological and cognitive status; safety status; and social and role status (Johnson & Maas, 1998; Johnson et al., 1996). Researchers then used a modified Delphi process to categorize the

282 outcome labels within the eight broad categories. Eight focus groups were conducted to develop the outcomes further (Johnson & Maas, 1998). A two-step process, using hierarchical clustering techniques was used to develop taxonomy classes and the following six domains:

1. Functional Health: Outcomes that describe capacity for and performance of basic tasks of life

2. Physiological Health: Outcomes that describe organic functioning

3. Psychosocial Health: Outcomes that describe psychological and social functioning

4. Health Knowledge and Behavior: Outcomes that describe attitudes, comprehension, and actions with respect to health and illness

5. Perceived Health: Outcomes that describe impressions of an individual's health

6. Family Health: Outcomes that describe health status, behavior, or functioning of the family as a whole or of an individual as a family member (Johnson & Maas, 1998).

The NOC Second Edition included a seventh domain: Community Health (University of Iowa, 2002). Content validity of the outcomes, definitions, and indicators were established by surveying nurse experts randomly selected from across the U.S. nursing community (Johnson & Maas, 1998). A sample of 200 nurses was mailed questionnaires that consisted of eight to 10 outcomes with their definitions and indicators. The respondents were asked to rate the importance of each indicator and nursing's contribution to each outcome on a five-point scale. Researchers used a modified Fehring technique to analyze the response. The assigned weights ranged from 0 for an answer of 1 to a weighted score of 1 for an answer of 5. Indicators with weighted scores of .80 or greater were identified as major indicators, and those with weighted scores between .60 to .79 as minor indicators (Johnson & Maas, 1998).

The NOC is currently being used in practice settings and computerized information systems. It is also being used internationally, and has been translated into Dutch, Japanese, Korean, and French. German and Spanish translations are underway (University of Iowa, 2002). To establish the NOC's reliability, validity, and sensitivity, more evaluation of the outcomes in clinical practice is necessary (Johnson & Maas, 1998). Currently, inter-rater reliability, criterion measures, and other methods are being used to assess the validity and reliability of the NOC in clinical practice settings (University of Iowa, 2002).

In summary, the use of NMDS and classification systems have implications for nursing research, clinical practice, education, administration, and health policy (Bowles & Naylor, 1996; Anderson & Hannah, 1993). To facilitate the extraction and identification of nursing practice, unified databases and standardized language need to be further developed and implemented.

9.4 Multidisciplinary Databases

9.4.1 *Resident Assessment Instrument (RAI) For Nursing Homes*

One of the most developed, tested, and utilized minimum data sets in the United States is the Resident Assessment Instrument (RAI) for nursing homes. A multidisciplinary database that includes nursing care data, the RAI was developed to provide a standardized assessment of nursing home residents, and improve the quality of care and outcomes for patients in nursing homes (Brunton & Rook, 1999; Rantz et al., 1996). The development of a uniform, comprehensive resident assessment system was one of the key recommendations of the 1986 report of the Institute of Medicine's Committee on Nursing Home Regulation (Hawes et al., 1995). In the committee's view, a comprehensive assessment of each resident is essential to the development of an individualized plan of care focusing on improving, maintaining, or minimizing the decline in the resident's functional status (Hawes et al., 1995).

The RAI development team included healthcare professionals from all disciplines, nursing home operators, resident advocates, and researchers (Hawes et al., 1997). The goal of the research team was to develop an instrument whose main focus was on clinical practice, and that assessed the "whole" person and fostered restorative and rehabilitative care (Hawes et al., 1997). The RAI was also created to promote communication and problem solving within a multidisciplinary team by developing a "common" language and understanding of the resident (Hawes et al., 1997). To develop the RAI, the research team reviewed over 80 existing geriatric instruments; identified the domains and items, definitions and response categories to be included; established reliability and validity of the instrument; and developed instruction and training manuals (Hawes et al., 1997).

One of the RAI's strengths is that it is considered a routine, interdisciplinary, standardized assessment process that is sensitive to changes in the residents' functional status and well-being (Rantz, Popejoy, et al., 1999). Developed as a minimum data set of items, definitions, and response categories designed to provide a comprehensive assessment of nursing home residents (Hawes et al., 1995; Rantz, Popejoy, et al., 1999), the RAI consists of the Minimum Data Set (MDS) and Resident Assessment Protocols (RAP).

The Minimum Data Set (MDS) is a core set of items that provides a comprehensive assessment of each resident's functional status, including his or her strengths, preferences, and needs (Hawes et al., 1997). The goal of the MDS is to capture indicators of a resident's clinical status that represent not only the pathologies inherent to very old age, but also the disabilities that can be minimized by high-quality care (Casten et al., 1998).

The MDS provides extensive standardized assessments to guide clinical practice, and serves as a mechanism for evaluating clinical care, measuring resident outcomes, and adjusting staffing ratios for acuity (Rantz, Popejoy et al., 1999). It also represents the clinical concerns of care providers responsible for the everyday care of residents and those who monitor their health status (Casten et al., 1998).

Full MDS assessments are performed on admission, and then at least annually or when there is a change in functional status (Rantz, Popejoy et al., 1999). To facilitate the monitoring of residents' conditions and capture subtle changes in the assessment that may indicate an alteration in status, quarterly MDS assessments are also performed using a subset of items from the full MDS (Rantz, Popejoy et al., 1999).

The most recently revised MDS scale is MDS 2.0. It consists of multiple domains and more than 400 individual items that describe residents' nursing needs, as well as their strengths and psychosocial needs (Clauser & Fries, 1992; Rantz, Zwygart-Stauffacher, et al., 1999). The domains are: background and customary routines, psychosocial well-being, communication/hearing patterns, physical functioning and structural problems, moods and behavior patterns, disease diagnoses, oral/nutritional status, skin condition, special treatments and procedures, cognitive patterns, vision patterns, continence, activity pursuit patterns, health conditions, oral/dentist status, and medication use (Hawes et al., 1997). Once the MDS is implemented, the data is assessed to determine "trigger" category scores. These triggers are individual items or combinations of MDS elements that fall within a range of values that lead the assessor to examine the resident's status in that category more carefully. This can then lead to a change in care provision or planning for the individual through the use of Resident Assessment Protocols (Clauser & Fries, 1992; Frederiksen et al., 1996).

The Resident Assessment Protocols (RAP) provide guidelines for a more in-depth assessment of 18 conditions related to the care of nursing home residents that influence their functional well being. They are: delirium, visual function, ADL functional/rehabilitative potential, psychosocial well-being, behavior problems, falls, feeding tubes, dental care, psychotropic drug use, cognitive loss/dementia, communication, urinary incontinence and indwelling catheter, mood state, activities, nutritional status, dehydration/fluid maintenance, pressure ulcers, and physical restraints (Clauser & Fries, 1992; Hawes et al., 1995; Hawes et al., 1997). Each RAP provides guidelines for developing care plans, including assessment protocols, summaries of options for care planning, and service provisions (Clauser & Fries, 1992).

9.4.2 *Reliability and Validity*

Content validity of the RAI was achieved through broad input from hundreds of clinicians, administrators, regulators, industry representatives, and consumer advocates (Clauser & Fries, 1992). Twenty-seven drafts were developed prior to the first clinical field testing of the MDS (Hawes et al., 1997). During field testing and re-testing, the RAI underwent another 15 revisions with clinical reviews (Hawes et al., 1997).

Three field tests have been implemented on the RAI. In the first, assessments were conducted on 383 residents of 10 nursing homes in two states (Hawes et al., 1995). The results led to dropping or revising more than half the items, changing procedures for gathering information, and revising the MDS format (Hawes et al., 1995). Two other clinical field trials using nursing staff trained in the MDS protocol occurred in 13 facilities across five states (Hawes et al., 1995; Snowden et al., 1999). Findings indicated that 89% of the items had an intraclass correlation score of 0.4 or higher, and 63% had a score of at least 0.6 (Hawes et al., 1995; Snowdon et al., 1999). Five of the MDS sections (background, physical functioning (ADLs) and structural problems, disease diagnoses, oral/nutritional status, and medication use) had excellent reliability of 0.7 or higher, and seven sections had average reliability levels of 0.6 or higher. The items in six other domains attained an average reliability of 0.5 to 0.59, while the remaining five domains achieved an average reliability of 0.4 to 0.49. Twenty-two items that did not attain adequate reliability were dropped from the instrument.

The RAI's reliability and validity have also been confirmed in multiple studies (Casten et al., 1998; Hawes et al., 1995; Hartmaier et al., 1995; Frederiksen et al., 1996; Hirdes et al., 1999; Morris et al., 1997, 1999).

9.4.3 *Effects of the RAI on Quality in Nursing Homes*

As a pre-/post-RAI evaluation test design, the quality of care and resident status for more than 4,000 residents in 10 states and 269 randomly selected nursing homes was assessed. This was done to examine changes in the process of care and longitudinal resident outcomes as measures of quality (Hawes et al., 1997). Statistically significant improvements were found in the following areas:

1. Increase in the comprehensiveness and accuracy of the information found in residents' medical records

2. Care plans post-RAI implementation addressed a greater percentage of residents' health problems, risk factors, and potential for improved function

3. Increased involvement of families and residents in care planning, use of advance directives, use of behavior management programs, involvement in activities, and decreased use of problematic interventions, such as indwelling catheters or physical restraints

4. Significant decrease in decline among residents in such areas as physical functioning in ADLs, cognitive status, and urinary continence

5. Significant reduction in the number of residents who required hospitalization with no increase in mortality (Fries et al., 1997; Hawes et al., 1995; Phillips et al., 1997).

9.4.4 *Quality Indicators (QI)*

The widespread use of the MDS 2.0 to assess nursing home residents permits comparisons between and among facilities of problem conditions in residents (Rantz, Zwygart-Stauffacher, et al., 1999). A team of researchers from the Center for Health Systems Research and Analysis at the University of Wisconsin-Madison and collaborators from the Multistate Nursing Home Case Mix and Quality Demonstration Project developed quality indicators (QI) from MDS 2.0 data. The QIs provide administrators and regulatory agencies with comparative benchmarks against which to measure potentially good or poor care practices (Rantz, Zwygart-Stauffacher et al., 1999; Wodchis & Nytko, 1998). The QIs were developed based on interdisciplinary input, empirical evidence, and field testing (Zimmerman et al., 1995).

The current QI instrument includes 30 different quality indicators measuring a variety of clinical problems and domains, such as accidents, behavioral/emotional patterns, cognitive patterns, and quality of life (Rantz, Zwygart-Stauffacher et al., 1999). Some QI items are risk-adjusted to explain differences in residents across organizations. Zimmerman et al. (1995) categorize the QI characteristics as: (1) resident- vs. facility-level; (2) prevalence vs. incidence; and (3) process vs. outcome.

1. Resident vs. Facility

At the resident level, QIs are classified as either the presence or the absence of a condition. The resident level QIs for the facility can be aggregated to determine the facility level QIs, which then can be used to compare with other facilities or the nursing home norms for the area.

At both the resident and the facility level, some QIs have associated risk factors in that an individual may have health or functional conditions that either increase or decrease the probability of having a specific QI. Risk factors are used to adjust for inter-facility variation in QI scores.

2. Prevalence vs. Incidence

At both the resident and facility level, prevalence QI is defined as the presence or absence of a condition at a single point in time. An incidence QI is when a condition is present on two or more consecutive assessments.

3. Process vs. Outcome

QIs examine both process and outcome measures of quality. Process indicators represent the content, actions, and procedures implemented by the caregiver in response to the resident's assessed condition. Outcome measures describe the results of the applied processes. The QIs can be a combination of both process and outcome measures, a process measure, or an outcome measure.

QIs are not absolute measures of quality. They are indicators of potentially good or poor practice and resident outcomes (Rantz et al., 2000). Organizations can receive quarterly reports that include their percentile rank compared to a larger pool of nursing homes. The score is the proportion of residents within the nursing home who have the problem identified by the QI. The numerator is the number of residents with the clinical indicator, and the denominator is the total number of residents who could potentially develop the problem, which could be the total number of residents in an organization (Rantz, Zwygart-Stauffacher et al., 1999). However, depending on the problem, some residents may be excluded from the denominator because the condition does not apply to them (Rantz, Zwygart-Stauffacher et al., 1999). A high score indicates a high incidence or prevalence of the problem and suggests possible problems with care. However, in some situations a high score does not represent an organizational problem. For example, if a nursing home has many patients who require urinary catheters or tube feeding, it will likely have high scores on the relevant QIs.

Reporting a facility's percentile compared to a standard, such as provincial standards, can be problematic, as the ranking can create a false impression of good quality (Rantz et al., 1996). For example, if many nursing homes have poor QI scores on an outcome measure, then the average score may actually reflect poor clinical outcomes and may lead homes with better-than-average scores to not try to improve their practice because they believe they exceed the acceptable level of quality. To prevent this, Rantz and her colleagues have begun to examine and identify absolute standards of thresholds that promote excellent performance, as well as potential quality issues. A panel of experts met and determined thresholds that reflect current practice. They reviewed relevant information related to individual QIs in order to determine a range of poor and good threshold scores, and verified their findings using a Delphi technique (Rantz et al., 2000). The thresholds provide a criterion for more meaningful interpretation of a facility's performance and are expected to be a better basis for identifying the need for quality improvement (Rantz et al., 2000).

In summary, QIs and the MDS 2.0 data are valuable sources of information that organizations can use to enhance clinical outcomes of residents in their quality improvement programs (Rantz, Popejoy et al., 1999). The process of comparing organizations and their residents' characteristics and outcomes can lead administrators and care providers to examine their practices and identify ways to improve them.

9.4.5 *Resource Utilization Groups (RUG-III)*

Data from the RAI are used to identify residents with complex medical or rehabilitative care needs, or with high disability in the activities of daily living (Hawes et al., 1997). The most recent version of the RAI contains all the items required for the Resource Utilization Groups (RUG) III, a resident-based case mix classification system used to determine the nursing home's payment and resource use (Hawes et al., 1997). The nursing home case mix systems generally focus on explaining daily resource use (Clauser & Fries, 1992). RUG-III explains resource use and effectively identifies resources provided to nursing home residents by describing what care is actually provided without addressing whether the levels of care and resources are appropriate (Clauser & Fries, 1992; Fries et al., 1994). The goal of RUG-III is to categorize nursing home residents by resident characteristics.

The RUG system encompasses up to three dimensions in describing a resident. The first examines one of seven major types of nursing home residents. The second is an index of activities of daily living that measures the functional capability of the resident in toileting, eating, bed-to-chair transfer, and bed mobility. The third identifies the particular services required by the resident or problems that exist (Clauser & Fries, 1992). Seven hierarchical categories—special rehabilitation, extensive services, special care, clinically complex, impaired cognition, behavioral problems, and reduced physical functions—describe types of residents in decreasing order of resource use. Residents are placed in one of 44 RUG-III groups found within the seven hierarchical categories (Clauser & Fries, 1992).

RUG-III was developed from a database of 7,658 residents in 203 nursing homes across seven states (Clauser & Fries, 1992). Data related to measures of resource use and resident characteristics were collected through staff reporting. Researchers then calculated the total time spent over a 24-hour period caring directly and indirectly for each resident from MDS 2.0 data. Findings indicate that, with groups that are relatively homogenous, the RUG-III system of 44 groups explained 55.5% of the variation among individual residents in 24-hour resource cost (Clauser & Fries, 1992). When facility or unit identifiers were included as covariates to the model, the RUG-III variance explanations increased to 68% and 71%, respectively (Clauser & Fries, 1992).

Bjorkgren et al. have begun to examine a home care classification system based on RUG-III. They developed a modified home care model by incorporating the Instrumental Activities of Daily Living into the nursing home RUG-III classification, and tested it on a sample of 804 individuals seeking home care in 14 regions across the state of Michigan. The model explained 33.7% of the variance of per diem cost using cost-weighted formal and informal care as the dependent variable. Bjorkgren et al. identified issues related to the large amount of informal care provided to an individual receiving home care that need to be explored, such as whether informal care is a substitute for formal care, or whether it should be treated as a separate input with specified costs. If informal care is recognized as having costs, then specific guidelines need to be developed to capture those costs.

9.4.6 RAI/MDS Series

Since the development and implementation of the RAI for nursing homes, RAIs have been developed for other practice settings. For example, the Resident Assessment Instrument–Home Care (RAI-HC) was developed as an assessment system in the home care environment, and is used to guide comprehensive assessments and planning for individuals cared for in their homes (Landi et al., 2000; Morris et al., 1999). Reliability and validity of the RAI-HC have been established through extensive testing in the United States, Canada, Japan, Czech Republic, and Australia (Hirdes et al., 1999; Landi et al., 2000; Morris et al., 1997). The two elements of the RAI-HC are the Minimum Data Set-Home Care (MDS-HC) and the Clinical Assessment Protocols (CAPs) (Morris et al., 1997).

The MDS-HC is based on and designed to be compatible with the MDS 2.0 for nursing homes (Morris et al., 1997). The functional, health status, social environment, and service items in the MDS-HC (114 items) are the same as the MDS 2.0 for nursing homes and reflect the needs of the frail elderly, regardless of where they reside (Morris et al., 1997; Wodchis & Nytko, 1998). Items that were created solely for the MDS-HC are in the areas that are experienced less frequently in nursing homes, such as the role of informal supports, indicators of abuse of the older person, instrumental activities of daily living (IADL) self-performance, environmental conditions, a variety of health conditions including preventative health measures, and a series of service indicators (Morris et al., 1997).

Similar to the RAPs, the Clinical Assessment Protocols (CAPs) use 30 triggers to guide the assessor through best practice in developing a care plan for an identified issue, risk, or potential (Morris et al., 1999). CAPs are "triggered" by clinical algorithms that identify whether there is evidence of a problem in health, function, or well-being, currently or in the future, and prompts the healthcare team to complete a more detailed assessment (Hirdes et al., 1999). The CAPs include general guidelines for further client assessment and individualized care planning (Landi et al., 2000).

RAI/MDSs are also being developed and tested in acute- and mental health-care settings, as well as in complex continuing care. The RAI for Acute Care (RAI-AC) has recently undergone reliability and validity testing in Canada, the United States, the United Kingdom, Norway, and Iceland (Hirdes et al., 1999). The RAI for Mental Health settings (RAI-MH) was developed by a research team representing Canada, the United States, the United Kingdom, Japan, the Netherlands, and Norway, and is being implemented voluntarily in Ontario, Canada (Hirdes et al., 1999). The RAI for Post-Acute Care is being developed for short-stay clinically complex participants and those requiring general rehabilitation (Hirdes et al., 1999).

With its consistent terminology, common core items, and common conceptual basis, the RAI/MDS series supports an integrated health information system that can be used across community, institutional, and acute-care settings (Hirdes et al., 1999). Using this series, an individual could move from one healthcare sector to another and have comparable information transferred between settings to promote continuity of care (Hirdes et al., 1999).

9.4.7 Benefits and Barriers to RAI Systems

There are a number of advantages to implementing the RAI systems for quality improvement efforts (Rantz et al., 1996). Individual data collected on a regular basis facilitates the monitoring of quality care indicators and evaluation of individual outcomes. The RAI can be used to determine staffing needs and for continuous quality improvement initiatives (Hawes et al., 1995). The data obtained can also support decision-making and evidence-based practice. Policy-makers can use the data to set nursing home payment and home care rates.

The RAI/MDS series was developed to establish an integrated health information system based on a common language, theoretical conceptual basis, clinical emphasis, and data collection methods (Hirdes et al., 1999). According to Hirdes et al., the benefits of this type of system include: the ability of different healthcare sectors to access the same information, which will lead to better continuity of care; decreased costs by avoiding redundant assessments and service provision; and better client outcomes because the use of a common language and the focus on the individual instead of the provider promote less ambiguity about the appropriate services required and more effective interventions.

The implementation of quality indicators will allow facilities and regulatory agencies to assess the quality of care and identify potential issues. They will also be able to compare directly the cost effectiveness of different facilities and agencies for specific types of individuals and practices, and policy-makers can use this information to allocate resources to maximize population health (Hirdes et al., 1999).

While there are many advantages to using the RAI, there are also some barriers. Staff have raised concerns about the amount of time it takes to complete the RAI, and report that completing the RAI adds to their documentation burden (Hawes et al., 1995). The lack of RNs in long-term care facilities may also limit the ability to perform consistent systematic assessments of residents and to follow through with resident care (Rantz, Popejoy, et al., 1999). Many facilities employ one nurse to implement all the RAI assessments. While this practice enhances reliability of data, the RAI process is more effective when integrated into the clinical practice of all professional staff working with residents (Rantz, Popejoy, et al., 1999). Staff who are working with the residents are in the best position to develop and implement the care plan (Rantz, Popejoy, et al., 1999). The use of multiple, largely untrained data collectors across sites also raises concerns about inter-rater reliability (Lipowski & Bigelow, 1996).

In implementing the RAI, consideration should be given to ethical and privacy issues. In the current technological environment, researchers could retrieve an individual's personal information without the person knowing or giving specific consent for that use of the data. Safeguards need to be put in place and policies established on who may have access to the data and how it will be used (Rittman & Gorman, 1992). (Canada has very strict informed consent rules, as do other countries.)

The timeliness of data access is another issue that must be addressed (Hirdes & Carpenter, 1997). Researchers, service providers, and policy-makers require information to guide decisions, so the turnaround time to receive data should not be excessive (Hirdes & Carpenter, 1997).

9.5 Outcome and Assessment Information Set (OASIS)

The Outcome Assessment and Information Set (OASIS) was developed approximately 10 years ago as part of an outcome-based quality improvement (OBQI) initiative in home care (Shaughnessy et al., 1998a). The OBQI is a continuous quality-improvement approach based on patient outcomes. Under the OBQI initiative, reports are produced for organizations based on systematic, uniform outcome measures (Shaughnessy et al., 1998a). The Health Care Financing Administration (HCFA) funded Shaughnessy et al. (1998a) and the Center for Health Services and Policy Research at the University of Colorado to develop a comprehensive system of home care quality measures for implementing the OBQI initiative. This resulted in the development of OASIS, which forms the basis for measuring patient outcomes in the community (OASIS Overview, 2002).

OASIS consists of a standard set of assessment questions for collecting data to determine the quality of home health care (Clark, 1998b). The OASIS data items provide information on the sociodemographic, environmental, support system, health status, and functional status attributes of adult patients. They can be used to monitor patient outcomes, perform clinical assessments, develop care plans, and support internal agency-level quality assessments (OASIS Overview, 2002). Each client is assessed first on admission, at each 60-day period that the client continues to receive home care, and at discharge (Clark, 1998b). OASIS has 98 questions, but not all questions are answered each time the client is assessed (Clark, 1998b). By measuring the client's status over time, care providers can assess and evaluate his or her improvement, stabilization, and regression in any number of specific areas (Clark, 1998b).

The first version, OASIS-A, was released in 1995, and the current version, OASIS-B, was launched in 1997 (Shaughnessy et al., 1998a). The data items were developed with the involvement of home care clinicians and experts, and went through several iterations based on clinical and empirical research. Shaughnessy et al. (1998a) developed OASIS specifically to measure and risk-adjust patient outcomes in home health care and, according to the reviewed literature, the researchers completed extensive validity and reliability tests on the OASIS items.

The OASIS project was piloted in 50 agencies across the United States and is a prototype for a project that the Health Care Financing Administration (HCFA) mandated under the Medicare Conditions of Participants (Polzien et al., 1998). HCFA requires all Medicare-certified agencies in the United States to complete comprehensive assessments using OASIS at specified time points during the client's home care experience (Koch, 1997). HCFA then uses the data obtained through OASIS to facilitate interdisciplinary care and coordination of services. The data can also inform and maintain an effective data-driven OBQI (Koch, 1997). The OASIS data set will become the primary source of information for guiding payments for home health care and will eventually be used for the purpose of quality control (Wilson & Twiss, 1997).

Shaughnessy, Crisler, Schlenker, and Hittle (1998b) discuss the types of reports that can be generated through the use of OASIS, which include: annual clinical outcomes such as physiologic, functional, and cognitive outcomes; utilization outcomes such as hospitalization and discharge to the community; case mix reports of clients admitted over a 12-month period to an agency (which describe the characteristics, circumstances, disabilities, and diseases of clients relative to both a national case mix reference sample and the case mix of the participating agency in the previous year); and reports on selected negative events, such as falls, that agencies can use to examine and improve their clinical practices.

9.5.1 Benefits and Limitations

The use of OASIS offers benefits to both agencies and patients. It can be used to establish benchmarks for care and assess performance from year to year, and to provide data that nurse researchers can use to explore best practices and improve quality of care for home care clients. In the United States, it can also be used in managed care contracting negotiations (Clark, 1998b).

OASIS also has some limitations, including the length of time required to complete an assessment. Cohen (1999) states that an OASIS assessment can add more than half an hour to the initial client visit and to the subsequent visits when the OASIS assessment is redone. However, once staff move beyond the initial learning curve, Koch (1997) notes that entering OASIS items takes approximately three to five minutes on average.

Researchers have also identified two critical elements missing from the standard OASIS data collection process: the link between outcomes and utilization, and outcomes and cost data, and the lack of tools to support "real-time" reporting that agencies can use in their day-to-day operations (Wilson & Twiss, 1997).

Staff training and commitment are critical to the successful collection of OASIS data. To achieve quality, accurate outcomes, home care staff must be properly educated about the importance of accurately assessing their clients using OASIS (Wilson, 1997). Adams, DeFrates, and Wilson (1998) explored whether a home health agency could use OASIS and the OBQI model to enhance improvement and stabilization scores for clients receiving home health services. This study was part of a larger research project exploring whether standardized data improved home health outcomes. The sample consisted of 817 patients referred for home health services. Data were collected using 17 items from the OASIS assessment form. The researchers assessed five global measures: ambulation/locomotion, bathing, management of oral medications, pain, and dyspnea. For each outcome measure, researchers analyzed variances to compare both improvement and stabilization scores over time. Reliability or validity measurements were not described. According to the results, the use of an OASIS subset and the OBQI model did not consistently increase the number of clients who improved or stabilized on the outcome measure explored. There were no statistically significant results.

The researchers also identified limitations in the use of OASIS. The ability to implement accurate assessments of clients performing the outcomes is critical to the quality of the data. To complete an accurate assessment, staff must observe the client performing the behavior. However, the clinicians often did not observe the client actually perform the outcome. Instead, many clinicians participating in the study rated their clients based on the client's self-report. When they observed the client performing the outcomes, they discovered that the client's self-report was not accurate. This highlights the importance of observing client behavior when assessing outcome measures. However, in the real world of home care, nurses may not observe the client performing such activities of daily living as bathing.

9.6 Discussion

In the changing healthcare environment, there is an increasing need to identify, measure, and evaluate quality outcomes. The development of relevant quality outcomes requires partnerships among service providers, government, and the research community, as well as a common language to link them together (Hirdes & Carpenter, 1997). In the past, it has been difficult to develop evidence-based practice and policy, because of ineffective communication mechanisms, limitations in knowledge, methodological issues, and the lack of data or the inability to access it (Hirdes & Carpenter, 1997). The use of databases, such as an NMDS, RAI series of instruments, or OASIS, may begin to resolve these issues.

Whichever database is chosen, it is important to recognize that the reliability and validity of databases is complex and often confused with the reliability and validity of the classification systems used within a minimum data set (Ryan & Delaney, 1995). Although the reliability and validity of the classification system will affect the reliability and validity of the data within a minimum data set, the reliability and validity of the actual data must also be considered. Incomplete records, unreliable or invalid coding, or missing variables may limit the value of the data (Ryan & Delaney, 1995). For the data to be reliable and valid, standardized classification systems must be used and the reliability of the data needs to be monitored regularly (Ryan & Delaney, 1995).

All NMDS systems have the benefit of making nurses' work visible and providing evidence-based knowledge to guide both nursing practice and the decisions made by policy-makers and healthcare providers. The information obtained through the use of a NMDS facilitates system-level planning and evaluation, as well as benchmarking within and against similar organizations. It also helps identify best practices. A growing body of evidence generated from a NMDS could provide the nursing profession with substantial benefits with respect to nursing effectiveness, quality assurance, mapping trends, and nursing research (Goossen et al., 1998). The challenge is to continue to implement clinical testing of the different components of a NMDS to determine their weaknesses, strengths, and applicability, and their validity and reliability in different clinical settings.

For NMDS systems to reach their full potential, developers must address the issue of whether the same variables are being compared, and how to deal with differences in scope, population, sample, actual data, abstraction, and aggregation (Goossen et al., 1998). If the underlying structures of the data sets are incompatible, then they cannot be compared. This raises the question of how to develop standardized data in different healthcare settings, countries, and healthcare delivery models. The issues of standardized language and classification systems continue to fuel the debate about whether there should be one acceptable classification system and, if so, which one it should be. One classification system would be advantageous, as everyone would be aware of the vocabulary and the classification, and would have to utilize it (McCormick & Jones, 1998). The data would also be comparable across setting, place, and country. However, the assumption that all practicing nurses would embrace one classification system and learn to use it in a consistent manner is unrealistic. Data needs to be captured in a way that permits integration across levels and sites of care, delivery models, providers, and management domains (McCormick & Jones, 1998). The mapping of classification systems appears to be a feasible alternative to implementing one classification system. The work of the ICNP demonstrates potential in this area.

Goossen et al. (1998) raised the question of whether a specific NMDS still has relevance in today's healthcare environment. This question is supported by the CINHAL literature search, which revealed that most of the literature describing NANDA, NIC, OCS, and HHCC was published prior to 1997. The NOC system is the only NMDS that has published most of its work over the past five years. The cost of implementing and supporting minimum data sets within organizations, and the fact that client care is provided mainly by multidisciplinary teams, suggest that the focus should be on developing multidisciplinary databases rather than discipline-specific ones.

Ideally, it would be advantageous to have a database that could capture clients' healthcare experiences as they move across the healthcare continuum. While the RAI/MDS series holds the most promise of eventually providing this capability, it is not currently feasible for one classification system to cover all factors relevant to a client's care in all settings (Shaughnessy et al., 1998a). Each database has been developed for a specific reason. For example, the NMDS systems were developed to capture and make nursing practice visible, the RAI was developed to deliver care to the elderly client, and OASIS is used in home care. The choice of which database to use depends on such factors as the type of clients, the purpose for measurement, the ease of data collection, the cost, and the degree of informatic technology within the organization. Regardless of this, the use of a minimum data set is necessary to identify best practices, nursing effectiveness, quality assurance, trends, and nursing research (Goossen et al., 1998). The challenge is to continue to identify methods of developing and using databases that are reliable and valid, and that best reflect nursing practice.

References

Adams, C. E., DeFrates, D., & Wilson, M. (1998). Data driven quality improvement for HMO patients: One agency's experience with OASIS and OBQI. *Journal of Nursing Administration, 28*(10), 20–25.

Anderson, B., & Hannah, K. J. (1993). A Canadian nursing minimum data set: A major priority. *Canadian Journal of Nursing Administration, 6*(2), 7–13.

Anonymous (2001). Determining cost of nursing interventions: A beginning. *Nursing Economics, 19*(4), 146–160.

Bakken Henry, S., Elfrink, V., McNeil, B., & Warren, J. J. (1998). A review of the International Classification of Nursing Practice and discussion of its relevance to current efforts in the United States. *Online* [http://www.amia.org/pubs/symposia/D004890.PDF].

Beyea, S., & Wilkinson, J. (1999). Nursing diagnosis or patient problem? *Nursing diagnosis, 10*(1), 32–34.

Björkgren, M. A., Fries, B. E., & Shugarman, L. R. (2000). A RUG-III Case-mix system for home care. *Canadian Journal on Aging, 19*(Supplement 2), 106–125.

Blewitt, D. K., & Jones, K. R. (1996). Using elements of the nursing minimum data set for determining outcomes. *Journal of Advanced Nursing, 26*(6), 48–56.

Bowker, G. C., Leigh Star, S., & Spasser, M. A. (2001). Classifying nursing work. *Online Journal of Issues in Nursing* [http://www.nursingworld.org/ojin/tpc7/tpc7_6.htm].

Bowles, K. H., & Naylor, M. D. (1996). Nursing intervention classification systems. *Image: The Journal of Nursing Scholarship, 28*(4), 303–308.

Brunton, B., & Rook, M. (1999). Implementation of the Resident Assessment Instrument: A Canadian experience. *Healthcare Management Forum, 12*(2), 49–53.

Canadian Nurses Association (2000). *Collecting data to reflect nursing impact.* Ottawa, Canada.

Casten, R., Powell-Lawton, M., Parmelee, P. A., & Kleban, M. H. (1998). Psychometric characteristics of the Minimum Data Set I: Confirmatory factor analysis. *Journal of the American Geriatrics Society, 46*, 726–735.

Clark, J. (1998a). The international classification for nursing practice project. *Online Journal of Issues in Nursing* [http://www.nursingworld.org/ojin/tpc7/ tpc7_3.htm].

Clark, L. (1998b). Incorporating OASIS into the Visiting Nurses Association. *Outcomes Management for Nursing Practice, 2*(1), 24–28.

Clauser, S. B., & Fries, B. E. (1992). Nursing home resident assessment and case-mix classification: Cross national perspectives. *Health Care Financing Review, 13*(4), 135–155.

Coenen, A., & Schoneman, D. (1995). The nursing minimum data set: Use in the quality process. *Journal of Nursing Care Quality, 10*(1), 9–15.

Cohen, J. (1999). Oasis: A welcoming patch of green? *Nursing & Health Care Perspectives, 20*(6), 328.

Daly, J. M., Maas, M. L., & Johnson, M. (1997). Nursing outcomes classification: An essential element in data sets for nursing and health care effectiveness. *Computers in Nursing, 15*(2), S82–S86.

Delaney, C., Herr, K., Maas, M., & Specht, (2000). Reliability of nursing diagnoses documented in a computerized nursing information system. *Nursing Diagnoses, 11*(3), 121–134.

Delaney, C., & Moorhead, S. (1995). The nursing minimum data set, standardized language, and health care quality. *Journal of Nursing Care Quality, 10*(1), 16–30.

Frederiksen, K., Tariot, P., & Jonghe, E. D. (1996). Minimum data set plus (MDS+) scores from five rating scales. *Journal of the American Geriatrics Society, 44*, 305–309.

Fries, B. E., Hawes, C., Morris, J. N., Phillips, C. D., Mor, V., & Park, P. S. (1997). Effect of the national resident assessment instrument on selected health conditions and problems. *Journal of the American Geriatrics Society, 45,* 994–1001.

Fries, B. E., Schneider, D. P., Foley, W. J., Gavazzi, M., Burke, R., & Cornelius, E. (1994). Refining a case-mix measure for nursing homes: Resource utilization groups (RUG-III). *Medical Care, 32*(7), 668–685.

Goossen, W. T. F., Epping, P.J. M. M., Van den Heuvel, W. J. A., Feuth, T., Frederiks, C. M. A., & Hasman, A. (2000). Development of the nursing minimum data set for the Netherlands (NMDSN): Identification of categories and items. *Journal of Advanced Nursing, 31*(3), 536–547.

Goossen, W. T. F., Epping, P. J. M. M., Feuth, T., Dassen, T. W. N., Hasman, A., & Van Den Heuvel, W. J. A. (1998). A comparison of nursing minimal data sets. *Journal of the American Medical Informatics Association, 5*(2), 152–163.

Hannah, K. J., & Anderson, B. J. (1994). Management of nursing information. In J. M. Hibberd and M. E. Kyle (Eds.) *Nursing administration: A micro/macro approach for effective nurse executives* (pp. 516–533). Norwalk, CT: Appleton & Lange.

Hartmaier, S. L., Sloane, P. D., Guess, H. A., Koch, G. G., Mitchell, M., & Phillips, C. D. (1995). Validation of the minimum data set cognitive performance scale: Agreement with the mini-mental state examination. *Journal of Gerontology, 50A*(2), M128–M133.

Hawes, C., Morris, J. N., Phillips, C. D., Mor, V., Fries, B. E., & Nonemaker, S. (1995). Reliability estimates for the minimum data set for nursing home resident assessment and care screening. *The Gerontologist, 35*(2), 172–178.

Hawes, C., Morris, J. N., Phillips, C. D., Fries, B. E., Murphy, K., & Mor, V. (1997). Development of the nursing home resident assessment instrument in the USA. *Age and Aging, 26*(S2), 19–25.

Hirdes, J. P., & Carpenter, G. I. (1997). Health outcomes among the frail elderly in communities and institutions: Use of the minimum data set (MDS) to create effective linkages between research and policy. *Canadian Journal on Aging* (Suppl.), 16, 53–69.

Hirdes, J. P., Fries, B. E., Morris, J. N., Steel, K., Mor, V., Frijters, D., LaBine, S., Schalm, C., Stones, M. J., Teare, G., Smith, T., Marhaba, M., Perez, E., & Jonsson, P. (1999). Integrated health information systems based on the RAI/MDS series of instruments. *Healthcare Management Forum, 12*(4), 30–40.

Iowa Intervention Project (1995). Validation and coding of the NIC taxonomy structure. *Image: The Journal of Nursing Scholarship, 27*(1), 43–49.

Johnson, M. (1998). Overview of the Nursing Outcomes Classification (NOC). *Online Journal of Nursing Informatics, 2*(2). http://cac.psu.edu/~dxm12.OJNI.html.

Johnson, M., & Maas, M. (1998). The nursing outcomes classification. *Journal of Nursing Care Quality, 12*(5), 9–20.

Johnson, S. J., Brady-Schluttner, K., Ellenbecker, S., & Johnson, M. (1996). Evaluating physical functional outcomes: One category of the NOC system. *MEDSURG Nursing, 5*(3), 157–162.

Koch, L. (1997). Using OASIS to teach OBQI. *Caring Magazine, 16*(8), 34–46.

LaDuke, S. (2000). NIC puts nursing into words. *Nursing Management, 31*(2), 43–44.

Landi, F., Tua, E., Onder, G., Carrara, B., Sgadari, A., Rinaldi, C., Gambassi, G., Lattanzio, F., & Bernabei, R. (2000). Minimum data set for home care: A valid instrument to assess frail older people living in the community. *Medical Care, 38*(12), 1184–1190.

Lipowski, E. E., & Bigelow, W. E. (1996). Data linkage for research on outcomes of long-term care. *The Gerontologist, 36*(3), 441–447.

Maas, M. L., Johnson, M., & Moorhead, S. (1996). Classifying nursing-sensitive patient outcomes. *Image: The Journal of Nursing Scholarship, 28*(4), 295–301.

Maas, M. L., & Wilkinson, J. (2000). Response to S. Beyea's "nursing diagnosis or patient problem?" *Nursing Diagnosis, 11*(2), 84–86.

Martin, K. S. (1999). The Omaha System: Past, present and future. *Online Journal of Nursing Informatics, 3*(1). http://cac.psu.edu/~dxm12/OJNI.html.

Martin, K., & Scheet, N. (1992). *The Omaha system: Applications for community health nursing.* Philadelphia: W. B. Saunders.

McCloskey, J., & Bulechek, G. (1998). Nursing Interventions Classification: Current status and new directions [On-Line], *Online Journal of Nursing Informatics, 2*(2). [http://cac.psu.edu/~dxm12/OJNI.html.]

McCormick, K. A., & Jones, C. B. (1998). Is one taxonomy needed for health care vocabularies and classifications? *Online Journal of Issues in Nursing* [http://www.nursingworld.org/ojin/tpc7/tpc7_2.htm].

Morris, J. N, Carpenter, I., Berg, K., & Jones, R. N. (1999). *Outcome measures for use with home care clients.* Unpublished manuscript.

Morris, J. N., Fries, B. E., Steel, K., Ikegami, N., Bernabei, R., Carpenter, I., Gilgen, R., Hirdes, J. P., & Topinkova, E. (1997). Comprehensive clinical assessment in community setting: Applicability of the MDS-HC. *Journal of the American Geriatrics Society, 45*, 1017–1024.

O'Brien Pallas, L., Giovannetti, P., Peereboom, E., & Marton, C. (1995). *Case costing and nursing workload: Past, present and future.* Hamilton, Canada: Quality of Nursing Worklife Research Unit. *OASIS Overview. On-line* [http://cms.hhs.gov/oasis/hhoview.asp].

Phillips, C. D., Morris, J. N., Hawes, C., Fries, B. E., Mor, V., Nennstiel, M., & Iannacchione, V. (1997). Association of the Resident Assessment Instrument (RAI) with changes in function, cognition, and psychosocial status. *Journal of the American Geriatrics Society, 45*, 986–993.

Polzien, G., Kendal, B. J., & Hindelang, M. (1998). The challenge of implementing OASIS. *Home Healthcare Nurse, 16*(12), 806–812.

Prophet, C. M., & Delaney, C. W. (1998). Nursing outcome classification: Implications for nursing information systems and the computer-based patient record. *Journal of Nursing Care Quality, 12*(5), 21–29.

Rantz, M. J. (2001). The value of a standardized language. *Nursing Diagnosis, 12*(3), 107–108.

Rantz, M. J., Mehr, D. R., Conn, V. S., Hicks, L. L., Porter, R., Madsen, R. W., Petrowski, G. F., & Maas, M. (1996). Assessing the quality of nursing home care: The foundation for improving resident outcomes. *Journal of Nursing Care Quality, 10*(4), 1–9.

Rantz, M. J., Petroski, G. F., Madsen, R. W., Mehr, D. R., Popejoy, L., Hicks, L. L., Porter, R., Zwgart-Stauffacher, M., & Grando, V. (2000). Setting thresholds for quality indicators derived from MDS data for nursing home quality improvement reports: An update. *Journal of Quality Improvement, 26*(2), 101–110.

Rantz, M. J., Popejoy, L., Zwygart-Stauffacher, M., Wipke-Tevis, D., & Grando, V. T. (1999). Minimum data set and resident assessment instrument. Can using standardized assessment improve clinical practice and outcomes of care. *Journal of Gerontological Nursing, 25*(6), 35–43.

Rantz, M. J., Zwygart-Stauffacher, M., Popejoy, L. L., Mehr, D. R., Grando, V., Wipke-Tevis, D. D., Hicks, L. L., Conn, V. S., Porter, R., & Maas, M. (1999). The minimum data set: No longer just the clinical assessment. *Annals of Long-Term Care, 7*(9), 354–360.

Rittman, M. R., & Gorman, R. H. (1992). Computerized databases: Privacy issues in the development of the nursing minimum data set. *Computers in Nursing, 10*(1), 14–18.

Ruland, C. M. (2001). Evaluating the beta version of the International Classification for Nursing Practice for domain completeness, applicability of its axial structure and utility in clinical practice: A Norwegian project. *International Nursing Review, 48*, 1–8.

Ryan, P., & Delaney, C. (1995). Nursing Minimum Data Set. *Annual Review of Nursing Research, 13*, 169–194.

Saba, V. K. (1993). Nursing diagnostic schemes. In *Papers from the nursing minimum data set conference* (pp. 54–67). Ottawa, Canada: Canadian Nurses Association.

Saba, V.K. (1994). *Home health classification (HHCC) of nursing diagnoses and interventions.* Washington, DC: Author.

Saba, V. K. (2001a). Home health care classification system (HHCC): Background. *Online* [http://www.sabacare.com].

Saba, V. K. (2001b). Nursing informatics: yesterday, today and tomorrow. *International Nursing Review, 48*(3), 177–189.

Shaughnessy, P. W., Crisler, K. S., & Schlenker, R. E. (1998a). Outcome-based quality improvement in home health care: The OASIS indicators. *Home Health Care Management & Practice, 10*(2), 11–19.

Shaughnessy, P. W., Crisler, K., Schlenker, R., & Hittle, D. (1998b). OASIS: The next 10 years. *Caring Magazine, 17*(6), 32–42.

Smith Higuchi, K. A., Dulberg, C., & Duff, V. (1999). Factors associated with nursing diagnosis in Canada. *Nursing Diagnosis, 10*(4), 137–147.

Snowden, M., McCormick, W., Russo, J., Srebnik, D., Comtois, K., Bowen, J., Teri, L., & Larson, E. B. (1999). Validity and responsiveness of the minimum data set. *Journal of the American Geriatrics Society, 47*, 1000–1004.

University of Iowa (2002). Nursing outcomes classification: Overview. *On-line* [http://www.nursing.uiowa.edu/noc].

Van Achterberg, T., Frederiks, C., Thien, N., Coenen, C., & Persoon, A. (2002). Using ICIDH-2 in the classification of nursing diagnoses: Results from two pilot studies. *Journal of Advanced Nursing, 37*(2), 135–144.

Whitley, G. G. (1999). Process and methodologies for research validation and nursing diagnoses. *Nursing Diagnoses, 10*(1), 5–14.

Wilson, A. (1997). Using outcomes and OASIS as strategic tools. *Home Healthcare Nurse Manager, 3*(1), 19–25.

Wodchis, W., & Nytko, B. (1998). Using the minimum data set. *Canadian Nursing Home, 9*(2), 15–20.

Zimmerman, D. R., Sarita, S., Arling, G., Ryther Clark, B., Collins, T., Ross, R., & Sainfort, F. (1995). Development and testing of nursing home quality indicators. *Health Care Financing Review, 16*(4), 107–127.

Index